Advances in Anesthesia®
Volume 10

Advances in Anesthesia®

Volumes 1 through 7 (Out of print)

Volume 8

Organization of an Acute Pain Management Service, *by Timothy R. Lubenow and Anthony D. Ivankovich*
Acute Pediatric Pain Management, *by Thomas R. Vetter*
Anesthetic Management of the Patient With Acute Spinal Cord Injury, *by Tod B. Sloan, Rosemary Hickey, and Maurice S. Albin*
Anesthetic Evaluation for the Reconstructed Heart, *by Paul R. Hickey*
The Role of α_2 Agonists in Anesthesia, *by Mervyn Maze*
Echocardiography in the Operating Room, *by Gerard McCloskey*
Implications of Nitrous Oxide Administration, *by Michael N. Skaredoff*
Alternatives to Perioperative Blood Transfusion, *by Gary Stack and Edward L. Snyder*
Calcium Action and General Anesthesia, *by Richard Prielipp and Gary P. Zaloga*
Intravascular Catheter-Related Infection in the Critically Ill Patient, *by Stephen O. Heard and Lori E. Circeo*
Evaluating Anesthetic Outcome, *by Kenneth J. Tuman*

Volume 9

Aspiration: An Overrated Risk in Elective Patients, *by Charles J. Coté*
Neonatal Surgical Emergencies, *by Steven C. Hall*
Postoperative Cardiac Consultation: The Art and Science, *by Bruce S. Kleinman*
Assessment of Perioperative Ischemia, *by Jane E. Carter, Lee A. Fleisher, and Paul G. Barash*
Quality Assurance and Anesthetic Outcome, *by Peter G. Duncan*
Prediction and Definition of Outcome, *by Joseph M. Civetta and Robert R. Kirby*
Monoclonal Antibody Therapy of Sepsis, *by Janice L. Zimmerman*
Hyperbaric Oxygen for the 1990s, *by Edward K. McGough*
Pharmacogenetics, *by David J. Byers and Morton C. Green*
Anesthesia Dental Complications, *by Sanford L. Klein*
Genetic Determinants of the Site of Action of Volatile Anesthetics, *by Margaret M. Sedensky and Philip G. Morgan*

Advances in Anesthesia®

Editor

Robert K. Stoelting, M.D.

Professor and Chairman, Department of Anesthesia, Indiana University School of Medicine, Indianapolis, Indiana

Associate Editors

Paul G. Barash, M.D.

Professor and Chairman, Department of Anesthesiology, Yale University School of Medicine; Dean of Academic Affairs, Yale University School of Medicine; Chief, Department of Anesthesia, Yale–New Haven Hospital, New Haven, Connecticut

T. James Gallagher, M.D.

Professor of Anesthesiology and Surgery, Department of Anesthesiology, University of Florida College of Medicine; Chief, Critical Care Medicine, Shands Hospital, Gainesville, Florida

Volume 10 • 1993

Mosby Year Book

St. Louis Baltimore Boston Chicago London Philadelphia Sydney Toronto

Mosby
Year Book
Dedicated to Publishing Excellence

Sponsoring Editor: Bernadette Buchholz
Associate Managing Editor, Manuscript Services: Denise M. Dungey
Editing Coordinator, Manuscript Services: Laura A. Pelehach
Senior Production Assistant: Sandy Rogers
Proofroom Manager: Barbara M. Kelly

Mosby–Year Book, Inc.
11830 Westline Industrial Drive
St. Louis, MO 63146

Editorial Office:
Mosby–Year Book, Inc.
200 North LaSalle St.
Chicago, IL 60601

International Standard Serial Number: 0737-6146
International Standard Book Number: 0-8151-8275-9

Contributors

Ronald Lea Akers, Jr., M.D.

Assistant Professor of Surgery, The Department of Surgery, Tulane University School of Medicine, New Orleans, Louisiana

Christina Campbell, M.D., Ch.B.

Associate Professor of Anesthesia, Indiana University School of Medicine, Indianapolis, Indiana

Aurel C. Cernaianu, M.D.

Assistant Professor of Surgery, University of Medicine and Dentistry of New Jersey, Robert Wood Johnson Medical School at Camden, Director, Research Programs, Division of Cardiothoracic Surgery and Department of Anesthesiology, Cooper Hospital/University Medical Center, Camden, New Jersey

Janet B. Clarke, Ph.D.

Research Associate in Anesthesiology, Department of Anesthesiology, College of Medicine, University of Arizona, Tucson, Arizona

Stephan Cohn, M.D.

Assistant Professor, Department of Anesthesia and Critical Care, University of Chicago Division of the Biological Sciences, Pritzker School of Medicine, Chicago, Illinois

Anthony J. DelRossi, M.D.

Associate Professor of Surgery, University of Medicine and Dentistry of New Jersey, Robert Wood Johnson Medical School at Camden; Chairman, Department of Surgery, Head, Division of Cardiothoracic Surgery, Cooper Hospital/University Medical Center, Camden, New Jersey

Thomas J. Ebert, M.D., Ph.D.

Associate Professor of Anesthesiology, Associate Adjunct Professor of Physiology, Department of Anesthesiology, Medical College of Wisconsin; VA Medical Center, Milwaukee, Wisconsin

Jay L. Falk, M.D.

Director, Emergency Medicine Residency Program, Orlando Regional Medical Center, Orlando, Florida

A. Jay Gandolfi, Ph.D.

Professor of Anesthesiology, Pharmacology, and Toxicology, Department of Anesthesiology, College of Medicine, University of Arizona, Tucson, Arizona

Arthur M. Lam, M.D., F.R.C.P.C.

Professor of Anesthesiology and Neurologic Surgery, University of Washington School of Medicine; Attending Anesthesiologist, Harborview Medical Center, Seattle, Washington

A. Joseph Layon, M.D.

Associate Professor, Departments of Anesthesiology and Medicine, University of Florida, College of Medicine, Gainesville, Florida

Richard C. Lind, M.S.

Senior Research Specialist, Department of Anesthesiology, College of Medicine, University of Arizona, Tucson, Arizona

Karen S. Lindeman, M.D.

Assistant Professor, Department of Anesthesiology/Critical Care Medicine, The Johns Hopkins Medical Institutions, Baltimore, Maryland

Michael E. Mahla, M.D.

University of Florida College of Medicine, Department of Anesthesiology, Gainesville, Florida

L. Michael Newman, Ph.D., M.D.

Assistant Professor of Anesthesiology and of Obstetrics and Gynecology, Rush Medical College, Director of Obstetric Anesthesia, Department of Anesthesiology, Rush-Presbyterian-St. Luke's Medical Center, Chicago, Illinois

Ammon B. Peck, Ph.D.

Professor, Department of Pathology and Laboratory Medicine, University of Florida, College of Medicine, Gainesville, Florida

Michael F. Roizen, M.D.

Chairman, Department of Anesthesia and Critical Care; Professor, Department of Medicine, University of Chicago Division of the Biological Sciences, Pritzker School of Medicine, Chicago, Illinois

John A. Youngberg, M.D.

Associate Professor of Anesthesiology, The Department of Anesthesiology, Tulane University School of Medicine, New Orleans, Louisiana

Publisher's Preface

This volume of *Advances in Anesthesia* represents the ninth and final volume to be led by Robert K. Stoelting, M.D., as editor. Since the publication of volume 2 in 1985, Dr. Stoelting and his colleagues, Paul G. Barash, M.D., and T. James Gallagher, M.D., have devised interesting and diverse collections of authoritative review articles that have established this series as an important resource for anesthesiologists.

Reading through the chapter titles of these nine volumes, one sees virtually every significant concern of anesthesia in the late '80s and the '90s and a veritable "Who's Who" of the North American anesthesia community among the authorship. Through their persuasive skills and their editorial talents, Drs. Stoelting, Barash, and Gallagher have elicited genuinely authoritative articles of lasting value.

We publishers appreciate Dr. Stoelting's professionalism and responsiveness in meeting a long succession of deadlines during this 9-year period. We also note that Dr. Gallagher actually founded the series, being the sole editor of volume 1. Hence, he will retire from this series following a full decade of fruitful effort.

For Volume 11 and beyond, the editor of *Advances in Anesthesia* will be Carol L. Lake, M.D., aided by Dr. Barash, who will continue to be involved with this series, and by Richard J. Sperry, M.D. We believe this new team will continue to serve our readers with well-selected and well-prepared information.

Mosby–Year Book, Inc.

Contents

Chemical Dependency and the Anesthesiologist

L. Michael Newman Ph.D., M.D.

Assistant Professor of Anesthesiology and of Obstetrics and Gynecology, Rush Medical College, Director of Obstetric Anesthesia, Department of Anesthesiology, Rush-Presbyterian-St. Luke's Medical Center, Chicago, Illinois

In 1990, the American Society of Addiction Medicine and the National Council on Alcoholism and Drug Dependence set forth a new definition of alcoholism (chemical dependency) that stated:

> Alcoholism (chemical dependency) is a primary, chronic disease with genetic, psychosocial, and environmental factors influencing its development and manifestations. The disease is often progressive and fatal. It is characterized by continuous or periodic impaired control over drinking (drug use), preoccupation with the drug alcohol (or drug of choice), use of alcohol (drug[s]) despite adverse consequences, and distortions in thinking, most notably denial.[1]

The commonly used/abused substances are the following: narcotics—heroin, meperidine, codeine, and china white or kitchen laboratory-produced fentanyl; stimulants—cocaine and amphetamines; psychedelics—phencyclidine (PCP or angel dust), lysergic acid diethylamide (LSD), and peyote; depressants—alcohol, benzodiazepines, barbiturates, and marijuana. It is rare for a person with chemical dependency to use only one drug. Current research indicates that a high percentage of persons with chemical dependency use multiple drugs. A recent survey of a single recovery program demonstrated that two thirds of the patients were using more than one drug in the 6 months prior to admission.[2]

A person is referred to as an addict if he or she exhibits the three Cs: Compulsive use, loss of Control, and Continued use in spite of adverse consequences. It is clear that there is a continuum from nonuser to addict. The term *drug dependence* is defined as either physical or psychological dependence on a drug. Drug or substance abuse is the use of drugs but not to the degree of addiction.[3] Thus, the spectrum from addict to nonuser is based on some index of chemical consumption and degree of interference with normal psychosocial functioning.

The concern of the anesthesiologist is what drugs are being used or were used by the patient, for how long and how frequently, and how much at a time. This allows one to make some inferences about tolerance and cross-tolerance to the anesthetics. Additionally, if the patient says he or she is currently abstinent, it is necessary to determine how this abstinence is maintained. It is rare for a person who had a history of chemical dependency or drug abuse to be able to quit without some sort of support system. One clue is to look for the presence of recovery programs in the patient's life and directly ask if he or she is going to Rational Recovery, Alcoholics Anonymous, Narcotics Anonymous, or Cocaine Anonymous meetings regularly. A detailed, accurate, current drug history is invaluable.

Substance abuse has reached epidemic proportions in the United States. In 1991, the Senate Judiciary Committee said there were 2.2 million hard-core cocaine addicts in the United States. This is a rate of 1 per 1,000 individuals.[4] There are more than 500,000 opiate addicts in the United States. The Department of Health and Human Services has estimated that although the consumption of alcohol has gradually declined during the 1980s, about 10% of adults in the United States are dependent on alcohol and at least three out of 100 deaths in the United States are alcohol-related.[5] By 1986, it was thought that 40% of the U.S. population had tried cocaine. In addition to the addicts, there is a large segment of the population that uses illicit drugs recreationally, as well as those who are not addicted but are classified as drug abusers or pre-addicts.

According to the 15th National Institute on Drug Abuse High School Senior Survey,[6] there doesn't seem to be much hope for the near future. Of the teens surveyed, 19.7% reported current use of illegal drugs. The statistics for drug use by the senior class of 1989 were as follows: cocaine 2.8%; daily alcohol use 4.2%; binge drinking 33%; and PCP 1.4%, which represents a fourfold increase from the survey when taken the previous year. Additionally, nearly 19% of those surveyed reported that they smoked cigarettes daily. On June 7, 1991, the results of a national survey were released by Antonia Novello, M.D., the Surgeon General of the United States.[7] Of the 20.7 million students across the nation in grades 7 through 12, 10.6 million (51%) drink alcoholic beverages: 8 million (39%) drink weekly, 5.4 million (26%) binge on occasion, and 454,000 (2.2%) binge on five or more drinks in a row at least once a week. Of those who binge, 58% said they drink when they are upset and 30% said they drink when they are bored.

Drug use in the parturient has been examined by the National Institute on Drug Abuse. In 1988, three of five women of child-bearing age drank alcoholic beverages. In their peak reproductive years (18 to 34 years), one in every ten American women drank an average of two or more drinks a day—an amount that could endanger an unborn baby. It was also reported that nearly 10% of women of child-bearing age used an illicit drug in the month prior to the survey. In 1987, the Office for Substance Abuse Prevention studied 36 hospitals across the country. They reported that 11% (range from 0.4% to 27%) of new mothers used cocaine, marijuana, heroin, methadone, PCP, and/or amphetamines while pregnant.

The problem of substance abuse is not one that is confined to the inner city or to patients in the public clinics. A recent study in Florida demonstrated that the urine of one in seven pregnant patients tested positive for alcohol, marijuana, cocaine, or opiates. There was no difference between the wealthier private patients and the less-fortunate parturients cared for in public clinics.[8] Other works concur with this finding and indicate that the problem of substance abuse is not limited to the socially disadvantaged.[9, 10]

If anesthesiologists were faced with a patient using a specific drug in specific amounts, life would be immeasurably easier. However, as previously mentioned, multiple drug use is the rule, not the exception. A typical scenario is for an individual to use cocaine or methamphetamine to get high and then alcohol or opiates to come down. Another picture is that when users of cocaine can't get their drug of choice, they use heroin, PCP, or marijuana instead. Denial is a cornerstone of the addictive process, so it is no surprise that patients will often deny current drug use. It would seem that this problem could be handled by use of urine drug screens. However, it has been shown that the agreement between laboratory tests and self-reports of drug use depends, in part, upon the characteristics of the drug taken and the pattern of use.[11] Drugs with short half-lives such as alcohol, nicotine, and caffeine may not be detected unless the use is frequent. Drugs with longer half-lives such as heroin, methadone, cocaine, methamphetamine, and marijuana will be detected unless the use is sporadic or infrequent.

In general, the problems faced by the anesthesiologists dealing with the drug user center on the interaction between the drug(s) used and the anesthetics. Specifically, the concern is with tolerance and cross-tolerance; physiological alterations secondary to drug use that affect the anesthetics; acute drug use and the anesthetics; and finally, what occurs when the patient is withdrawn from the drug and an anesthetic is added. There is a paucity of well-controlled experimental literature dealing with these phenomena. Additionally, there are problems caused by the interaction of the drugs abused and the normal functioning of the body, such as the cardiovascular effects of cocaine or ethanol.

Clearly, users of illicit drugs administer them via different routes: oral, inhalational, and parenteral or through some mixture of these routes, depending on the drug used. It is not news that hepatitis and human immunodeficiency virus (HIV) are rampant in the drug-using culture. HIV cannot only be transmitted via needle stick, but also via contaminated blood transferred through the mucous membranes of the eyes, nose, and mouth. A survey by the Centers for Disease Control found that anesthesiologists and nurse anesthetists had 3.6 blood contacts per 100 surgical procedures.[12] A blood contact was defined as getting stuck with a needle or cut with a sharp object that had been in contact with the patient's blood; getting splashed with blood in the eyes, nose or mouth; or having one's skin touched with blood. The message is short and simple: *Be careful out there and take protective measures!* Wear gloves especially when starting intravenous lines, wear glasses and masks, and immediately wash any blood off of yourself.

Finally, the effects of substance abuse are particularly devastating to the unborn. Accordingly, attention will be given to the effects of drugs and drug abuse on pregnancy as well as on fetal and neonatal life. Anesthesiologists are not only called on to provide anesthesia to these infants but may also participate in the perinatal resuscitation of these neonates. Babies born of addicted mothers may evidence a neonatal withdrawal syndrome. The syndrome is not drug-specific but occurs during the withdrawal of any drug that has created a degree of physical dependence in the fetus/neonate. The syndrome is characterized by signs and symptoms of central nervous system (CNS) excitation, altered gastrointestinal (GI) tract function, respiratory distress, and autonomic symptoms. Irritability is the most common symptom, followed by tremors and hypertonicity. Seizures may also appear in the withdrawing neonate. The treatment of the neonatal withdrawal syndrome is symptomatic and supportive. The syndrome is self-limiting and will subside over time. The duration of withdrawal symptoms depends on the drug(s) used by the parturient, how she used the drug, and in what quantity.[13]

Alcohol

Pharmacology and Physiology

Ethanol is a small, simple, mildly polar molecule that readily crosses cell membranes. Alcohol is not known to bind to any specific receptor site like narcotics or benzodiazepines. Some of the effects of alcohol are thought to be mediated by increasing the inward flux of the chloride ion at the gamma aminobutyric acid-a (GABAa) chloride channel.[14] The GABAa receptor is also referred to as the GABA-benzodiazepine receptor. Hence, a probable mechanism for the cross-tolerance is noted between benzodiazepines and ethanol. Another site of the action of alcohol in the central nervous system is the NMDA receptor of the glutamate system.[15] Alcohol has also been shown to have effects on the adenylate cyclase system.[16] Alcohol is an inducer of the cytochrome P-450 system; therefore, it will speed up the metabolism of compounds that are processed by this oxidative system. Since ethanol induces its own metabolism, the tolerance seen is both pharmacokinetic and pharmacodynamic. There is evidence that neuronal calcium channels are involved in ethanol tolerance. The administration of calcium channel blockers during ethanol ingestion prevented the development of tolerance to the behavioral effects of ethanol.[17] Cross-tolerance has been demonstrated between ethanol and benzodiazepines,[18, 19] potent inhalational agents,[20, 21] marijuana,[22] and ketamine.[23] The use of the calcium channel blockers nitrendipine and nimopdipine prevented alcohol withdrawal-induced seizures more effectively than diazepam.[24] It is common folklore that alcoholics require a greater dose of sodium thiopental (pentothal) for induction of anesthesia. However, careful studies have failed to confirm the existence of cross-tolerance between ethanol and a number of short-acting barbiturates (in a rat model).[25] Additionally, it has been recently demonstrated that chronic alcohol intake does not change thiopental anesthetic requirement, pharmacokinetics, or pharmacodynamics in abstinent patients.[26]

Some of the specific organ damage seen in alcoholics are the following: fatty liver, cirrhosis of the liver, Korsakoff's syndrome secondary to brain damage, peripheral neuropathy, impaired nutritional status, and cardiomyopathy. It is not known why a specific target organ is selected preferentially in one person and another organ in another person. It is estimated that cirrhosis occurs in 10% to 20% of heavy drinkers.[27] The effects of ethanol on the liver that are of concern to anesthesiologists include alterations in coagulation status, reduced albumin production resulting in increased potency of drugs due to decreased protein binding, and decreased metabolic clearance of drugs. It has been demonstrated that alcoholic patients with no cardiac history and a normal electrocardiogram will have a flattened Starling curve in response to an increased afterload.[28] That is, the heart of a seemingly normal sober alcoholic or recovering alcoholic may not be able to respond to stress by increasing its output or work. Additionally, it has recently been demonstrated that alcohol intoxication has a depressant effect on left ventricular function in non-alcoholic volunteers.[29] The increased sympathetic nervous system activity that is associated with acute intoxication appears to be a toxic, rather than a compensatory, effect. Of interest is that up to 50% of people with idiopathic cardiomyopathy in the United States are alcohol dependent.[30] Finally it has been demonstrated (in a canine) that after crystalloid volume resuscitation from hemorrhagic shock, the cardiac dysfunction persists in animals chronically fed alcohol.[31] Thus the alcoholic patient is apt to decompensate in response to stress, have a greater cardiac depressant response to anesthetics, and is less likely to rapidly recover from hypovolemic/hemorrhagic shock as would be seen in trauma patients. These patients may need pharmacologic cardiotonic support, such as dopamine or dobutamine, during the anesthetic or prior to induction and for some time in the recovery phase. They are also candidates for early intervention with invasive cardiac monitoring, depending on the clinical picture. It is suggested that signs of cardiac decompensation in the alcoholic population be responded to aggressively with invasive monitoring and pharmacologic support.

The alcoholic patient will often be dehydrated, hypokalemic, hypomagnesemic, and hypoglycemic. These derangements can all be easily corrected. However, caution must be used in giving large amounts of glucose in possibly thiamine-deficient patients since this can lead to encephalopathy.

Finally, first-pass metabolism of orally adminstered ethanol is significantly lower in women than in men. The result of this is that both alcoholic and nonalcoholic groups of women have higher blood ethanol concentrations than men after an equivalent dose of ethanol.[32] It is thought that these data may be the basis for the observation of unusual vulnerability of women who abuse alcohol to early onset of liver and/or brain damage.[33, 34] Based on these data, it is reasonable to assume that the same will hold true for the cardiac effects of ethanol ingestion. That is, the left ventricular dysfunction may manifest sooner in women who abuse alcohol. Ergo, anesthesiologists should be prepared to see cardiac decompensation in the alcoholic parturient in response to stress; for example, rapid sequence induction for cesarean section.

There is a well-defined withdrawal syndrome that begins 12 to 48 hours after cessation of ethanol ingestion. The mild withdrawal syndrome includes tremor, weakness, sweating, hyperreflexia, and GI symptoms. Occasionally a patient may have a grand mal seizure, which currently is treated with a benzodiazepine. A more severe withdrawal syndrome, delirium tremens, may also develop. This syndrome is characterized by autonomic lability, increased pulse rate, and hyperthermia.

Obstetric, Fetal, and Neonatal Effects

Alcoholic women have significantly higher rates of spontaneous abortion, miscarriage, and stillbirth. Low birth weight and intrauterine growth retardation (IUGR) are the most consistently observed effects of fetal exposure to ethanol.[35] The leading known cause of mental retardation is fetal alcohol syndrome (FAS). FAS occurs in between one and three cases of 1,000 live births. The diagnosis of FAS requires evidence of: 1) growth retardation; 2) neuropsychological impairment; and 3) craniofacial anomalies as well as other abnormalities such as heart murmurs, and liver and kidney problems. Only 10% of fetuses that are exposed to large doses of ethanol exhibit FAS.[13] Smoking and other drugs may augment the toxicity of alcohol on the fetus.

Anesthetic Considerations

Regional anesthesia/analgesia is preferred in the nonintoxicated patient when appropriate for the surgery. Chronic alcohol abusers may be relatively hypovolemic due to inhibition of antidiuretic hormone. Consequently, volume loading and careful incremental dosing is safest, whether regional or general anesthesia is used. The presence of peripheral neuropathy is not a contraindication to regional analgesia/anesthesia. There is no evidence that peripheral neuropathy is exacerbated by spinal or epidural anesthesia. Only in multiple sclerosis has there been any implication of anesthesia interacting with a neurological disease. Parturients who had multiple sclerosis and received 0.5% bupivacaine suffered an increased incidence of relapse.[36] However, those who received 2% lidocaine or 0.25% bupivacaine had no problem. The use of regions anesthesia requires careful documentation and discussion with the patient.

Be aware of the coagulation status of the patient. A prothrombin time (PT) and partial thromboplastin time (PTT) should be available as well as a bleeding time to assess platelet function. If the PT is elevated secondary to alcoholic liver disease, there is an increased risk of epidural or subdural hematoma with regional block. If the PT were just mildly increased (25% to 50%) and the bleeding time and PTT were normal, a regional anesthetic may be used in specific clinical situations, such as cesarean section.

It recently has been demonstrated in rats that 15 days of ongoing administration of ethanol has no significant effect on the dose of intrathecal lidocaine to produce sensory blockade. However, 14 hours after withdrawal of ethanol, the dose of lidocaine was increased by 80% for sensory block and by 53% for motor block and the duration of the motor blockade was significantly reduced.[37] The authors have demonstrated cross-tolerance between alcohol and intrathecal lidocaine in rats. However, it is a far jump from rats to humans, but it would be no surprise to have an alcoholic patient who requires more local anesthetic than a nonuser of ethanol. Given the possible unknown volume status and the possibility of tolerance of the local anesthetic, a continuous regional anesthetic technique that allows for a more precise, slow, controlled block is preferred. The only caution is with the use of spinal microcatheters. There have been 11 cases of cauda equina syndrome reported that have all involved larger doses of local anesthetic than one might expect to use normally to achieve a block.[38] Thus, in the alcoholic patient, avoidance of the intrathecal microcatheter may be prudent. If more local anesthetic is needed, it would be difficult to know whether it is due to the cross-tolerance previously described or to the catheter being in the area of the cauda equina.

The hazards of general anesthesia in the alcoholic patient are many. There is, of course, the problem of volume status, electrolyte imbalances, and subclinical left ventricular dysfunction manifest by stress. The alcoholic patient ought to be told about the possibility of awareness during surgery since it is more likely in this group secondary to cross-tolerance with the potent inhalationals. The use of scopolamine may help to produce adequate amnesia for the operation. Low pseudocholinesterase levels in the patient, as a consequence of liver dysfunction, may lengthen the action of succinylcholine. Recent data indicate that the clearance, steady-state volume of distribution, and elimination half-time for vecuronium, in a dose of 0.1 mg/kg, were unchanged in patients with alcoholic liver disease.[39] The dose of thiopental should be low if there is severe liver dysfunction or any suspicion of myocardial instability since reduced binding of the thiobarbiturates will increase their depressant properties. If the liver and heart are reasonably normal, use of a normal (3 to 5 mg/kg) dose of sodium thiopental is recommended since there is no need to increase the dose secondary to cross-tolerance. Should some element of left ventricular dysfunction be suspected, propofol may be the drug of choice. It has recently been demonstrated that propofol does not have negative inotropic effects.[40] Anesthesiologists are sometimes faced with an intoxicated patient for emergency surgery. Such patients are often uncooperative and there is concern about the myocardial depressant effect of the chronic ethanol abuse, as well as the direct depressant effect of the current circulating ethanol. Intoxicated patients are very labile and may easily be given too much anesthesia. Therefore, anesthesiologists should proceed slowly and carefully. Since a postoperative withdrawal syndrome may manifest, administration of a long-acting benzodiazepine during the anesthetic should be considered. Finally, two cases of difficult intubation have been reported in children with FAS.[41] In one of these cases, the child could not be intubated and the airway was quite difficult to maintain for a hernia repair. External examination of the airway of both of these infants revealed a normal appearance.

Cocaine

Pharmacology and Physiology

Cocaine is a naturally occurring alkaloid derived from the plant *Erythroxylon coca*. Cocaine is taken by intranasal insufflation, injection, or freebase smoking, or by the inhalation of the vaporized alkaloidal rock (crack) cocaine. Cocaine, which is metabolized in the plasma and liver by cholinesterase, has potent local anesthetic properties and is a potent central nervous system stimulant. Its mechanism of action is to prevent the re-uptake of norepinephrine, dopamine, and other catecholamines secreted at the nerve endings and to block the sodium (fast) conduction channels.[42] Ergo, cocaine may be thought of as both a sympathomimetic and a local anesethetic. Cocaine acts to accelerate and desynchronize the electroencephalogram. It increases blood pressure, heart rate, respiration, and uterine tone. It causes cardiac arrhythmias and convulsions and may also cause hyperglycemia and hyperpyrexia due to the enhanced sympathetic tone.

The deleterious cardiac effects of cocaine are becoming increasingly well-known and documented in literature. Twenty-one patients who used cocaine for at least 6 months were studied with holter monitors and treadmill tests an average of 9 days after admission to a withdrawal center. Eight of the patients who evidenced spontaneous ST segment elevation did so at a time other than during the treadmill testing.[43] Cocaine in a dose of 2 mg/kg was given intranasally to patients undergoing cardiac catheterization and produced an increase in heart rate and arterial pressure as well as an 8% to 12% decrease in the diameter of the left coronary artery.[44] These effects were mediated by alpha-adrenergic stimulation since they were reversed by the administration of the alpha blocker phentolamine. Similar results were found in canines; that is, cocaine administration produced decreased myocardial perfusion.[45] In addition to reduction of myocardial perfusion, cocaine has a direct depressant effect on the left ventricle.[46] Cocaine has been found to produce marked conduction impairment in both the His-Purkinje system and in the ventricular myocardium.[47] Based on the effects of cocaine, it has been postulated that the "adrenergic and anesthetic properties of cocaine could act synergistically to elicit and maintain ventricular fibrillation. Adrenergic receptor activation would trigger the event whereas sodium channel blockade would create the re-entrant substrate to perpetuate the malignant arrhythmias."[48] Finally, in 20% of patients who died with detectable cocaine in their body fluid, myocarditis was present and attributed to microvascular injury from cocaine.[49] Potentially catastrophic cardiac events are possible, not only in patients currently using cocaine, but also in recent users. Pregnant patients may be at even more risk since the cardiovascular toxicity to cocaine is increased in parturients.[50] The use of beta-adrenergic blocking agents has been suggested for cocaine-induced arrhythmias and calcium channel blockers for cocaine-induced ischemia.[51]

Obstetric, Fetal, and Neonatal Effects

Chasnoff and his coworkers,[52, 53] as well as others,[54, 55] have reported increases in the incidence of spontaneous abortion, abruptio placentae, prematurity, and intrauterine growth retardation after intrapartum exposure to cocaine. There has been a report of the rupture of an unscarred uterus in a primigravid woman associated with cocaine abuse.[56] A case report of a maternal and fetal death secondary to cocaine use to enhance sex was postulated to be secondary to hemodynamic overload, cardiac ischemia, and arrhythmia. The authors concluded that the unexpected cardiac and neurologic disasters associated with cocaine abuse provide compelling evidence that it is the most lethal drug abused.[57] Cocaine-exposed infants have asymmetrical fetal growth retardation (i.e., disproportionately small head circumference for body weight at birth), which is similar to that seen in ethanol exposed infants.[58] There have been reported cases of cerebral infarction in infants whose mothers had used cocaine just prior to labor and delivery.[59] It has been reported that on the first postnatal day, infants exposed to intrauterine cocaine have significantly increased peak systolic, end diastolic, and mean blood flow velocities in the pericallosal, internal carotid, and basilar arteries.[60] These hemodynamic alterations may increase the chance of intracranial hemorrhage in the infant.

The rate of cardiac anomalies among cocaine-positive infants is nearly four times higher than that in drug-free infants. It was concluded that cocaine exposure during prenatal life appears to predispose infants to structural cardiovascular malformations and electrocardiographic abnormalities, as well as to possible cardiopulmonary autonomic dysfunction.[61] Finally, there is an increased incidence of respiratory pattern abnormalities in cocaine exposed babies. Fortunately, the abnormal cardiorespiratory pattern can be normalized by treatment with theophylline. There also is an increased incidence of sudden infant death syndrome (SIDS) in cocaine-exposed neonates; SIDS is reported to be as high as 17% in these infants compared to 4% in narcotic-addicted infants and approximately 0.5% in the general population.[62] There is a withdrawal syndrome seen in the cocaine-exposed infants that consists of jitteriness, hyperreflexia, hypertonicity, irritability, and GI disturbances. The syndrome may persist months longer than that in methadone or heroin addicted babies.

Anesthetic Considerations

There is a depletion of catecholamines in the cocaine-abusing patient; hence, a phlegmatic response to ephedrine given to counteract hypotension may be seen. Should hypotension occur, the use of a direct-acting sympathomimetic such as phenylephrine 100 μg or epinephrine 5 to 10 μg intravenously (IV), is recommended. Due to a depletion of catecholamines, cocaine-abusing patients may exhibit an increased sensitivity to depressants evidenced by a decrease in the minimum alveolar concentration (MAC) of the potent inhalational agents. Anesthesiologists should probably avoid the use of nitrous oxide, halothane, and ketamine if a general anesthetic is given since these agents may exacerbate cocaine toxicity. Labetalol[63] and esmolol[64] are the drugs of choice when dealing with the acutely toxic patient. Anesthesiologists should be wary of nonselective beta blockers since they can produce unopposed alpha-adrenergic tone. Esmolol is an ultra-short beta1-selective blocker that works well in the face of acute cocaine toxicity. Additionally, the use of a calcium channel blocker should be considered for treatment of cardiac dysrhythmias.[65]

A new cause for unexplained tachycardia and hypertension is the use of speedballs—heroin laced with cocaine[66]—prior to hospital admission or operation. As previously mentioned, the likelihood of adverse cardiac events is high. Ergo, the key to treatment of these patients is to be prepared. Labetalol, esmolol, a calcium channel blocker, as well as cardiotonic drugs should be readily available. Lastly, severe thrombocytopenia has been reported to be associated with cocaine abuse.[67] Accordingly, it is prudent to check a platelet count prior to starting a regional anesthetic.

The neonate of a cocaine-abusing mother coming to the hospital for surgery should be watched for the aforementioned cardiac and neurological problems. Additionally, these neonates may exhibit a withdrawal syndrome or have a high incidence of SIDS and therefore must be closely monitored in the postoperative period.

Amphetamines

Amphetamines have a pharmacology and physiology similar to cocaine; that is, enhancing the release of catecholamines. A cause for concern is a new form of methamphetamine—ice,[68] which is a purer and more crystalline form that is smoked. Ice is highly addictive and its prolonged use is associated with fatal lung and kidney disorders. Other effects of ice are paranoia, aggressive behavior, and hallucinations. A major difference between cocaine and ice is that the effects of smoking crack last 20 to 30 minutes, whereas the effects of smoking ice last 8 to 24 hours. From an anesthetic point of view, problems with amphetamine abusers will respond well if they are treated as cocaine abuse problems. Research involving canines has shown that acute amphetamine administration will increase the MAC of halothane while chronic administration will decrease the MAC of halothane.[69] Cardiac arrest[70] during a cesarean section and pulmonary edema after a cesarean section[71] in amphetamine users have been reported. These catastrophic events were attributed to the effects of the amphetamine use.

Opiates

Physiology and Pharmacology

Opiates affect the central nervous system neurons involved in respiration, pain perception, and affective behavior. Peripherally the opiates act to decrease gastrointestinal tract motility. The opiates exert their action by interacting with specific receptors found in the brain, spinal cord, and gut. The opiates have little, if any, direct effect on the cardiovascular system. However, the cardiovascular response to postural change is blocked by opiates, and consequently, orthostatic hypotension may occur. Additionally, the results of necropsies on 169 opiate addicts showed that only 4% had normal hearts. Forty percent died due to infective endocarditis or its consequences, 24% died of an overdose, and 68% of the patients had cardiomegaly.[72]

There is a great degree of tolerance produced to the various effects of the opiates. The greatest tolerance produced is to the euphoriant effects, followed by pain and respiratory depression. There is little, if any, tolerance to the GI effects of opiates. There is a withdrawal syndrome seen after cessation of opiate use. After the last dose, the syndrome will manifest itself within 2 to 4 hours for meperidine, 8 to 12 hours for morphine and heroin, and 24 to 48 hours for methadone. The symptoms include anxiety, restlessness, lacrimation, tremors, hot and cold flashes, tachycardia, tachypnea, muscle spasms, and GI disturbances. The withdrawal is rarely fatal in adults. Unlike cocaine and ethanol, narcotics have few deleterious effects on the human physiology. Other than overdose or behavioral problems, the devastating effects of the narcotic occurs as a infective consequence of poor hygiene and dirty needles.[73]

Obstetric, Fetal, and Neonatal Effects

As with other drugs of abuse, the effects of narcotics on the unborn are devastating. Fetal exposure to heroin or methadone is associated with lower birth weight, shorter body length, and smaller head diameter than nonexposed infants.[74] Another problem that occurs is meconium-stained amniotic fluid, which is taken as indicative of intrauterine fetal distress and/or hypoxia. Other complications of pregnancy that are increased in the heroin addict include: abruptio placentae, pregnancy-induced hypertension, premature rupture of membranes, antenatal bleeding, and premature labor. In late pregnancy, abrupt maternal withdrawal may be accompanied by fetal withdrawal, which is characterized by hyperactivity, hypoxia, passage of meconium, and death. The use of narcotic antagonists should be reserved for the maternal life-threatening overdose. The most serious and disturbing complication is the five to tenfold increase in SIDS seen in infants of opiate-addicted mothers. There is, of course, a neonatal withdrawal syndrome that is characterized by signs and symptoms of CNS excitation, altered GI tract function, respiratory distress, and autonomic symptoms. In short, the same irritability, tremors, hypertonicity, and etcetera that are seen in other neonatal withdrawal syndromes occur in infants born to opiate-abusing women. Between 2% and 11% of addicted neonates may experience a seizure between the third and 34th postnatal day. Methadone-exposed neonates seem more prone to seizures than heroin-addicted neonates. Treatment is symptomatic, and the opioid paregoric is more effective than other nonopiate sedatives in ameliorating the withdrawal syndrome.

Anesthetic Considerations

The patient should either be continued on methadone maintenance therapy or placed on methadone maintenance to avoid the complications of a superimposed withdrawal syndrome. The withdrawal syndrome may manifest itself as unexplained hypotension during an otherwise uneventful general anesthetic.[75] The blood pressure will be restored to control levels by cautious administration of morphine (10 mg IV) or the equivalent dose of the specific narcotic being used by the patient, if the narcotic is known. Regional anesthesia is the choice for the opiate-abusing patient. Spinal and epidural opiates should be avoided in this population, as the respiratory depressant effects may be enhanced by the narcotic maintenance therapy. Agonist-antagonists should not be administered as part of an epidural or subarachnoid regimen since there is a reported case of epidural butorphanol producing withdrawal symptoms in a patient.[76] If a general anesthetic is required, there is no problem with the use of potent inhalationals, since there is no cross-tolerance between them and the opiates.

Marijuana

The activity of marijuana is attributed to delta^9-tetrahydrocannabinol (THC). Centrally, THC produces euphoria and sleeplessness while peripherally it is a beta adrenergic agonist. Thus, marijuana increases heart rate, myocardial work load, and plasma volume. These effects can be blocked by propranolol. There is some cross-tolerance between THC and alcohol, but not between THC and opiates.[77] THC has a long serum half-life and is a potent inducer of hepatic microsomal enzymes. There is a suggestion of a neonatal withdrawal syndrome among infants of heavy marijuana users that is characterized by tremulousness and withdrawal-like crying.

The anesthetic concerns are few, but the major one concerns the chronic bronchitis seen in heavy marijuana users. Other problems may be caused by potentiating the beta adrenergic agonist properties of THC with drugs such as ephedrine. There are theoretical grounds for cross-tolerance to the potent inhalationals; however, acute use of marijuana decreases the MAC of the potent inhalationals. The metabolism of halothane is increased[78] in marijuana users.

Phencyclidine

Phencyclidine (PCP) is a ketamine-like drug that has psychotomimetic and sympathomimetic effects. PCP produces increases in blood pressure, heart rate, and temperature. Unlike ketamine, however, PCP also produces seizures.[79] Prenatal exposure to PCP is associated with a high incidence of IUGR (32%), precipitate labor (43%), meconium-stained amniotic fluid (30%), symptoms of a moderate (38%) or severe (16%) neonatal withdrawal syndrome, and prolonged neonatal hospitalization[80] with possible compromise of the fetus. The temperature elevation can be treated with standard antipyretics. Acute intoxication can be expected to potentiate sedatives, narcotics, and sympathomimetic agents. There may be cross-tolerance to potent inhalational anesthetics, as well as to benzodiazepines. PCP inhibits psuedocholinesterase and thus will potentiate the effects of succinylcholine.

Nicotine

Nicotine is the active, addictive substance in tobacco that stimulates the central nervous system and the autonomic ganglia. The result is a release of epinephrine from the adrenal medulla and generalized vasoconstriction. Nicotine readily crosses the placenta. Pregnant smokers have an increased incidence of abruptio placentae, placenta previa, vaginal bleeding, ruptured membranes, intrauterine growth retardation, and preterm delivery. Infants of mothers who smoke are 25% to 50% more likely to die prior to their first birthday due to respiratory difficulties and SIDS. A preliminary report demonstrated a relationship between the number of cigarettes smoked by the mother and the development of cancer in the offspring. The risk was higher for Hodgkin's disease, acute lymphoblastic leukemia, and Wilms' tumor.[35]

Smoking on the day of surgery increases gastric volume and thus may increase the risk of aspiration. Cigarette smoking plays havoc with the airway as it produces increased levels of carboxyhemoglobin that can lead to hypoxia during intubation. Additionally, smoking produces chronic bronchitis and hyperreactive airways so that instrumentation can lead to bronchospasm. These problems are easily avoided with the use of regional anesthesia, where appropriate.

Summary

Drug use, abuse, and dependency are rampant in all social strata of our society. Given the statistics obtained from surveys of high school children, the problem will be here for some time to come. It is naive to think that the patients anesthesiologists deal with are not using and/or abusing drugs. Not only is it necessary to obtain a careful drug history, but it is crucial to be prepared to react to any abnormal response to anesthetic interventions. Since multiple-substance use is the rule, it should not be expected with any surety how the patient will react to anesthetic interventions. Regional anesthesia, where appropriate, is the choice in cooperative unintoxicated patients. General anesthesia may be necessary for behavioral control of the intoxicated patient. Whatever anesthetic technique is used, it is important to keep in mind the following: give small amounts of the drug(s) to see if there is an exaggerated response; don't be surprised if there is a greatly reduced response to the drug(s) administered; be prepared to switch techniques and pressors; prepared for resuscitation if major cardiac depression occurs; protect yourself—AIDS and hepatitis are ubiquitous in this population; and finally, be aware that babies of substance-dependent/abusing mothers are at high risk for adverse outcomes, especially when an anesthetic is added to the already unfavorable mix.

The Chemically Dependent Anesthesiologist

Physicians, like all human beings, are not immune to impairment secondary to psychiatric disease, chemical dependency, aging, and medical disorders. The remainder of this chapter will cover physician impairment due to substance abuse. It should be noted that the principles of intervention, treatment, and return to practice apply to all forms of impairment.

Prevalence

The percentage of anesthesiologists entering treatment programs (12% to 13%) is three to four times the percentage of anesthesiologists in the physician population of the United States (3% to 3.9%).[81, 82] Based on this percentage, it has been assumed that among anesthesiologists, chemical dependency is more common[83] than for other medical specialties or that anesthesiologists are at high risk for the development of chemical dependence.[84] The presumption that the incidence of chemical dependency is higher in anesthesiology is false. It is true, however, that substance abuse by anesthesiologists is detectable sooner than for other physicians due to the nature of the drugs to which anesthesiologists have access and also that anesthesiologsts are more likely to receive inpatient hospitalization as their initial therapy.[85] The 1991 report of the Committee on Occupational Health of Operating Room Personnel to the American Society of Anesthesiologists' House of Delegates indicated that from January 1986 to January 1991, there were 135 confirmed first-time substance abusers among the anesthesiology residents and fellows from 142 of 158 training programs. These data represent an incidence of 0.7% per year. Two previous studies of drug abuse in anesthesia personnel concur with the current data, showing the incidence to be 1.2% to 1.8%[86] and 1.1% for confirmed drug abuse.[87] This incidence is similar to the 1.1% incidence of hard core cocaine addicts and opiate addicts in the United States. Thus, anesthesiology is not a specialty rampant with addicts, but most likely a mirror of the American population. This information is not intended to minimize the problem, but rather to put it into perspective. The death rate in substance-abusing anesthesiologists, however, is alarming—ranging from 8% to 15% in previously cited studies.

For treatment, the current trend is for a person entering to be younger, to use fentanyl or sufentanil as the drug of choice, and to use multiple drugs.[75] A question that arises is whether anesthesiology causes the disease or if physicians with the disease choose anesthesiology as a specialty. Of the residents admitted to major impaired professional treatment programs, 32% were anesthesiology trainees.[75] Residents and junior staff being treated for chemical dependency stated that their recreational use of chemicals started when they were only 13 or 14 years old![76] Thus, the pattern of chemical use was established long before anesthesiology training. It is suggested that individuals who use chemicals as one of their major coping mechanisms (or as the only major coping mechanism) and choose medicine as a career frequently choose the specialty that requires physicians to administer psychoactive drugs by their own hand on a daily basis. Accessibility may attract the chemical dependent rather than cause the manifestation of the disease. In truth, probably both of these variables are influential—the disease chooses anesthesiology and the availability of drugs provides a mechanism for the disease to express itself.

Diagnosis

Diagnosis is most often dependent on the observation of a change in behavior and occurs in the following five areas[88]: (1) community—withdraws from community activities, driving under the influence violations, embarrassing social behavior; (2) employment—multiple jobs, geographical changes, unexplained gaps in the curriculum vitae; (3) family—withdrawal from family activities, divorce, child abuse, sexual problems; (4) physical—personal hygiene, dress habits, frequent illness, frequent accidents; and (5) hospital—usually the last place that the disease becomes manifest and normally occurs later in the course of the disease. Some of the signs of substance abuse in anesthesiologists include unusually heavy narcotic techniques, frequent breakage (thievery) of narcotic vials, unexplained and frequently occurring illness or absences, sloppy and/or incomplete anesthetic records, frequent need for bathroom (shootup) breaks, and unusual happiness (high) after returning from a break. There is no single symptom or pathognomonic sign displayed by substance-abusing physicians, but a change in behavior should always be considered as a possible manifestation of chemical dependency or psychiatric disease. If controlled substance use is monitored and it is noted that a physician uses 25 mL of fentanyl for sedation on a hip replacement on a 80-year-old patient under epidural anesthesia, a chemical dependency should be considered. Likewise, changes in quantity of drug use may be a tip that there is a drug abuse problem. While control of scheduled drugs in the operating suite is not the answer, it does accomplish a number of things. It sends the message that drug abuse is a serious problem, it raises awareness of the problem of chemical dependency, it may discourage recreational users from trying fentanyl or sufentanil, and it may uncover someone who is chemically dependent.[89]

Treatment

The mainstays of treatment and recovery are the following: (1) intervention; (2) diagnosis and treatment by an appropriate professional (i.e., an addictionologist); (3) participation in appropriate support groups (i.e., R.R., A.A., N.A., C.A., etc.); and (4) monitoring. The best thing to do if a staff member is suspected of having a problem with chemicals is to contact the State Medical Societies' Physicians Assistance Committee. The individuals in this group have the expertise to orchestrate and produce the intervention—they are aware of appropriate treatment programs and can be helpful in initiating a program to monitor the recovering physician. It is important to realize that the Impaired Physicians Committee is an advocacy group without disciplinary functions; it is not the state licensing authority and it handles all communications and cases with the highest degree of confidentiality. The Physicians Assistance Committee may be officially called the Wellness Committee, Physicians Health Committee, Physicians Aid Committee, or the Impaired Physicians Committee—regardless of the title, it is a committee of the State Medical Society whose purpose is to help sick physicians, not punish them.

The only firm rule about intervention is never do it alone. There should always be at least two trained intervenors and it can be very helpful if one of the intervenors is a recovering/recovered chemical dependant. The purpose of intervention is to break through the strong denial system that an impaired physician has built. Intervention should lead to appropriate evaluation and enrollment in a treatment program if necessary. A guide to competent professionals for treatment of chemical dependency is certification by the American Society of Addictive Medicine (ASAM). Be prepared to do whatever is necessary to get persons abusing chemicals into treatment. Time off work, assurance of employment on completion of treatment, and escorting of the physician to the treatment center are just a few of the things that may be necessary.

On return from treatment, the impaired physician will need to be monitored. The monitoring is critical for the physician to be successful in the recovery process and it must have all of the following components: (1) random monitoring for the absence of psychoactive compounds and the presence of prescribed drugs involving the use of breathalyzers or urine and/or blood samples. When using urinalyses, it is essential that the urine is seen leaving the person's urethra and going into the specimen bottle, so there is no question of substitution. Physicians on blockers such as naltrexone or disulfiram (Antabuse) should have these drugs present in the samples. It has been suggested that the most successful treatment outcomes for addicted physicians have been associated significantly with random urine monitoring.[90] (2) Monitoring the attendance of the recovering individual at the prescribed therapy sessions. (3) Monitoring the participation in the self-help groups such as R.R., A.A., N.A., or C.A. An early sign of a relapse or slip may be a decrease in the number of meetings attended. Facilitation of this monitoring may be all that is required since most states and/or treatment programs have a contract that recovering physicians must sign and then the state or program assumes responsibility for the monitoring. Just as knowing a patient's digoxin level is part of appropriate treatment, so is the monitoring of a person in recovery. There should be a contract spelling all of this out and signed by the recovering physician and the department chairman or his/her designate. It has been sugested that the presence of a contract and the enforcement of it will lead to a high rate of recovery.[91]

Prognosis

The data would suggest that the chemically dependent physician has about a 65% change of returning to practice and remaining abstinent.[73] When a structured follow-up program is instituted, the success rate rises to 75% to 83%.[81, 92] Slips do occur, and the greatest number occur within the first 2 years of sobriety. A slip should neither be ignored nor taken lightly, but rather be handled in concert with the treatment program. These events are not a sign of a poor prognosis.

Classical teaching has been that the disease of chemical dependency is never cured, only managed. However, a new alternative treatment philosophy based on the Rational Emotive Therapy of Albert Ellis suggests that chemical dependency is a condition/disease from which one may recover.[93] Chemical dependency or substance abuse is more aptly viewed, in this paradigm, as a condition analogous to hemorrhoids rather than a life-long disease such as asthma or diabetes mellitus. The emphasis is on the individual being responsible for his or her substance abuse. This approach may be more appealing to control-oriented anesthesiologists than the turn-it-over, spiritual programs such as A.A. Whatever the approach, the close monitoring of the recovering physician is imperative.

The big question is whether a person who was chemically dependent on fentanyl or sufentanil should return to the practice of anesthesiology. Farley (personal communication, 1988) states that residents have a very high relapse rate (20 out of 28 [71%]) and of these 20 major relapses, 19 were opiate users. These data are in agreement with the work of Menk et al.,[94] who report a relapse rate for parenteral narcotic users of 66%. A chilling finding by Menk et al. was that of the 52 relapsers, 13 died. Thus death from overdose (11/13) or suicide (2/13) was the relapse symptom in 25% of the cases. Current opinion is that re-entry into the practice of anesthesiology, especially at the resident level, is very hazardous. During treatment, serious consideration should be given to switching specialties. However, the cited data leave much to be desired on a scientific basis. The most important question concerns the nature of the monitoring in the relapsers and is unanswered in the published data. The current policy in the Department of Anesthesiology at Rush-Presbyterian-St. Luke's Medical Center (Kershberger JP, Newman LM: Unpublished manuscript, 1989) is to allow the person who is chemically dependent to return to work after treatment. This policy, which is modeled after the policies of the University of Pennsylvania[95] and Yale University (Swift CA: Personal communication), applies to both residents and staff physicians. All of the following factors must be in place for the recovering narcotic abuser to return to work: (1) agreement of the director of the treatment program that this is a good course of action; (2) naltrexone intake for 6 to 12 months; (3) monitored recovery program; and (4) agreement that any future use of psychoactive drugs will result in the physician leaving the field of anesthesiology and finding some other medical specialty. The American Society of Anesthesiologists has published Chemical Dependence Guidelines for Departments of Anesthesiology.[96]

Stress and Malpractice

Stress reduction programs and teaching of coping skills reduce the incidence of impairment among health care professionals.[97] There are further benefits in the areas of cost reduction. Another result is a reduction in malpractice lawsuit occurrence and payout per malpractice suit. Steffy et al.[98] have published data demonstrating that the establishment of an organization-wide stress management program resulted in a reduction in the number of workmen's compensation claims made as well as a drop in the cost per claim. The stress reduction programs were targeted to individuals and to departments as a whole. The average number of claims before the institution of a stress reduction program in a midwestern hospital with 1,000 employees was 3.1 claims per month with an average monthly cost of claims of $7,329. After the program was implemented, the claims per month decreased to 0.6 with an average monthly cost of $324. Jones et al.[99] presented data that demonstrates: (1) hospital departments with the highest stress levels accounted for 80% of the malpractice occurrences; (2) stress management programs reduced malpractice claims for an average of 1.64 per hospital in 1985 to 0.41 in 1986; (3) a significant reduction in cost per claim; and (4) a reduction in medication errors from ten per month to five per month after the stress management program. They further showed that the frequency of malpractice claims was significantly correlated to job stress, job dissatisfaction, and organizational stress. Personal stress, however, was not correlated with the frequency of malpractice claims. A recent article in American Medical News[100] detailed the preliminary results of a Rand Corporation study of malpractice claims in New Jersey. There were 20 claims filed and seven paid per 100 physician practice years for impaired physicians compared to 16 filed and four paid for a control group of unimpaired physicians. The same article gave results of a study of 224 physicians treated through the Oklahoma State Medical Association's Physician Wellness Committee. Before treatment, 108 claims were filed against 58 doctors for a total of $4.5 million paid between 1980 and 1990. For the same doctors after treatment, the numbers dropped to 15 claims filed against 15 doctors that paid a total of $6,000 with another $6,000 for pending judgments. Based on these data, it makes sense to institute stress management programs to reduce the incidence of impairment and malpractice. Intervention and treatment of impaired physicians ought to occur as soon as possible—primarily for the preservation of their lives, but also to significantly reduce the malpractice burden.

Summary

Addiction and substanace abuse occur in anesthesiologists at about the same rate as that for the general population. However, the mortality rate is disproportionally high regardless of control group used. The paramount, and perhaps only, sign of substance abuse is a change in behavior or increased behavioral lability. Early intervention, treatment, and monitored recovery can produce excellent results. The rate of occurrence and the amount paid for malpractice suits is higher in the impaired physician population. Stress management programs may be a prevention for substance abuse and malpractice.

Acknowledgments

The author acknowledges the invaluable editorial assistance of Jennifer Romero.

References

1. Zimmerman R: Redefining alcoholism stirs controversy. *US J Drug Alcohol Depend* 15:3, 1991.
2. Chapman-Walsh D et al: A randomized trial of treatment options for alcohol-abusing workers. *N Engl J Med* 325:775–782, 1991.
3. Rinaldi RC et al: Clarification and standardization of substance abuse terminology. *JAMA* 259:555–557, 1988.
4. Kelley J: New drug figures stir debate on treatment. *USA Today* May 10:7A, 1990.
5. Gordis E: Seventh special report to the U.S. Congress on Alcohol and Health. Washington DC, National Institute on Alcohol Abuse and Alcoholism, 1990.
6. Jones L: U.S. Teen drug use dropped in 1989, survey finds. *Am Med News* 23:5, 1990.
7. *The Chicago Tribune,* June 7, 1991, Section 1, p 18.
8. Chasnoff IJ, Landress HJ, Barrett ME: The prevalence of illicit-drug or alcohol use during pregnancy and discrepancies in mandatory reporting in Pinellas County, Florida. *N Engl J Med* 322:1202–1206, 1990.
9. Ney JA et al: The prevalence of substance abuse in patients with suspected preterm labor. *Am J Obstet Gynecol* 162:1562–1567, 1990.

10. Sloan LB et al: Substance abuse during pregnancy in a rural population. *Obstet Gynecol* 79:245–248, 1992.
11. Little RE et al: Agreement between laboratory tests and self-reports of alcohol, tobacco, caffeine, marijuana and other drug use in post-partum women. *Soc Sci Med* 22:91–98, 1986.
12. Panlilio AL et al: Blood contacts during surgical procedures. *JAMA* 265:1533–1537, 1991.
13. Levy M, Koren G: Obstetric and neonatal effects of drug abuse. *Emerg Med Clin North Am* 8:633–652, 1990.
14. Allan AM, Harris RA: Gamma-aminobutyric acid and alcohol actions: Neurochemical studies. *Life Sci* 39:2005–2015, 1986.
15. Hoffman PL et al: N-Methyl-D-Aspartate receptors and ethanol: Inhibition of calcium flux and cyclic GMP production. *J Neurochem* 52:1937–1940, 1989.
16. Bode DC, Molinoff PB: Effects of ethanol in vitro on the beta adrenergic receptor-coupled adenylate cyclase system. *J Pharmacol Exp Ther* 246:1040–1047, 1988.
17. Dolin SJ, Little HJ: Are changes in neuronal calcium channels involved in ethanol tolerance? *J Pharmacol Exp Ther* 250:985–991, 1989.
18. Newman LM et al: Regional blood flow and cerebral metabolic changes during alcohol withdrawal and following midazolam therapy. *Anesthesiology* 63:395–400, 1985.
19. Newman LM, Curran MA, Becker GL: Effects of chronic alcohol intake on anesthetic responses to diazepam and thiopental in rats. *Anesthesiology* 65:196–200, 1986.
20. Han YH: Why do chronic alcoholics require more anesthesia? *Anesthesiology* 30:341–342, 1969.
21. Johnstone RE, Kulp RA, Smith TC: Effects of acute and chronic ethanol administration on isoflurane requirement in mice. *Anesth Analg* 54:277–281, 1975.
22. Newman LM et al: delta9-tetrahydro-cannabinol and ethyl alcohol: Evidence for cross-tolerance in the rat. *Science* 175:1022–1023, 1972.
23. Newman LM, Curran MA, Becker GL: Alcoholism alters the anesthetic potency of ketamine. *Alcohol Clin Exp Res* 9:90, 1985.
24. Little HJ, Dolin SJ, Halsey MJ: Calcium channel antagonists decrease the ethanol withdrawal syndrome. *Life Sci* 39:2059–2065, 1986.
25. Curran MA, Newman LM, Becker GL: Barbiturate anesthesia and alcohol tolerance in a rat model. *Anesth Analg* 67:868–871, 1988.
26. Swerdlow BN et al: Chronic alcohol intake does not change thiopental anesthetic requirement, pharmacokinetics, or pharmacodynamics. *Anesthesiology* 72:455–461, 1990.
27. Grant BF, Dufour MC, Hartford TC: Epidemiology of alcoholic liver disease. *Semin Liver Dis* 8:12–25, 1988.
28. Regan TJ et al: Ventricular function in noncardiacs with alcoholic fatty liver: Role of ethanol in the production of cardiomyopathy. *J Clin Invest* 48:397–407, 1969.
29. Kelbaek H et al: Left ventricular function during alcohol intoxication and autonomic nervous blockage. *Am J Cardiol* 59:685–688, 1987.
30. Wang R et al; Alcohol and dilated cardiomyopathy: Incidence and correlation with clinical outcome. *J Subst Abuse Treat* 4:209–213, 1987.
31. Horton JW: Hemorrhagic shock complicated by chronic ethanolism. *Am J Physiol* 257:198–208, 1989.

32. Frezza M et al: High blood alcohol levels in women. *N Engl J Med* 322:95–99, 1990.
33. Morgan MY, Sherlock S: Sex-related differences among 100 patients with alcoholic liver diseases. *Br Med J* 1:939–941, 1977.
34. Jacobsen R: Female alcoholics: A controlled CT brain scan and clinical study. *Br J Addict* 81:661–669, 1986.
35. Cook SP et al, editors: *Alcohol, tobacco, and other drugs may harm the unborn.* Rockville, Md, US Department of Health and Human Services, DHHS Publication No (ADM) 90-1711, 1990.
36. Bader AM, Hunt CO, Datta S: Anesthesia for the obstetric patient with multiple sclerosis. *J Clin Anesth* 1:21–24, 1988.
37. Fassoulaki A, Drasner K, Eger EI: Is chronic ethanol consumption associated with tolerance to intrathecal lidocaine in the rat? *Anesth Analg* 70:489–492, 1990.
38. Rigler ML et al: Cauda equina syndrome, after continuous spinal anesthesia. *Anesth Analg* 72:275–281, 1991.
39. Arder JR et al: Vecuronium in alcoholic liver disease: A pharmacokinetic and pharmacodynamic analysis. *Anesthesiology* 68:771–776, 1988.
40. Lepage J-YM et al: Left ventricular performance during propofol or methohexital anesthesia: Isotopic and invasive cardiac monitoring. *Anesth Anal* 73:3–9, 1991.
41. Finucane BT: Difficult intubation associated with the foetal alcohol syndrome. *Can Anaesth Soc J* 27:574–575, 1980.
42. Laposata EA: Cocaine-induced heart disease: Mechanisms and pathology. *J Thorac Imaging* 6:68–75, 1991.
43. Nademanee K et al: Myocardial ischemia during cocaine withdrawal. *Ann Intern Med* 111:876–880, 1989.
44. Lange RA et al: Cocaine-induced coronary-artery vasoconstriction. *N Engl J Med* 321:1557–1562, 1989.
45. Oster ZH et al: Imaging of cocaine-induced global and regional myocardial ischemia. *J Nucl Med* 32:1569–1572, 1991.
46. Fraker TD et al: Mechanism of cocaine-induced myocardial depression in dogs. *Circulation* 81:1012–1016, 1990.
47. Kabas JS et al: Cocaine-mediated impairment of cardiac conduction in the dog: A potential mechanism for sudden death after cocaine. *J Pharmacol Exp Ther* 252:185–191, 1990.
48. Billman GE: Mechanisms responsible for the cardiotoxic effects of cocaine. *FASEB J* 4:2469–2475, 1990.
49. Virmani R et al: Cardiovascular effects of cocaine: An autopsy study of 40 patients. *Am Heart J* 115:1068–1076, 1988.
50. Woods JR, Plessinger MA: Pregnancy increases cardiovascular toxicity to cocaine. *Am J Obstet Gynecol* 162:529–533, 1990.
51. Gradman, AH: Cardiac effects of cocaine: A review. *Yale J Biol Med* 61: 137–147, 1988.
52. Chasnoff IJ et al: Cocaine use in pregnancy. *Cocaine use in pregnancy. N Engl J Med* 313:666–669, 1985.
53. Chasnoff IJ et al: Temporal patterns of cocaine use in pregnancy. *JAMA* 261:1741–1744, 1989.
54. Mastrogiannis DS et al: Perinatal outcome after recent cocaine usage. *Obstet Gynecol* 76:8–11, 1990.
55. Dombrowski MP et al: Cocaine abuse is associated with abruptio placentae

and decreased birth weight but not shorter labor. *Obstet Gynecol* 77:139–141, 1991.
56. Gonsoulin W, Borge D, Moise KJ: Rupture of unscarred uterus in primigravid woman in association with cocaine abuse. *Obstet Gynecol* 163:526–527, 1990.
57. Burkett G et al: Cocaine-related maternal death. *Am J Obstet Gynecol* 163:40–41, 1990.
58. Little BB, Snell LM: Brain growth among fetuses exposed to cocaine in utero: Asymmetrical growth retardation. *Obstet Gynecol* 77:361–364, 1991.
59. Chasnoff IJ et al: Perinatal cerebral infarction and maternal cocaine use. *J Pediatr* 108:456–459, 1986.
60. van de Bor M, Walther FJ, Sims ME: Increased cerebral blood flow velocity in infants of mother who abuse cocaine. *Pediatrics* 85:733–736, 1990.
61. Lipshultz SE, Frassica JJ, Orav EJ: Cardiovascular abnormalities in infants prenatally exposed to cocaine. *J Pediatr* 118:44–51, 1991.
62. Chasnoff IJ et al: Prenatal cocaine exposure is associated with respiratory pattern abnormalities. *Am J Dis Child* 143:583–587, 1989.
63. Gay GR, Loper KA: Control of cocaine-induced hypertension with labetalol. *Anesth Analg* 67:92, 1988.
64. Pollan S, Tadjziechy M: Esmolol in the management of epinephrine- and cocaine-induced cardiovascular toxicity. *Anesth Analg* 69:693–694, 1989.
65. Trouve R, Nahas G: Nitrendipine: An antidote to cardiac and lethal toxicity of cocaine. *Proc Soc Exp Biol Med* 183:392–397, 1986.
66. Samuels J, Schwalbe SS, Marx GF: Speedballs: A new cause of intraoperative tachycardia and hypertension. *Anesth Analg* 72:397–398, 1991.
67. Orser B: Thrombocytopenia and cocaine abuse. *Anesthesiology* 74:195–196, 1991.
68. Lerner MA: The fire of "ice". *Newsweek,* Nov 27, 1989, pp 37–40.
69. Johnston RR, Way WL, Miller RD: Alteration in anesthetic requirement with amphetamines. *Anesthesiology* 34:357–363, 1972.
70. Samuels SI, Maze A, Albright G. Cardiac arrest during cesarean section in a chronic amphetamine abuser. *Anesth Analg* 58:528–530, 1979.
71. Smith DS, Gutsche BB: Amphetamine abuse and obstetrical anesthesia. *Anesth Analg* 59:710–711, 1980.
72. Dressler FA, Roberts WE: Modes of death and types of cardiac diseases in opiate addicts: Analysis of 168 necropsy cases. *Am J Cardiol* 64:909–920, 1989.
73. Estroff TW, Gold MS: Chronic medical complications of drug abuse. *Psychiatr Med* 3:267–285, 1987.
74. Chasnoff IJ: Effects of maternal narcotic vs non narcotic addiction on neonatal neurobehavior and infant development. In Pinkert TM, editor: *Consequences of maternal drug abuse.* Washington DC, 1985, National Institute on Drug Abuse, pp 84–95.
75. Mark LC et al: Hypotension during anesthesia in narcotic addicts. *NY State J Med* 66:2685–2686, 1966.
76. Weintraub S et al: Acute narcotic withdrawal syndrome precipitated by epidural butorphanol. *Anesth Analg* 64:452–453, 1985.
77. Newman LM, Lutz MP, Domino EF: Delta^9-tetrahydrocannabinol and some CNS depressants: Evidence for cross-tolerance in the rat. *Arch Int de Pharmacodynam Ther* 207:254–259, 1974.
78. Berman ML, Bochantin JF: Effect of delta-9 tetrahydrocannabinol (mariuana)

on liver microsomal dechlorinase activity: A preliminary report. *Anesth Analg* 51:929–932, 1972.

79. Leccese AP et al: The convulsant and anticonvulsant effects of phencyclidine (PCP) and PCP analogues in the rat. *Behav Brain Res* 19:163–169, 1986.
80. Tabor BL, Smith-Wallace T, Yonekura ML: Perinatal outcome associated with PCP versus cocaine use. *Am J Drug Alcohol Abuse* 16:337–348, 1990.
81. Herrington RE, et al: Treating substance-use disorders among physicians. *JAMA* 247:2253–2257, 1982.
82. Talbot GD et al: The medical association of Georgia's impaired physicians program. *JAMA* 257:2927–2930, 1987.
83. Arnold WA III: Environmental safety including chemical dependency. In Miller RD, editor: *Anesthesia,* ed 3. New York, 1990, Churchill Livingstone, pp 2407–2420.
84. Gallegos KV, Browne CH, Veit FW: Addiction in anesthesiologists: Drug access and patterns of substance abuse. *QRB* 14:116–122, 1988.
85. Ward CF, Newman LM: National conference on the impaired physician. Longnecker DE, editor: Report on scientific meeting. *Anesthesiology* 68:979–980, 1988.
86. Gravenstein JS, Kory WP, Marks RG: Drug abuse by anesthesia personnel. *Anesth Analg* 62:467–472, 1983.
87. Ward CF, Ward GC, Saidman LJ: Drug abuse in anesthesia training programs. *JAMA* 250:922–925, 1983.
88. Talbot DG, Benson EB: Impaired physicians: The dilemma of identification. *Postgrad Med J* 68:56–64, 1980.
89. Newman LM et al: A departmental approach to the prevention and detection of substance abuse by anesthesia personnel. Scientific Exhibit, American Association of Anesthesiologists Meeting, 1990.
90. Shore JH: The Oregon experience with impaired physicians on probation: An eight year follow-up. *JAMA* 257:2931–2934, 1987.
91. Polk SL: Substance abuse in anesthesia: Patient safety among issues. *Anesth Patient Safety Found Newsletter* 6:1–3, 1991.
92. Morse RM et al: Prognosis of physicians treated for alcoholism and drug dependence. *JAMA* 251:743–746, 1984.
93. Trimpey J: *The small book: Rational recovery from alcoholism,* ed 3. Lotus, Calif, 1989, Lotus.
94. Menk EJ et al: Success of reentry into anesthesiology training programs by residents with a history of substance abuse. *JAMA* 263:3060–3062, 1990.
95. Lecky JH et al: A departmental policy addressing chemical substance abuse. *Anesthesiology* 65:414–417, 1986.
96. Hug CC Jr, et al: *Chemical Dependence Guidelines for Departments of Anesthesiology.* Park Ridge, Ill, American Society of Anesthesiology, 1991.
97. Scott CD: Stress management can lead to reduced malpractice. *Physician Executive* Jan-Feb:18–20, 1988.
98. Steffy BD et al: A demonstration of the impact of stress abatement programs on reducing employees' accidents and their cost. *Am J Health Promotion* 1:25–32, 1986.
99. Jones JW et al: Stress and medical malpractice: Organizational risk assessment and intervention. *J Appl Psychol* 73:727–735, 1988.
100. Larkin H: Impaired colleagues: Add liability to list of reasons to get them help. *Am Med News* Nov 11, 1991, pp 13–14.

Preoperative Evaluation for Elective Surgery—What Laboratory Tests Are Needed?*

Michael F. Roizen, M.D.

Chairman, Department of Anesthesia and Critical Care; Professor, Department of Medicine, University of Chicago Division of the Biological Sciences, Pritzker School of Medicine, Chicago, Illinois

Stephan Cohn, M.D.

Assistant Professor, Department of Anesthesia and Critical Care, University of Chicago Division of the Biological Sciences, Pritzker School of Medicine, Chicago, Illinois

The first goal of preoperative evaluation is to reduce the morbidity of surgery. This goal encourages the use of tests to uncover hidden conditions that may contribute to perioperative morbidity. To accomplish this goal, preoperative medical assessment from the 1940s to the 1960s relied primarily on accurate history-taking and physical examination. Then in the early 1960s, Kaiser and Technicon introduced batteries of tests for multiphasic screening. The hypothesis was that if a disease could be identified with multiphasic screening before it became clinically evident, morbidity could be prevented. The ease and low cost of ordering and obtaining many tests made the process seem logical and desirable. As a result, many anesthesia departments made rather arbitrary rules—recommendations that became requirements—regarding the tests that should be performed before elective surgery. When, with good intentions, anesthesiologists and surgeons tried to follow the rules, problems arose. Physicians believed that with inexpensive batteries of tests they could efficiently screen for disease. Instead, they were often still trying to determine which tests to order before surgery, what to do about an unexpectedly abnormal result on the morning of surgery, or how abnormal a result had to be before seeking the ad-

*Much of this chapter is modified from Roizen MF, Hurd M: Preoperative patient evaluation, in Rogers MC (ed): *Current Practice in Anesthesiology,* ed 2. St Louis, Mosby–Year Book, 1990, pp 14–22.

vice of a consultant. The system of preoperative multiphasic screening with multiple nonselective tests proved impractical.

Soon the hypothesis that nonselective testing benefits patients by uncovering hidden conditions was challenged. Data indicated that testing without regard to risk group or likelihood of an abnormality leads to harm from pursuit of false-positive results, to information overload that may result in failure to pursue significant abnormalities, and to inefficient operating room schedules. In the past decade, several other factors also have affected the ordering of preoperative tests: the publication of practice guidelines to identify risk groups for whom specific tests are warranted; increased cost-consciousness; the proliferation of outpatient surgery; medicolegal issues; and most recently, practice marketability and surgeon profiling. To these factors may be attributed a reduction of almost 20% in unwarranted (nonselective) testing from 1977 to 1987.[1]

In the current cost-conscious medical environment, more than 60% of surgical patients come to the hospital on the morning of surgery, even at our tertiary care institution. At most community hospitals, 80% of surgical patients are either outpatients or morning-of-surgery admissions. Cost efficiency has created a preoperative assessment environment that severely limits time for test selection or discussions with patients about risk or the alternatives of perioperative care. We seem to be rushing from operating room to operating room to save operating room expense; the time of surgeons, anesthesiologists, and nurses; and capital costs. Thus, time and other constraints tempt us to return to ordering batteries of tests preoperatively. But such a solution increases physician risk. Inadequate or inappropriate care may result from the time-consuming follow-up of abnormal test results ultimately meaningless for patient care. The practice of ordering batteries of tests unnecessarily is not cost-effective and decreases funds that would otherwise be available to care for others.

The link between adequate preoperative evaluation and improved outcome is corroborated by some data and may be strongest when unsuspected cardiovascular disease is discovered, but the link is by no means proved. Because perioperative mortality and morbidity increase with the severity of preexisting disease,[2–8] careful evaluation and treatment should reduce their occurrence.[4, 9, 10] We will first review the scientific evidence that shows that with history and physical examination, one can select appropriate preoperative tests for patients that can reduce perioperative morbidity.

Routine Laboratory Testing Is Not the Most Effective Way to Evaluate Patients Preoperatively

Leonard and coworkers[11] reported that biochemical screening tests had no significant value in the preoperative screening of pediatric patients expected to be hospitalized for less than 1 week. In another study, Korvin and associates[12] reviewed biochemical tests given routinely to 1,000 patients on hospital admission. None of the tests produced a new diagnosis that was unequivocally beneficial to the patient. In an ambitious, controlled trial of multiphasic screening in 1,500 patients, Olsen and coworkers[13] found no difference in morbidity between control groups and groups having screening tests. Durbridge and colleagues[14] compared 1,500 patients who were randomly assigned to undergo or not to undergo screening tests on admission. No benefit resulted from the 8,363 tests that were performed with respect to duration of hospital stay or patient outcome. Narr et al.[15] found that more than 3,000 patients of American Society of Anesthesiologists (ASA) class I or II who underwent elective surgical procedures at the Mayo Clinic did not benefit from laboratory testing. Apfelbaum et al.[16] reviewed data from a multicenter study showing that asymptomatic individuals were more likely to be harmed by, than to benefit from, unwarranted tests and physicians' actions in response to the abnormal results of those tests.

Some testing is indicated to uncover disease in high-risk groups (i.e., the electrocardiogram [ECG] in men older than 40 years or women older than 50 years of age, the chest x-ray for a smoker with a productive cough) or to optimize therapy (glucose levels in a patient with diabetes mellitus, prothrombin time for a patient receiving sodium warfarin).[17, 18] But even for the elderly, for whom testing is likely to be of most benefit, nonselective screening has not been of great value. Domoto et al.[19] examined the yield and effectiveness of a battery of 19 screening laboratory tests performed routinely in 70 functionally intact elderly patients (average age, 82.6 years) who resided at a chronic care facility. The 70 patients underwent 3,903 screening tests. New abnormal results primarily occurred in five of the 19 screening tests; most of these new abnormalities were only minimally outside the normal range. Only four (0.1% of all tests ordered) led to change in patient treatment, none of which, Domoto and colleagues concluded, benefited any patient in an important way.

Wolf-Klein and colleagues[20] retrospectively studied the results of annual laboratory screening on a population of 500 institutionalized and ambulatory elderly patients (average age, 80 years). From the 15,000 tests performed, 756 new abnormalities were discovered, 690 of which were ignored. Sixty-six of the new abnormalities were evaluated; 20 new diagnoses resulted, 12 of which were treated. Two patients of the 500 ultimately may have benefited from eradication of asymptomatic bacteriuria (although eradication of asymptomatic bacteriuria has not been shown to improve the quality of life or extend the life span).[21–24]

Studies show that the history and physical examination are the best measures for screening for disease. Delahunt and Turnbull[25] evaluated patients who were assessed preoperatively for varicose vein stripping or inguinal herniorrhaphy. For 803 patients who underwent 1,972 tests, only 63 abnormalities were uncovered in those patients whose history or physical findings had not indicated the need for tests, but in no instance did the discovery of these abnormalities influence patient treatment. Rosselló and associates[26] retrospectively evaluated 690 admissions for elective pediatric surgical procedures. The history and physical examination indicated the probability of abnormalities in all 12 patients in whom an abnormality was found through laboratory testing. Clinical diagnosis, and not laboratory testing, was the apparent basis for any change in operative plans.

Several studies have compared outcome for groups of hospitalized patients who underwent laboratory screening tests to supplement the history and physical examination with that of patients who did not undergo routine screening tests. Wood and Hoekelman[27] found that 28 of 1,924 children examined had changes in preoperative clinical courses (all had surgery postponed) because of abnormal history, physical examination, or laboratory examination results. Three of those 28 patients for whom surgery was postponed had abnormal laboratory tests that were not indicated by history or physical examination findings. Thus, history or physical examination dictated appropriate laboratory testing for all but 3 of 1,924 patients. The abnormalities discovered for these 3 patients pertained to their chest radiographs. (These children were part of a study comparing perioperative outcome at two hospitals, one of which required chest radiographs as a screening test for elective surgery in children and one of which did not.) There were no differences noted in anesthetic or perioperative complications between the two groups. Wood and Hoekelman, therefore, recommended that chest radiographs not be obtained routinely for apparently healthy children.

Even in a referral population, history and physical examination determine more than 90% of the clinical course after consultation about cardiovascular, neurologic, or respiratory diseases.[28] Other studies also have demonstrated that the history and physical examination accurately indicate all areas in which subsequent laboratory testing proves beneficial to patients. For example, Rabkin and Horne[29, 30] examined the records of 165 patients having new (i.e., a change from a previous tracing) abnormalities on the ECG that were potentially surgically significant (i.e., that might affect perioperative management or outcome). In only two instances were the anesthetic or surgical plans altered by the discovery of new abnormalities on an ECG that were not indicated by history. Thus, for these 165 patients, for whom the benefits of a laboratory test should have been maximal (because a new abnormality was detected during the course of preoperative assessments), the history or physical examination determined case management most of the time. Even in one of the two instances of altered case management—a patient having atrial fibrillation—the physical examination should have indicated that an ECG needed to be performed. A history or physical examination was not available for the other patient.

Repeating laboratory tests when results were normal within the previous 2 months does not appear to benefit patients. Macpherson et al.[31] found that only 13 tests of more than 3,000 repeated within 1 year of surgery yielded new information, and the 13 new results could have been predicted from a new event in each patient's history.

In summary, the studies previously cited point to the inadequacy of routine laboratory tests as an independent means of assessing patients preoperatively. Most of these laboratory tests are superfluous to patient care management. The evidence supports the primacy of history and physical examination to screen for disease; laboratory tests can be used to screen for disease when such tests have proven effective but are better used to confirm clinical diagnoses or to optimize a patient's condition before surgery.

Random Testing May Introduce Additional Risk to the Patient

Unnecessary testing may lead physicians to pursue and treat abnormalities based on borderline positive and false-positive results. Few studies have examined whether increased tests and the follow-up of false-positive tests adversely affect patients. Roizen[32] retrospectively examined the adverse effects of chest x-ray examinations on patients. In this study population of 606 patients, 386 extra chest radiographs were ordered without indication. In those 386 patients, 1 elevated hemidiaphragm and probable phrenic nerve palsy was found that may have resulted in improved care for that patient. In addition, 3 lung shadows were found that resulted in three sets of invasive tests, including one thoracotomy without discovery of any disease. These procedures caused considerable morbidity, including 1 pneumothorax and 4 months of disability, for those patients. Tape and Mushlin[33] found that chest x-rays performed without indication or symptoms of disease, even in an elderly population, resulted in less benefit than harm.

In another study, Turnbull and Buck[34] examined the charts of 2,570 patients undergoing cholecystectomy to determine the value of preoperative tests. The history and physical examinations successfully indicated all tests that ultimately benefited the patients with 4 possible exceptions. But again, in those 4 patients it is doubtful if any benefit actually occurred. Among them was 1 patient whose emphysema was detected only with chest x-ray; he underwent preoperative physical therapy without subsequent postoperative complication. Two patients had unsuspected hypokalemia (3.2 and 3.4 mEq/L, respectively) and received potassium treatment prior to surgery. Data in the literature now indicate that no harm occurs to patients undergoing an operation with this degree of hypokalemia, and severe potential harm may be caused by treating such patients with oral or intravenous potassium.[35–39] The fourth patient in whom possible benefit occurred received a blood transfusion before cholecystectomy for an asymptomatic hemoglobin concentration of 9.9 g/dL. Since cholecystectomy is not normally associated with major blood loss, it is concluded that this patient also received no benefit and only the risk of transfusion from that preoperative laboratory test and its pursuit.

In another study, only 2 patients at most (who had eradication of asymptomatic bacteriuria) benefited from the 9,270 screening tests that were obtained.[40] At least 1 patient was seriously harmed from the pursuit of abnormalities on screening tests and their treatment; this woman developed atrial fibrillation and congestive heart failure after thyroid therapy was instituted for borderline low thyroxine and free thyroxine index tests. It is unclear if these investigators examined other patients for potential harm arising similarly from the pursuit and treatment of abnormalities.

When Batteries of Laboratory Tests Yield Abnormal Results That Are Neither Pursued nor Noted, Medicolegal Risk for Physicians Increases

Extra testing—testing that is not warranted by findings on a medical history—does not serve as medicolegal protection against liability. A series of studies (see Roizen[41]) shows that 30% to 95% of all unexpected abnormalities found on preoperative laboratory tests are not noted on the chart preoperatively. Many reports of preoperative radiographs, for example, are not on the chart before anesthesia is administered. This lack of notation occurs not only at university medical centers, but in community hospitals also. Data show that failure to pursue an abnormality that has been detected poses a greater risk to medicolegal liability than does failure to detect an abnormality.[42] In this way, extra testing results in extra medicolegal risk to physicians. Three true cases illustrate the pitfalls.

1. An asymptomatic woman scheduled for a tubal ligation with no indication for a chest x-ray received one on the morning of surgery. The x-ray showed a solitary left hilum. Three months later, after removal of the upper left lobe of her lung, she returned to work. She did not receive a tubal ligation nor any benefit from the removal of this benign cyst. The anesthesiologist and surgeon were successfully sued.
2. A patient employed as a litigator underwent a series of preoperative laboratory tests. No history of bleeding diathesis existed, but test results showed an abnormal prothrombin time. The anesthesiolgist discussed the abnormal result with the surgeon's first assistant and with the patient. It was decided that the abnormality posed no significant risk. Before the procedure but after anesthesia had been administered, the surgeon, fearing potential bleeding around a facial nerve in a litigator, requested a hematology consult. Surgery was postponed for 2 weeks, and the litigator underwent $1,900 worth of factor assays. His prothrombin time remains a laboratory test abnormality without explanation.
3. A patient received a preoperative chest x-ray that showed a cancer. The x-ray result was not sought by the anesthesiologist or the surgeon. The surgeon was successfully sued because he failed to pursue that abnormality.

Random Preoperative Testing Is Inefficient for Operating Room Schedules

According to hospital administrators in the United States, surgeons say that they order preoperative tests to satisfy the anesthesiologist: they find it easier just to order all the tests and let the anesthesiologist sort them out. Surgeons also believe that it is much more efficient to order batteries of tests than to have the anesthesiologist, who sees the patient the night before or the morning of surgery, try to get the tests on an emergency basis. These surgeons apparently do not realize that abnormalities detected by tests done in this battery fashion are not discovered until the night before or the morning of surgery, if at all. Then abnormal results on these tests delay or postpone schedules, as extra effort and time are wasted in obtaining consultant reviews of false-positive or slightly abnormal results.

This approach may soon change with the advent of profiling. Profiling, which requires the use of a unique personal identification number, is the detailed, computerized recording of all resources used by a physician for a procedure for the purpose of comparison against the resources used by other physicians for the same procedure. The medicolegal effects of profiling may be perverse—lawsuits may be filed against physicians who, in their efforts to keep cost per patient down, fail to order appropriate tests. Then the problem regarding preoperative test selection in the next 5 years may not be too many unnecessary tests, but rather too few warranted tests.

Guidelines and Patient Questionnaires Can Expedite the Process of Test Selection

At the University of California, San Francisco, Kaplan et al.[43] found that even a partial history, combined with the expert rules in Tables 1 and 2,

TABLE 1.
Current (1992) Minimal (? Maximal) Laboratory Test Recommendations Based on Benefit Exceeding Risk in Asymptomatic Patients Scheduled for Peripheral Surgical Procedures

Age (yr)	Men and Women	Men Only	Women Only
≤40			? pregnancy test*
40–49	Hematocrit (HCT)	ECG	? pregnancy test*
50–64	HCT, ECG		
65–74	HCT, blood urea nitrogen (BUN), ECG, ?chest x-ray†		
≥75	HCT, BUN, glucose, ECG, chest x-ray†		

*If patient cannot rule out pregnancy definitely.
†Benefit-risk ratio of chest x-ray for asymptomatic individuals over the age of 60 is not clear, but it appears that risk exceeds benefit until over age 74.

TABLE 2.
Simplified Strategy for Preoperative Testing*†

Preoperative Condition‡	HGB		WBC	PT/PTT	PLT BT	Elect	Creat BUN	Blood Gluc	SGOT/Alk PTAse	X-ray	ECG	Preg	T/S
	M	F											
Procedure with blood loss	X	X											X
Procedure without blood loss													
Neonates	X	X											
Age <40		X											
Age 40–49		X									m		
Age 50–64		X									X		
Age ≥65	X	X								±	X		
Cardiovascular disease							X			X	X		
Pulmonary disease										X	X		
Malignancy	X	X	L	L						X			
Radiation therapy			X							X	X		
Hepatic disease				X					X				
Exposure to hepatitis									X				

Renal disease	X	X				X	X				
Bleeding disorder				X	X						
Diabetes mellitus						X	X	X		X	
Smoking ≥20 pack-yr	X	X							X		
Possible pregnancy											X
Diuretic use						X	X				
Digoxin use						X	X			X	
Steroid use						X		X			
Anticoagulant use	X	X		X							
CNS disease			X			X	X	X		X	

*Modified from Roizen et al: *Anesthesiol Clin North Am* 5:15-34, 1987. Kaplan EB et al: *JAMA* 253:3576-3581, 1985. Blery C et al: *Lancet* 1:139–141, 1986.

†± = perhaps obtain; * = obtain for leukemias only; X = obtain; m = men only; HGB = hemoglobin; WBC = white blood cell count; PT = prothrombin time; PTT = partial thromboplastin time; PLT = platelet count; BT = bleeding time; Elect = electrolytes (i.e., sodium, potassium, chloride, carbon dioxide, and proteins); Creat/BUN = creatinine or blood urea nitrogen; SGOT/Alk PTAse = serum glutamic-oxaloacetic transaminase and alkaline phosphatase; T/S = blood typing and screen for unexpected antibodies.

‡Not all diseases are included in this table. The physician's own judgment is needed regarding patients with diseases not listed.

conveyed enough information to indicate correctly all but 22 abnormalities (none of which affected patient outcome) in more than 2,785 preoperative blood tests obtained (counting the complete blood count and simultaneous multichannel analysis of six variables [SMA 6] as one test). Knowing only the admission diagnosis, previous discharge diagnoses, and scheduled operation, and using previously determined indications for laboratory testing enabled detection of virtually all abnormalities that would have been detected with routine screening.

Several groups have tested the effects and sensitivity of orally administered or written questionnaires as a means of linking the selection of laboratory tests with a patient's medical history.[41, 44] In 1987, McKee and Scott[45] used an orally administered set of 17 questions and patient demographics to select preoperative tests for 400 patients. They found that age was the best predictor of abnormalities on preoperative tests. Complications occurred most commonly in patients who reported positive symptoms on the questionnaire and who were older.

A recent study determined that the responses of patients to written questions can be used to predict which laboratory tests will yield abnormal results for those patients. After the patient answers the questionnaire, a plastic overlay reveals what tests are indicated. If the patient cannot answer the questions, a standard group of tests is ordered. Even in a tertiary care hospital that admits very sick patients, more than 60% of those laboratory tests now routinely obtained could be eliminated. The elimination of such tests could result in more than an 80% reduction in patient charges and hospital costs (Finkler[46] and personal communication, S.N. Cohen).

The protocols outlined in Tables 1 and 2 offer guidelines for using clinical judgment in ordering laboratory tests. A careful history and physical examination of the patient are required with special attention to testing whenever indicators of disease entities listed in the tables are discovered. The protocol clearly places the burden on an accurate history.

We do not say that all standard screening tests should be discontinued. Some are beneficial: the ECG for the patient with diabetes mellitus, for men older than 40 years, and for women older than 50 years of age; the fecal occult blood test for individuals older than 40 years of age (every 2 years, every year in high-risk groups); the Papanicolaou smear (every 3 years for sexually active women, every year for women at high risk); and the mammogram (every year for women 50 years of age and for women older than 40 years in high-risk groups).[17, 18, 47, 48] That is the point of the screening history, to identify individuals likely to benefit from testing. The rationale for the choice of some specific tests deserves further comment.

Hemoglobin, Hematocrit, and White Blood Cell Counts

How many asymptomatic patients have a degree of abnormality on hematocrit or the white blood cell (WBC) count that alters perioperative management? I would define the following values as not meriting intervention perioperatively: a hematocrit of 27 to 54 for patients undergoing operations during which major blood loss is unlikely and a WBC count of 2,400 to 16,000 per cubic millimeter for individuals not undergoing insertion of a prosthesis. When values fall outside these ranges, we recommend seeking alternative diagnoses before the institution of anesthesia or surgery. The data available in the literature[41] indicate that either preoperative hematocrit or hemoglobin levels should be determined for all surgical patients older than 60 years of age. Hematocrit and red blood cell antigen screening is warranted for all patients undergoing procedures involving possible loss of more than 2 U per 70 kg of body weight. WBC counts appear to be rarely indicated in asymptomatic individuals but might be considered when a prosthesis is to be inserted.

Blood Chemistries and Urinalysis

What blood chemistries would have to be abnormal, and how abnormal would they have to be, to justify changing the perioperative management? Abnormal hepatic or renal function might change the choice and dose of anesthetic or adjuvant drugs. About one in 700 supposedly healthy patients is actually harboring hepatitis, and one in three of those will become jaundiced. However, our group found no asymptomatic patient who denied exposure to hepatitis who then became jaundiced after uneventful surgery (Apfelbaum et al.[16] data from 3,500 patients in a prospective study). These data imply that either the screening history suffices or the incidence of asymptomatic hepatitis is decreasing. Unexpected abnormalities are reported for 2% to 10% of patients with multiphasic screening, and these abnormalities lead to many additional tests that usually (in approximately 80% of cases) have no significance for the patient. Unexpected abnormalities that are significant arise in 2% to 5% of patients studied. Of these abnormalities, approximately 70% are related to blood glucose and blood urea nitrogen (BUN) levels. The 2 to 20 additional tests on the screening SMA 6-21 panels lead to very few important discoveries affecting anesthesia. In fact, the false-positive rate is so high (96.5% for the test for calcium) that the value representing cost vs. benefit for most of these tests (even when the initial tests are free) is negative, as is the value representing benefit vs. risk.

If a screening test for hepatitis is desired because the incidence of hepatitis is 0.14% and/or because one wishes to avoid the potential legal problems of postanesthetic jaundice, only three tests appear to be justified: serum glutamic-oxaloacetic transaminase, blood glucose, and BUN. Even then, the last two are indicated only for patients older than 64 years of age. In fact, if the data from our group on asymptomatic liver disease can be generalized, no blood chemistry tests are warranted for patients younger than 64 years of age. Furthermore, if the antibody test that detects non-A, non-B hepatitis (now called hepatitis C) proves as useful after infection has occurred, the medicolegal risk posed by postanesthetic jaundice will be even less.

Abnormalities are commonly found on urinalysis.[41] The quality of urinalysis results obtained with dipstick technique has been variable at best. In addition, these abnormal results usually do not lead to beneficial changes in management unless an implant operation is planned. Most of the results that do lead to beneficial changes could have been obtained by history or determination of BUN and glucose levels, tests that are already recommended for all patients older than 64 years of age. Thus, urinalysis, although initially inexpensive, becomes an expensive test to justify on a cost-benefit or benefit-risk basis.

Chest X-ray Examination

What abnormalities on chest radiographs would influence management of anesthesia? Certainly, it may be important to know about the existence of tracheal deviation; mediastinal masses; pulmonary nodules; a solitary lung mass; aortic aneurysm; pulmonary edema; pneumonia; atelectasis; new fractures of the vertebrae, ribs, or clavicles; dextrocardia; or cardiomegaly before proceeding to anesthesia and surgery. However, a chest radiograph probably would not detect the degree of chronic lung disease requiring a change in anesthetic technique any better than would the history and physical examination. The data reviewed by Roizen[41] show that abnormalities are rare in the asymptomatic individual. In fact, if the patient is asymptomatic and younger than 74 years of age, the risks of chest x-ray examination probably exceed the potential benefits. This analysis is, of course, predicated on maximizing benefit to society in general, as one cannot predict in advance which patients will benefit or which will be harmed.

Screening for Cardiac Disease

Although individual episodes of myocardial ischemia may not produce symptoms, almost all patients (excluding diabetics and patients with autonomic insufficiency) have symptoms that lead one to screen for myocardial disease. Identifying patients with coronary artery disease, aortic valvular disease, or low left ventricular ejection fraction to alter their perioperative care may improve outcome. Identification of these cardiac conditions with low-risk tests is often followed by percutaneous transluminal coronary angioplasty (PTCA), coronary artery bypass graft (CABG), or recommendation for increased perioperative monitoring and more aggressive pain management to improve outcome and the chance of survival. While such reasoning is logical, it has not been tested by rigorous prospective trial. Rao et al.[49] found that scrupulously maintaining hemodynamics of patients in an intensive care unit for 3 days after surgery reduced the reinfarction and mortality rates by more than 60%. Hertzer et al.[50, 51] followed up 1,000 vascular surgery patients who either did or did not undergo coronary revascularization preoperatively. Initially mortality rates increased for the former, but that group had a lower 5-year cardiac death rate (Table 3). Similar results have emerged from the multicenter Coronary Artery Surgical Study (CASS, reviewed in Roizen[52]) and from a study of patients who

TABLE 3.
A Comparison of Mortality after Vascular Surgery with and without Preoperative Myocardial Revascularization*

Surgical Indication	PTCA or CABG, %	Vascular Surgery Alone, %	Combined Immediate Mortality, %	Combined 5-year Cardiac Deaths, %
Abdominal aortic aneurysm following CABG	5.0	1.6	6.6	17.5
Abdominal aortic aneurysm alone		3.3	3.3	26
Lower extremity ischemia following CABG	5.5	0.0	5.5	
Lower extremity ischemia alone		1.8	1.8	
Cerebrovascular disease following CABG	5.5	0.0	5.5	
Cerebrovascular disease alone		0.3	1.8	

*Data from Hertzer NR et al: *Ann Surg* 199:223–233, 1984; and Hertzer NR et al: *Clev Clin Q* 53:133–143, 1986.

underwent PTCA before noncardiac surgery.[53] Thus, attempts have been made to identify factors in the history that lead to increased risk. The 12 factors in history that correlate with ECG abnormalities and the 5 factors, including ECG abnormalities, that have been correlated with outcome after vascular surgery appear in Figure 1.[52] The following generalizations can be made from the data: ECG is not needed preoperatively for women younger than 50 years and men younger than 40 years of age who are without chest pain, congestive heart failure, hypertension, diabetes mellitus, dysrhythmia, or shortness of breath if they do not need vascular sur-

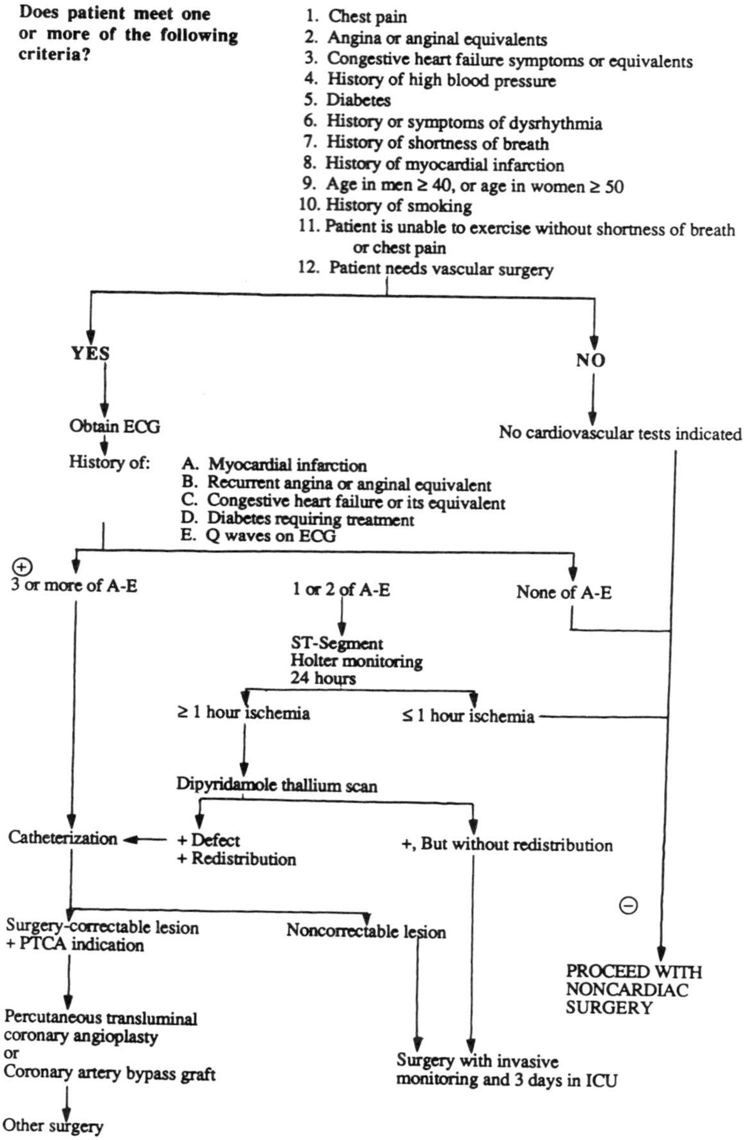

FIG 1.

Flowsheet shows how to decide which tests to perform: use history to segregate patients into groups to test and/or monitor invasively. (From Roizen MF, Hurd M: Preoperative patient evaluation. In Rogers M, editor: *Current practice in anesthesiology*. New York, 1990, Decker, pp 14–22. Used by permission.)

gery, do not smoke, and are able to exercise. For procedures more likely to be associated with cardiovascular events, men and women with three of the following should undergo cardiac catheterization: a history of myocardial infarction, congestive heart failure, hypertension, diabetes mellitus, or angina. Individuals with one or two of these conditions probably would benefit from Holter monitoring to determine their risk group.

A simple approach to preoperative cardiac evaluation is the use of Holter monitoring for detection of ischemia during daily life. After ambulatory Holter monitoring of patients for 24 hours, Raby et al.[54] documented complications in one third of those with 1 hour or more of preoperative ischemia and in only 1% of nonischemic patients. There is some evidence[55] that Holter monitoring may be an inexpensive way of evaluating patients before proceeding to the tests to be described.

Determination of systolic left ventricular function may provide prognostic information for major surgery, given the association of congestive heart failure with morbid postoperative events. Radionuclide angiography can define systolic and diastolic function. Most investigators attempting to predict operative risk have evaluated only systolic function; however, we are becoming increasingly aware that diastolic failure is also a problem, particularly for patients with hypertension.

Kazmers et al.[56] studied 60 patients undergoing abdominal aortic aneurysm repair. Although patients with a low ejection fraction survived the operation and had no higher incidence of perioperative myocardial infarction (a tribute to modern perioperative management), their long-term survival was poor (50% vs. 86% at 20 months).

Pasternack et al.[57] showed that patients with an ejection fraction above 55% had no myocardial infarctions, whereas four of five patients with an ejection fraction below 35% suffered a myocardial infarction postoperatively within 48 hours. Their patients did not fare as well in the perioperative period as did those of Kazmers' group; still, a previous myocardial infarction predicted a 26% probability of re-infarction, and 50% of patients older than 80 years sustained an infarction perioperatively.

Del Guercio et al.[58] studied 148 elderly patients who had been cleared for major surgery by their internists. Preoperatively, patients were admitted to the intensive care unit (ICU) for insertion of a pulmonary artery catheter. Cardiac output, pulmonary capillary wedge pressure, and O_2 delivery were measured. Patients were classified into one of four stages, from normal to having severe, uncorrectable deficits. In 34 patients, severe hemodynamic abnormalities were detected and, for most of these, surgery was canceled. Of 8 high-risk patients who underwent the planned surgical procedure, all died, whereas the mortality was 0% for stage 1 and 8.5% for stage 2 and stage 3 patients.

Another method advocated for preoperative risk assessment is dipyridamole-thallium scanning (DTS). Dipyridamole is a potent coronary vasodilator, which produces a coronary steal by increasing blood flow to normal areas and diminishing collateral flow to poststenotic areas. Areas that are prone to ischemia are hypoperfused after dipyridamole administration;

several hours later when the "steal" has subsided, the areas are perfused normally. Such areas are said to have a redistribution defect. Fixed defects represent old myocardial infarctions.

The Massachusetts General Hospital experience[59] with DTS has yielded two important observations: an old myocardial infarction is not a risk factor in itself and an area of redistribution (i.e., myocardium at risk) is associated with an adverse outcome. The most recent results of this group[60] suggest that DTS is most helpful in risk stratification of patients at intermediate risk based on clinical evaluation. If a patient has a negative DTS or a low clinical risk, based on patient factors and type of operation, we might choose, given the low rate of adverse cardiac events, to forego extensive invasive monitoring and extended ICU care with the potential for reducing costs and iatrogenic complications.

Patients who are at high risk because of individual and surgical risk factors should probably not undergo DTS. They should undergo coronary angiography and revascularization or give informed consent that addresses the high risk of their surgery. Preoperative CABG or coronary angioplasty may be useful, although some dismiss them as survival tests and debate their capacity to decrease perioperative mortality.

Patients with a markedly positive DTS should probably undergo myocardial revascularization. Lette et al.[61] demonstrated in a study of 66 patients that those with markedly positive scans (16 patients) tended to die (7 of 10 patients operated on) if surgery was not canceled. Recently, Mangano et al.[62] challenged the effectiveness of DTS for the preoperative screening of vascular surgery patients, but the limitations of their study (noted in an accompanying editorial[63]) make their challenge less compelling. Furthermore, patients with diabetes mellitus undergoing vascular surgery commonly (80%) have positive dipyridamole scans; only by quantifying the degree of redistribution is it possible to stratify the risk of these patients by means of DTS. Lane et al.,[64] who studied 101 patients with diabetes mellitus, found that neither the type of anesthesia (regional vs. general) nor the use of pulmonary artery catheters, nor the site of surgery (aortic vs. femoral), nor the use of nitroglycerin infusions predicted outcome. The presence of angina and a high Goldman classification[65] predicted cardiac complications as did the presence of more than two reversible effects and defects in distribution in the left anterior descending artery. Thus, when patients are segregated preoperatively for either more invasive monitoring, CABG, or PTCA before vascular surgery, it is not clear that such procedures are just a survival test accompanied by increased short-term morbidity. In Figure 1, we present an algorithm for pursuing laboratory testing for cardiovascular disease.[41] The data do not support the use of the algorithm as a guideline or a standard but only as one option. Until these procedures gain widespread acceptance and until extensive trials show that they reduce overall mortality, the goal of optimizing care and minimizing myocardial morbidity seems logical.

Pulmonary Function Testing

These expensive tests are rarely needed but are useful for determining those who may benefit from bronchodilator therapy and to predict risk for thoracic operations before obtaining informed consent. The indications for pulmonary function tests in Table 4 seem justified by the data.[41]

Clotting Function Studies

Virtually no asymptomatic patient in the literature has had unequivocal benefit from clotting function studies preoperatively. Most show symptoms or have a medication history suggesting that clotting function tests may be necessary. Aspirin at 60 mg per 70 kg of body weight per day does not seem to pose a risk for bleeding, but the data are not available for 300 mg or more within 12 hours of surgery. Since the pharmacology of aspirin changes when more than 2 g per 70 kg is consumed per day, patients should be evaluated if they cannot stop aspirin early enough to have no appreciable acetylsalicylic acid level for 24 hours before surgery (the period without aspirin necessary to generate the approximately 50,000 new platelets per cubic millimeter needed for normal platelet aggregation), if surgical hemostasis cannot be assured or if a regional procedure into a closed space is planned. Figure 2 presents an algorithm for determining whether coagulation tests are indicated.

Other Tests: Pregnancy and Acquired Immunodeficiency Syndrome Screening

Tests for acquired immunodeficiency syndrome (AIDS) and pregnancy and screening for hemoglobinopathy and malignant hyperthermia raise ethical issues that may require close attention to institutional policy and the immediate availability of counseling services. Moreover, all of these tests

TABLE 4.
Indications for Pulmonary Function Tests

History of at least one of the following:
- Chronic obstructive pulmonary disease
- Shortness of breath
- Orthopnea

Or at least one of the following needs to be determined:
- Reversibility of bronchospasm
- Baseline condition if intubation is expected preoperatively
- Risk for lung resection (maximal midexpiratory flow rate, maximum breathing capacity, diffusing capacity for carbon monoxide).

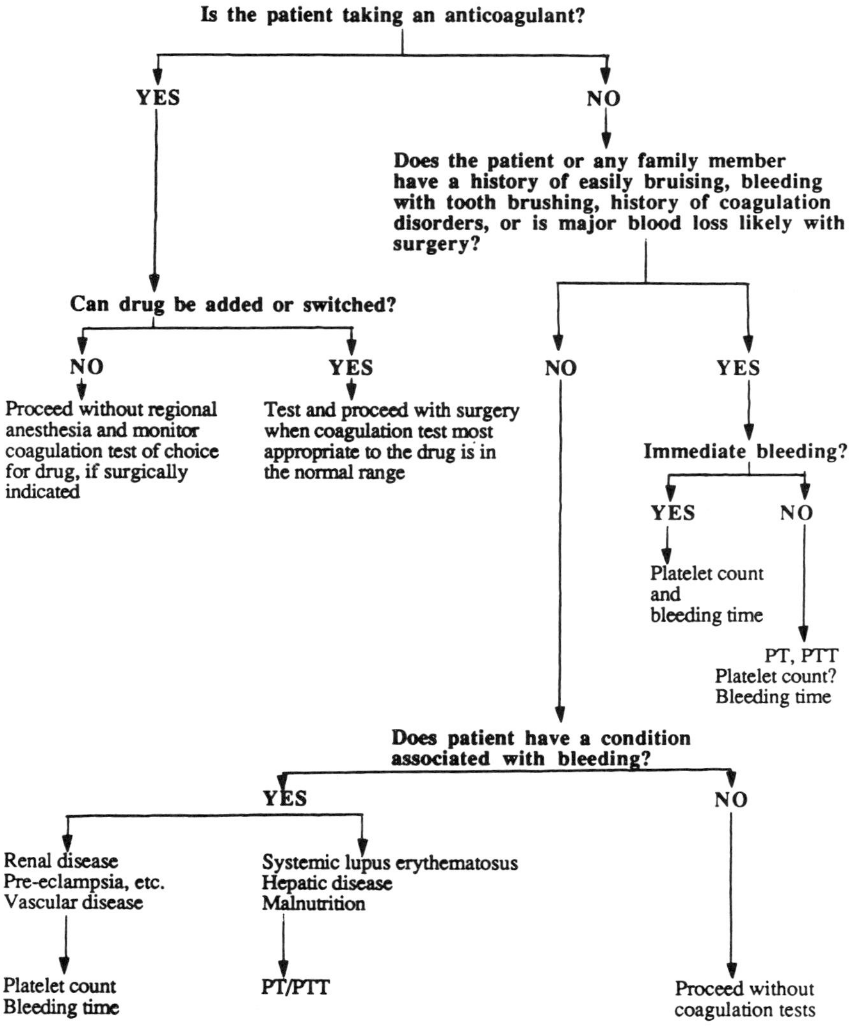

FIG 2.
Flowsheet shows how to decide if coagulopathy exists or coagulation tests are indicated. (From Roizen MF, Hurd M: Preoperative patient evaluation. In Rogers M, editor: *Current practice in anesthesiology*. New York, 1990, Decker, pp 14–22. Used by permission.)

have associated risks. The physician may therefore decide to limit testing to only at-risk populations (e.g., for pregnancy testing, only female patients who believe they may be pregnant).

Testing of the asymptomatic population for AIDS is not likely to be the most effective way of uncovering the disease. Of the more than 70,000 people in the United States who had AIDS as of 1990, only 1 person has not been gay, had sex with a prostitute, used intravenously administered drugs and shared needles, been stuck with a needle, cared for a family member with AIDS, or received a blood transfusion after 1979. One program screening for human immunodeficiency virus (HIV) in asymptomatic individuals was able to produce an acceptably low false-positive rate by diagnosing HIV infection only after one sample of blood produced positive results on four different tests and after a second sample of blood had been used for verification. Thus, for pregnancy, hemoglobinopathies, malignant hyperthermia, and AIDS, the history is still best at identifying those at risk for the condition.

We believe that because we biased the analysis to favor laboratory testing, the guidelines in Table 1 provide the upper limits of tests to be performed in asymptomatic individuals. Just as good an argument could be made for no testing of asymptomatic individuals in low-risk groups.

How To Choose Preoperative Tests Based on History

I firmly believe that a clinic can be set up to perform preoperative assessment cost-effectively. In the clinic, history-taking can be accomplished in one of several ways. Patients may complete a questionnaire or a check-off list on paper, enter their responses by computer,* or respond orally to questions asked by a health professional. Whatever the method, the goal is a thorough history that the anesthesiologist can then use to determine necessary tests and perioperative care. The charge for the physician's time for assessment will be offset by elimination of the cost of unwarranted tests and of operating room expense when surgery is delayed.[66] For cost savings alone, hospitals and payors should favor a clinic for preoperative assessment.

Finally, I believe the anesthesiologist is the most logical choice to perform preoperative assessment, to ensure follow-up of the initial assessment, and to discuss with the patient the risks and benefits of the tests and the risks associated with anesthesia, the procedure, and postoperative care. In a good system for assessment, risk is discussed in light of abnormal test results. Knowing which abnormal results are likely to affect patient treatment is, therefore, of great importance. Tables 1, 2, and 4 and Figures 1 and 2 present the most appropriate choices for testing based on published evidence. These recommendations were made after an examination of the potential for abnormalities in each risk group and after assumptions about the benefits and harms proceeding from the abnormalities.[47, 48] Randomized trials proving the benefits and harms, however, are rare. To institute

*Dr. Roizen developed a preoperative health questionnaire at the University of Chicago to help solve the problem of inefficient preoperative assessments and test selection methods. The University owns the patent rights to develop and market this product. If the product is successful, Dr. Roizen will benefit financially since the University distributes to its faculty a royalty and partial ownership right from such inventions.

selective testing and to avoid the four hazards of batteries of tests requires either a preoperative clinic or provision for an assessment system in the offices of the surgeon or primary care physician. The rewards for such a system are not only fewer tests, but reduced medicolegal risk, and improved patient outcome. They will also be evident in the physician's pride in delivering quality care and, ultimately, in the patient's satisfaction.

References

1. Macario A et al: A tale of three cities: has reassessment of preoperative laboratory testing changed the test-ordering patterns of physicians? *Surg Gynecol Obstet* (in press).
2. Vacanti CJ, VanHouten RJ, Hill RC: A statistical analysis of the relationship of physical status to postoperative mortality in 68,388 cases. *Anesth Analg* 49:564–566, 1970.
3. Lewin I et al: Physical class and physiologic status in the prediction of operative mortality in the aged sick. *Ann Surg* 174:217–231, 1971.
4. Goldman L et al: Multifactorial index of cardiac risk in noncardiac surgical procedures. *N Engl J Med* 297:845–850, 1977.
5. Keats AS: The ASA classification of physical status—a recapitulation. *Anesthesiology* 49:233–236, 1978.
6. Rehder K: Clinical evaluation of isoflurane: Complications during and after anaesthesia. *Can Anaesth Soc J* 29:S44–S48, 1982.
7. Cohen MM, Duncan PG. Physical status score and trends in anesthetic complications. *J Clin Epidemiol* 41:83–90, 1988.
8. Ziffren SE, Hartford CE: Comparative mortality for various surgical operations in older versus younger age groups. *J Am Geriatr Soc* 20:485–489, 1972.
9. Okelberry CR: Preadmission testing shortens preoperative length of stay. *Hospitals* 49:71–74, 1975.
10. Duckett JB: Preoperative assessment of the patient for outpatient anesthesia. In Brown BB Jr, editor: *Outpatient anesthesia.* Philadelphia, 1978, Davis, pp 21–29.
11. Leonard JV, Clayton BE, Colley JRT: Use of biochemical profile in children's hospital: Results of two controlled trials. *Br Med J* 2:662–665, 1975.
12. Korvin CC, Pearce RH, Stanley J: Admission screening: Clinical benefits. *Ann Intern Med* 83:197–203, 1975.
13. Olsen DM, Kane RL, Proctor PH: A controlled trial of multiphasic screening. *N Engl J Med* 294:925–930, 1976.
14. Durbridge TC et al: Evaluation of benefits of screening tests done immediately on admission to hospital. *Clin Chem* 22:968–971, 1976.
15. Narr BJ, Hansen TR, Warner MA: Preoperative laboratory screening in healthy Mayo patients: Cost-effective elimination of tests and unchanged outcomes. *Mayo Clin Proc* 66:155–159, 1991.
16. Apfelbaum J et al: How frequently do asymptomatic patients benefit from the pursuit of abnormalities in their preoperative test results? *Anesthesiology* 73:A1254, 1990.
17. Sox HC Jr, editor: *Common diagnostic tests: Use and interpretation.* Philadelphia, 1987, American College of Physicians.
18. Hayward RSA et al: Guideline for periodic preventive care. In Eddy DM, edi-

tor: *Common screening tests.* Philadelphia, 1991, American College of Physicians.
19. Domoto K et al: Yield of routine annual laboratory screening in the institutionalized elderly. *Am J Public Health* 75:243–245, 1985.
20. Wolf-Klein GP et al: Efficacy of routine annual studies in the care of elderly patients. *J Am Geriatr Soc* 33:325–329, 1985.
21. Dontas AS et al: Bacteriuria and survival in old age. *N Engl J Med* 304:939–943, 1981.
22. Boscia JA et al: Epidemiology of bacteriuria in an elderly ambulatory population. *Am J Med* 80:208–214, 1986.
23. Boscia JA et al: Therapy vs no therapy for bacteriuria in elderly ambulatory nonhospitalized women. *JAMA* 257:1067–1071, 1987.
24. Nordenstam GR et al: Bacteriuria and mortality in an elderly population. *N Engl J Med* 314:1152–1156, 1986.
25. Delahunt B, Turnbull PRG: How cost effective are routine preoperative investigations? *NZ Med J* 92:431–432, 1980.
26. Rosselló PJ, Cruz AR, Mayol PM: Routine laboratory tests for elective surgery in pediatric patients. *Bol Assoc Med P R* 72:614–623, 1980.
27. Wood RA, Hoekelman RA: Value of the chest x-ray as a screening test for elective surgery in children. *Pediatrics* 67:447–452, 1981.
28. Sandler G: Costs of unnecessary tests. *Br J Med* 2:21–24, 1979.
29. Rabkin SW, Horne JM: Preoperative electrocardiography: Its cost-effectiveness in detecting abnormalities when a previous tracing exists. *Can Med Assoc J* 121:301–306, 1979.
30. Rabkin SW, Horne JM: Preoperative electrocardiography: Effect of new abnormalities on clinical decisions. *Can Med Assoc J* 128:146–147, 1983.
31. Macpherson DS, Snow R, Lofgren RP: Preoperative screening: Value of previous tests. *Ann Intern Med* 113:959–973, 1990.
32. Roizen MF et al: The relative roles of the history and physical examination, and laboratory testing in preoperative evaluation for outpatient surgery: The Starling curve of preoperative laboratory testing. *Anesthesiol Clin North Am* 5:15–34, 1987.
33. Tape TG, Mushlin AI: The utility of routine chest radiographs. *Ann Intern Med* 104:663–670, 1986.
34. Turnbull JM, Buck C: The value of preoperative screening investigations in otherwise healthy individuals. *Arch Intern Med* 147:1101–1105, 1987.
35. Hirsch IA et al: The overstated risk of preoperative hypokalemia. *Anesth Analg* 67:131–136, 1988.
36. Vitez TS et al: Chronic hypokalemia and intraoperative dysrhythmias. *Anesthesiology* 63:130–133, 1985.
37. Harrington JT, Isner JM, Kassirer JP: Our national obsession with potassium. *Am J Med* 73:155–159, 1982.
38. Lawson DH: Adverse reactions to potassium chloride. *Q J Med* 43:433–440, 1974.
39. Lawson DH, Hutcheon AW, Jick H: Life threatening drug reactions amongst medical inpatients. *Scott Med J* 24:127–130, 1979.
40. Levinstein MR et al: Yield of routine annual laboratory tests in a skilled nursing home population. *JAMA* 258:1909–1915, 1987.
41. Roizen MF. Preoperative evaluation. In Miller RD, editor: *Anesthesia,* ed 3, vol 1. New York, 1990, Churchill Livingstone, pp 743–772.
42. Robertson WM: *Medical malpractice: A preventive approach.* Seattle, 1985, University of Washington.

43. Kaplan EB et al: The usefulness of preoperative laboratory screening. *JAMA* 253:3576–3581, 1985.
44. Roizen MF et al: Elimination of unnecessary laboratory tests by preoperative questionnaire. *Anesthesiology* 61:A455, 1984.
45. McKee RF, Scott EM: The value of routine preoperative investigations. *Ann R Coll Surg Engl* 69:160–162, 1987.
46. Finkler SA: The distinction between cost and charges. *Ann Intern Med* 96:102–109, 1982.
47. US Preventive Services Task Force (Lawrence RS, chairman): *Guide to clinical preventive services. An assessment of the effectiveness of 169 interventions.* Baltimore, 1990, Williams & Wilkins.
48. Hayward RSA et al: *Preventive care guidelines; 1991.* Ann Intern Med 114:758–783, 1991.
49. Rao TLK, Jacobs KH, El-Etr AA: Reinfarction following anesthesia in patients with myocardial infarction. *Anesthesiology* 59:499–505, 1983.
50. Hertzer NR et al: Coronary artery disease in peripheral vascular patients: A classification of 1000 coronary angiograms and results of surgical management. *Ann Surg* 199:223–233, 1984.
51. Hertzer NR et al: Late results of coronary bypass in patients with peripheral vascular disease. *Clev Clin Q* 53:133–143, 1986.
52. Roizen MF, Ellis JE: Anesthesia for vascular surgery. In Barash PG, Cullen BF, Stoelting RK, editors: *Clinical anesthesia,* ed 2. Philadelphia, 1992, JB Lippincott, pp 1059–1094.
53. Huber KC et al: Outcome of noncardiac operations in patients with severe coronary artery disease successfully treated preoperatively with coronary angioplasty. *Mayo Clin Proc* 67:15–21, 1992.
54. Raby KE et al: Correlation between preoperative ischemia and major cardiac events after peripheral vascular surgery. *N Engl J Med* 321:1296–1300, 1989.
55. Fleisher LA et al: The predictive value of preoperative silent ischemia for postoperative ischemic cardiac events in vascular and nonvascular surgery patients. *Am Heart J* 122:980–986, 1991.
56. Kazmers A, Cerqueira MD, Zierler RE: The role of preoperative radionuclide ejection fraction in direct abdominal aortic aneurysm repair. *J Vasc Surg* 8:128–136, 1988.
57. Pasternack PF et al: The value of radionuclide angiography as a predictor of perioperative myocardial infarction in patients undergoing abdominal aortic aneurysm resection. *J Vasc Surg* 1:320–325, 1984.
58. Del Guercio LRM, Cohn JD: Monitoring operative risk in the elderly. *JAMA* 243:1350–1355, 1980.
59. Eagle KA et al: Dipyridamole-thallium scanning in patients undergoing vascular surgery: Optimizing preoperative evaluation of cardiac risk. *JAMA* 257:2185–2189, 1987.
60. Eagle KA et al: Combining clinical and thallium data optimizes preoperative assessment of cardiac risk before major vascular surgery. *Ann Intern Med* 110:859–866, 1989.
61. Lette J et al: Postoperative myocardial infarction and cardiac death: Predictive value of dipyridamole-thallium imaging and five clinical scoring systems based on multifactorial analysis. *Ann Surg* 211:84–90, 1990.
62. Mangano DT et al: Dipyridamole thallium-201 scintigraphy as a preoperative screening test: A reexamination of its predictive potential. *Circulation* 84:493–502, 1991.

63. Pohost GM: Dipyridamole thallium test. Is it useful for predicting coronary events after vascular surgery? *Circulation* 84:931–932, 1991.
64. Lane SE et al: Predictive value of quantitative dipyridamole-thallium scintigraphy in assessing cardiovascular risk after vascular surgery in diabetes mellitus. *Am J Cardiol* 64:1275–1279, 1989.
65. Goldman L et al: Cardiac risk factors and complications in non-cardiac surgery. *Medicine* 57:357–370, 1978.
66. Rupani G et al: Can a system change improve operating room efficiency? *Anesthesiology* 71:930, 1989.

Preoperative Evaluation of the Autonomic Nervous System

Thomas J. Ebert, M.D., Ph.D.

Associate Professor of Anesthesiology, Associate Adjunct Professor of Physiology, Department of Anesthesiology, Medical College of Wisconsin, Milwaukee, Wisconsin; VA Medical Center, Milwaukee, Wisconsin

It is my perception that the evaluation of the autonomic nervous system during the preoperative bedside visit is nearly nonexistent in today's practice of anesthesiology. Although the majority of anesthesiologists are aware that the patient with diabetes mellitus frequently has autonomic dysfunction, the general implications of autonomic dysfunction in terms of perioperative management and postoperative sequelae are poorly understood at best. This lack of understanding is in part attributed to the fact that the relationship between autonomic dysfunction and anesthetic outcome is still emerging. As an example, consider the following new knowledge. Balanced autonomic outflow to the heart appears to play a critical role in cardiac well-being. Recent data suggest that impaired parasympathetic activity to the heart predisposes to malignant arrhythmias and sudden death,[1–3] while intact cardiac baroreflexes appear to be importantly involved in terminating a myocardial ischemic episode.[4, 5] We have recently demonstrated in patients with diabetes mellitus that the degree of impairment of the autonomic reflexes is directly related to the degree of hemodynamic instability after induction of anesthesia.[6] Moreover, impaired preoperative autonomic function may predict postoperative cardiac dysfunction.[7] Thus, it appears that an intact and functional autonomic nervous system plays an important role in limiting the likelihood of cardiac morbidity and mortality in patients undergoing anesthesia and surgery. It is because of these emerging relationships that the anesthesiologist must begin to consider the functional status of the autonomic nervous system during the preoperative visit.

In this chapter, I will review some of the basic physiology related to the regulation of autonomic neural outflow and provide information about some of the routine autonomic tests that can be applied to patients to evaluate the integrity of the autonomic nervous system. Finally, I will review the literature that suggests that autonomic function has an important relationship to cardiac well-being in patients recovering from anesthesia and surgery.

Autonomic Physiology

The efferent component of the autonomic nervous system consists of sympathetic and parasympathetic (vagal) divisions, both of which are tonically active. Their activity and the relative balance between these two divisions are regulated moment-to-moment by afferent input directed primarily to the medullary vasomotor center (Fig 1). By far the most important of these inputs is that derived from the arterial and low-pressure, cardiopulmonary baroreceptors. There are other neural inputs that can substantially modify autonomic outflow, but will not be considered in this chapter. These include input from thermal and somatic receptors, nociceptors, chemoreceptors, and descending signals from higher cortical centers.

Arterial Baroreceptors

Mechanoreceptors located in the arch of the aorta and in the carotid sinus continually sense the prevailing blood pressure and send inhibitory information to the vasomotor center (see Fig 1).[8] Efferent responses are directed to the heart, kidney, adrenal medulla, and the peripheral vascula-

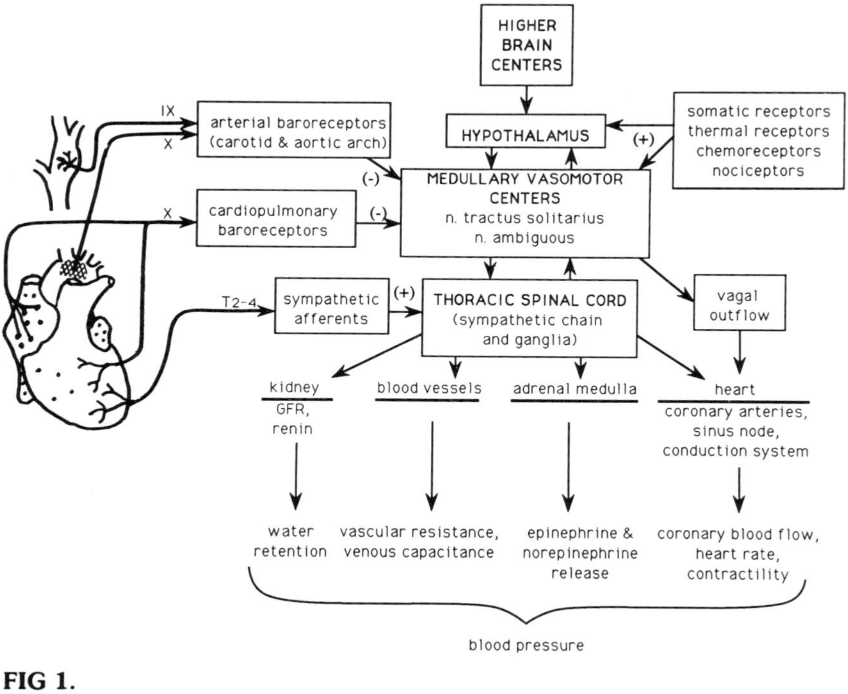

FIG 1.
Schematic that depicts the afferent, central, and efferent projections of the autonomic nervous system. The majority of sensors respond to blood pressure perturbations and initiate reflex responses to maintain blood pressure homeostasis.

ture. Reflex changes in vascular resistance are strictly mediated by efferent sympathetic nerve activity, while baroreflex heart rate responses are primarily mediated through the parasympathetic nervous system. For example, reflex heart rate changes in response to blood pressure perturbations in man can be virtually abolished with atropine[9] but are minimally altered during pharmacological cardiac sympathectomy (i.e., propranolol or high epidural anesthesia).[10, 11] In addition, there is evidence in humans that the carotid baroreceptor reflex is primarily involved in controlling heart rate while the aortic baroreceptor reflex preferentially regulates peripheral sympathetic outflow.[12]

Low-pressure, Cardiopulmonary Baroreceptor Reflex

Receptors in the atria and ventricles of the human heart (especially the veno-atrial junction) send afferent signals through the vagal nerves that mediate a tonic restraint on sympathetic outflow (see Fig 1). For example, when central venous pressure is reduced by hemorrhage or orthostatic stress, these receptors are unloaded and sustained reflex increases in sympathetic outflow are directed to the skeletal muscle and splanchnic vascular beds.[13] Heart rate does not change, in part, because this low-pressure baroreflex is initiated before there is any detectable decrease in systemic blood pressure, suggesting that the arterial baroreceptors are not involved in the efferent response. This selective peripheral sympatho-excitation from unloading of low-pressure baroreceptors provides the first line of defense against hypotension when blood volume is reduced and therefore, plays an important role in maintaining blood pressure homeostasis.

In addition, there are chemosensitive receptors in the ventricle that send information to the central nervous system via vagal pathways and elicit an inhibition of cardiac-vagal and peripheral sympathetic nerve traffic. This reflex is classically termed the Bezold-Jarisch reflex.[13, 14] However, ventricular receptors are not entirely chemosensitive because stimulation of ventricular mechanoreceptors can also trigger a reflex bradycardia and hypotension. These mechanoreceptors are believed to be involved in the syncope associated with exertion in patients with severely stenotic aortic valves.

Finally, there are sensory receptors in the ventricle that send sympathetic afferents to the spinal cord that initiate reflex increases of heart rate and arterial pressure.[13, 14] These receptors may be responsible for the perceived pain of angina pectoris, but their role in circulatory control is less well-defined than those of the vagally mediated atrial and ventricular reflexes.

Evaluating Autonomic Function

History

On initial evaluation of patients prior to surgery, routine information derived by careful history-taking can raise suspicion concerning autonomic dysfunction. Clinical symptoms of autonomic neuropathy are generally nonspecific and may be mimicked by other visceral diseases or various medical therapies. Thus, the problem in evaluating the autonomic nervous system by history alone is determining whether symptoms are due to irreversible autonomic neuropathy or due to other reversible processes (Table 1).

Important information that should be obtained while taking the patient's history relates to orthostatic tolerance. Does the patient have problems when arising in the morning? Is there dizziness or faintness, nausea, or diaphoresis while upright? Has the patient fainted? Is fainting associated with emotional stress? Is it a common occurrence? Is there any relationship to meals (postprandial fainting is a frequent occurrence in patients with autonomic impairment)? In patients with diffuse autonomic derangements, bladder sphincter disturbances and impotence may precede symptomatic orthostatic intolerance. Occasionally, patients with autonomic dysfunction will have night blindness or nasal stuffiness. This is presumably due to a loss of sympathetic control of pupil dilation and loss of vasoconstrictor activity of the mucosal vessels. Occasionally, there will be an impaired ability to sweat (anhydrosis). The history must include details of all medications being taken by the patient with particular attention to antihypertensive, antidepressant, tranquilizer, and diuretic agents (see Table 1). Alcohol intake should be quantitated, and the presence or absence of peripheral neuropathy must be determined. In patients with positive findings on history or with disease processes that are commonly associated with autonomic dysfunction such as diabetes mellitus, chronic alcoholism, and chronic renal failure, additional bedside tests of autonomic function should be carried out. These will be described.

Laboratory Evaluation

There are a number of laboratory tests used to evaluate autonomic function and to determine the site of the lesion influencing autonomic competency; that is, an afferent, central, or efferent site. These tests can be carried out if an equipped laboratory is available in the hospital. I refer the reader to Chapter 16 in the textbook *Autonomic Failure,* edited by Sir Roger Bannister,[15] that details the type of equipment that is necessary to establish an autonomic testing unit and also details some of the precise clinical tests that can be carried out. These tests include: measurements of plasma levels of catecholamines and other vasoactive hormones, such as renin, angiotensin, and vasopressin; measurement of forearm blood flow with plethysmography, arterial blood pressure, cerebral electroencephalography and blood flow studies, and bladder and sphincter function; tests of temperature regulation, sweating, and baroreflex function; and cardiac electrophysiological investigations. Many of these measurements and tests are not practical during the bedside examination. Clearly, however, such tests should be carried out in a logical order as part of the evaluation in patients with a history of syncope.

TABLE 1.
Reversible Causes of Postural Hypotension Mimicking Autonomic Dysfunction

Reduced circulatory blood volume
Hemorrhage
Dehydration
Burns
Varicose veins
Posthemodialysis
Postexercise
Impaired reflex responses
Prolonged bed rest
Space flight
Hyperthermia
Pharmacological agents
Antihypertensives
Diuretics, adrenergic blockers
Ca^{2+} channel blockers, central acting
Phenothiazines
Tricyclics
Nitrates
Alcohol
Insulin
Benzodiazepines
Others
Arrhythmias
Electrolyte imbalance, especially low K^+
Adrenal insufficiency
Malignancy
Infectious neuronitis (Gullian-Barré)

Bedside Autonomic Tests

In patients with a positive history or disease processes associated with autonomic dysfunction, a number of simple tests can be performed by the anesthesiologist during the bedside visit. These tests can be divided into tests of cardiac-vagal function and tests of sympathetic function (Table 2). I will briefly describe the procedures for carrying out each of these tests with the goal that standardization be achieved to better interpret the degree of autonomic impairment.

Postural Stress: Supine to Standing (Sympathetic Function)

The easiest and most commonly performed bedside test to evaluate autonomic function is to record the blood pressure and heart rate response to

TABLE 2.
Routine Tests of Autonomic Function

Tests of cardiac-vagal function
- Respiratory sinus arrhythmia*
- Valsalva ratio (phase IV/II)
- Bradycardia during phenylephrine challenge
- Absence of tachycardia with atropine

Test of sympathetic function
- Cardiac
  - Tachycardia during standing or head-up tilt*
  - Tachycardia during Valsalva strain (phase II)
- Peripheral
  - Blood pressure overshoot after Valsalva release (phase IV)
  - Blood pressure increase with cold pressor test*
  - Diastolic blood pressure increase with isometric handgrip exercise
  - Systolic and diastolic blood pressure response to upright posture*

*Tests that can be carried out during preoperative evaluation at bedside.

assumption of the upright posture. One simply needs a watch with a second hand, a sphygmomanometer, and a stethoscope. Following a supine resting period of at least 10 minutes, heart rate and blood pressure should be measured. The patient then rises unaided, in a timely fashion, to the upright position and stands absolutely still. After 50 seconds in the upright position, the blood pressure cuff should be inflated and both systolic and diastolic components of blood pressure obtained during the ensuing cuff deflation. This should immediately be followed by the determination of heart rate (which can also be done simultaneous to the blood pressure measurement if a second observer is available). Some investigators have taken measurements during the second minute of upright posture,[16] while others have determined the ratio of the heart rate at 15 and 30 seconds after assuming the upright posture.[17, 18] However, simply obtaining a blood pressure and heart rate approximately 1 minute after assuming the upright posture appears to be adequate.

When taking the blood pressure in a standing subject, the cuff should be approximately at the phlebostatic axis. This is often done by having the patient rest an arm on the investigator's shoulder while in the upright position. The decline in systolic pressure that occurs during standing is due to a reduction in cardiac preload and cardiac output despite a reflex tachycardia and arterial vasoconstriction. A decline in systolic pressure of greater than 20 mm Hg is generally used as a critical value suggestive of autonomic dysfunction. However, anywhere from 5% to 20% of normal individuals between 20 and 80 years of age will have a drop in blood pressure equal to or slightly greater than 20 mm Hg without subjective signs or symptoms of impending syncope.[19,20] Thus, a 30 mm Hg decline in systolic pressure is a more appropriate response suggestive of autonomic dysfunction. Similarly, diastolic blood pressure should not decrease by more than 10 mm Hg during 1 minute of standing (it normally increases slightly in healthy individuals). Greater decreases in diastolic blood pressure suggest impaired peripheral sympathetic vasoconstriction. The absence of tachycardia during standing has also been interpreted as an impairment of sympathetic drive to the heart. Heart rate should increase at least 10 beats/minute in the upright position (unless patients are receiving beta-adrenergic blockers).

There are numerous causes of hypotension during upright posture that are not related to autonomic dysfunction (see Table 1). These must be considered when interpreting the patient's response to orthostatic stress.

Cold Pressor Test (Sympathetic Function)

A second simple bedside test used to evaluate peripheral sympathetic vasoconstrictor mechanisms is to record the blood pressure response to a 1-minute immersion of the hand in ice water.[6] This is called the cold pressor test. Both systolic and diastolic blood pressures at the 60th second of immersion should increase at least 10 mm Hg. Generally there is a concomitant tachycardia associated with this test, but it can be variable in nature and thus does not yield useful information.

Isometric Handgrip Exercise (Sympathetic Function)

If one has a calibrated handgrip dynamometer available, then the blood pressure response to a sustained isometric contraction at 30% of the patient's maximum strength can be obtained.[17] The diastolic blood pressure increase at the end of the 3-minute static contraction should be at least 10 mm Hg above that measured during a precontraction baseline period. The failure to record a diastolic blood pressure increase of greater than 10 mm Hg is suggestive of deficient efferent sympathetic mechanisms.

Respiratory Sinus Arrhythmia (Parasympathetic Function)

Perhaps the most sensitive test of cardiac-vagal function is to determine the maximum-to-minimum heart rate variation that occurs during forceful breathing (Fig 2). This is most easily quantitated by obtaining a continuous record of the electrocardiogram at the bedside, although a finger on the pulse during deep breathing might be sensitive enough to detect a respectable respiratory sinus arrhythmia (RSA). Seated or lying subjects should breathe in and out maximally at a rate of six breaths/minute (5 seconds in, 5 seconds out). The average maximum-to-minimum heart rate during three consecutive breaths should be greater than 10 beats/minute.[17,21,22] A recent study in our laboratory determined that patients with diabetes mellitus and with R-R interval variations less than 30 milliseconds during forceful breathing were at increased risk of hypotension following induction of anesthesia compared to those with a greater degree of RSA.[6]

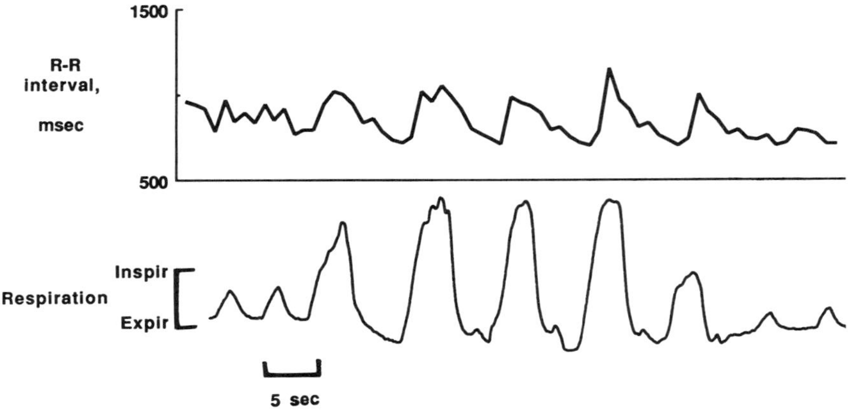

FIG 2.
A representative tracing from a healthy volunteer demonstrating respiratory sinus arrhythmia during both quiet breathing and during forceful breathing. The average maximum-to-minimum heart rate (R-R interval) changes that occur during three consecutive large breaths has been used as an index of cardiac-parasympathetic function.

Valsalva's Maneuver (Sympathetic and Parasympathetic Function)

This test of autonomic function is a bit more complex than other tests but has been used extensively in the past and considerable information is available regarding normal and abnormal responses to this maneuver.[6, 17, 18, 23] This test requires a pressure manometer connected to a mouthpiece, a continuous recording of the electrocardiogram, and (ideally) intraarterial blood pressure. The subject sits quietly or lies supine and blows into a mouthpiece with an open glottis and holds an airway pressure of 40 mm Hg for 15 seconds. The heart rate normally increases during phase II of the maneuver. This is 10 to 15 seconds after initiating the blowing but prior to release of the strain (Fig 3). The tachycardia is due to arterial baroreflex responses to the reduction in transmural pressure at intrathoracic baroreceptors and the reduction in blood pressure due to a reduced venous return and cardiac output. During the strain, peripheral sympathetic activity is reflexly augmented and peripheral vasoconstriction occurs (see Fig 3). On release of the strain, preload is restored, cardiac output increases, and blood is pumped into a highly constricted peripheral vasculature. Thus, there is a blood pressure overshoot that occurs after release (phase IV). This hypertension stimulates the baroreceptors and initiates a rapid reflex bradycardia. The ratio of the longest R-R interval during phase IV of this maneuver, to the shortest R-R interval during phase II of the maneuver, has been used as an index of cardiac-vagal function (Table 3). If recordings of intraarterial blood pressure (or beat-to-beat blood pressure with a noninvasive device) are taken during this maneuver, addi-

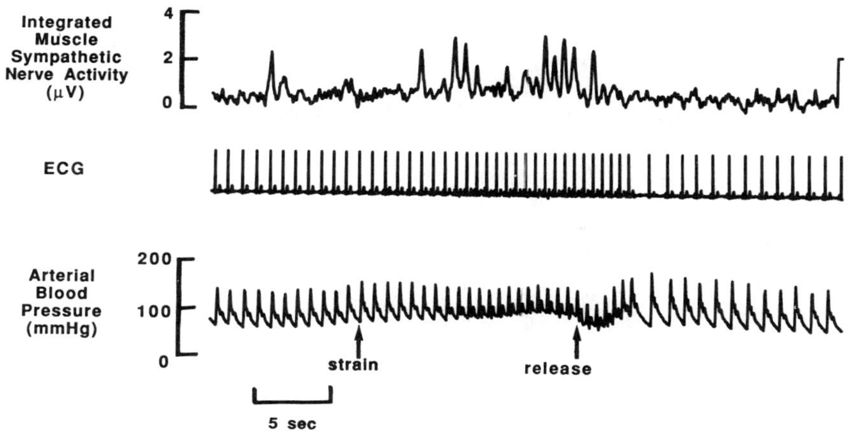

FIG 3.
A representative tracing from one healthy volunteer performing a Valsalva maneuver (40 mm Hg blowing pressure maintained for 15 seconds). In this individual, direct recordings of efferent sympathetic nerve activity directed to skeletal muscle were obtained with microneuropathy. The tachycardia and augmentation in sympathetic vasoconstrictor traffic that occurs during the Valsalva strain is due to a reduction in transmural pressure at intrathoracic baroreceptors. The bradycardia and inhibition of sympathetic outflow that occurs on release of the Valsalva maneuver is due to a blood pressure overshoot that augments inhibitory baroreceptor afferent traffic. The blood pressure overshoot is a result of improved cardiac output into a highly constricted peripheral vascular bed.

tional insights can be obtained. For example, the failure to observe a blood pressure overshoot following release of the strain suggests that peripheral sympathetic vasoconstriction has not occurred. The failure to observe a blood pressure overshoot during phase IV may lead to calculation of a low Valsalva ratio because of the absence of a hypertensive stimulus to the baroreceptors.

State of the Art: Power Spectral Analysis of Heart Rate Variability

The breath-to-breath fluctuation in heart period that has been traditionally referred to as RSA consists of oscillations that are in phase with respiration and due primarily to cardiac-vagal mechanisms. However, there are other periodic (and occasionally aperiodic) oscillations in heart period that are unrelated to respiration and are usually slower than the respiratory frequency. By applying Fourier transformation to a time series of heart periods (for example, 256 consecutive heart beats of data), the heart period oscillations can be mathematically decomposed into a series of sine waves with different amplitudes and frequencies.[24] This frequency domain approach (where frequency is represented on the x-axis and the squared amplitude of the sine wave on the y-axis) reveals a consistent peak (or power)

TABLE 3.
Critical Values of Bedside Autonomic Tests Suggestive of Autonomic Impairment

Max-min R-R interval during forceful breathing	<30 msec* <10 bpm†
Valsalva ratio*	<1.2
Systolic blood pressure increase during cold pressor test*	<10 mm Hg
Systolic blood pressure decrease during standing†‡	>30 mm Hg
Diastolic blood pressure decrease during standing†‡	>10 mm Hg

*Burgos et al.[6]
†Ewing et al.[17]
‡Moore, Newton.[16]

at the breathing frequency between 0.2 to 0.3 Hz, which is due primarily to intact parasympathetic innervation of the sino-atrial node of the heart (Fig 4). There are two slower oscillations that show spectral peaks at less than 0.03 Hz and between 0.05 and 0.15 Hz, respectively. The extremely slow oscillations (less than 0.03 Hz) have significant power and may be related to thermoregulatory phenomena or gradual fluctuations in circulating hormone concentration.[24] This slow frequency band is frequently omitted in analyses. The remaining low-frequency oscillations (0.05 to 0.15 Hz) are thought to be primarily due to changing levels of cardiac sympathetic activity[25, 26] (although contamination from parasympathetic input cannot be excluded[27]). There is reasonable experimental evidence that this low-frequency component is augmented by stressors known to increase sympathetic drive; for example, head-up tilt, mental arithmetic, and hypotension.[24] Moreover, this component is reduced in quadriplegic patients with interrupted sympathetic pathways[25] and is also reduced during syncopal episodes.[27]

Thus, the future in autonomic testing may be as simple as a hand-held computer interfaced with an electrocardiogram from which 5 minutes of quiet resting data can be obtained from supine patients at the bedside. A quick determination of the relative power in the low- and high-frequency ranges may provide the anesthesiologist with an index of relative sympathetic and parasympathetic function. Such insight has already proved to be extremely interesting. For example, reduced heart rate variability in the high-frequency range (parasympathetic region) occurs after myocardial infarction.[1, 3] This loss of power is thought to be related to an increased risk of ventricular fibrillation and sudden cardiac death.[1, 28, 29] Efforts to improve cardiac-vagal activity such as exercise training[30] and transdermal scopolamine[31] have reduced the incidence of cardiac dysrhythmias. In addition, an acute increase in power in the low-frequency (sympathetic) range and a decrease in high-frequency power has been observed during brief coronary artery occlusion in conscious dogs.[26] A predominance of low-frequen-

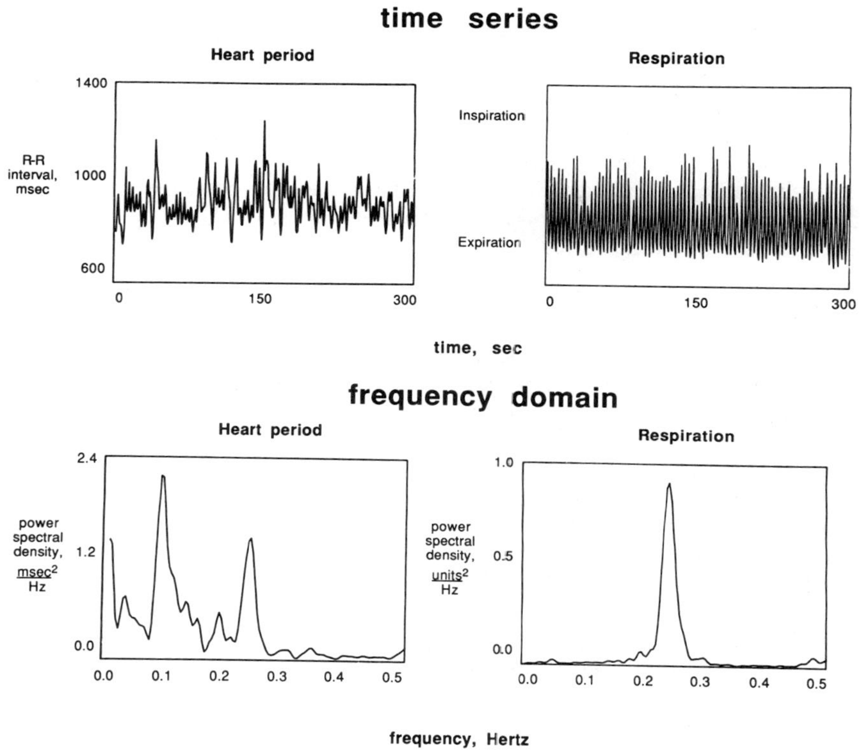

FIG 4.
Power spectral analysis of heart rate oscillations during 5 minutes of quiet breathing in one subject. Time domain (upper figures) and frequency domain (lower figures) are shown for the heart period and respiration signal. The breathing frequency is clearly depicted in the frequency domain and is centered about 0.25 Hz. The corresponding power peak noted in the heart period spectral analysis is also centered at 0.25 Hz. This is termed the high-frequency oscillation and it is believed to be a result of cardiac-vagal activity. The lower frequency power centered at 0.1 Hz has been related to cardiac sympathetic influences. Quantification of the relative power in these two peaks can be obtained by determining the area under the corresponding peaks. (Adapted from Ebert TJ: *Curr Opinions Anesth* 5, 1992.)

cy power and a reduction in high-frequency power has also been noted in patients shortly after myocardial infarction.[2, 3] These data raise the possibility that power spectral analyses of heart period oscillations could serve as an early marker of myocardial ischemia. Might such measurements in the perioperative and postoperative period serve a predictive value as well?

Autonomic Dysfunction: Who is at Risk?

As previously mentioned, there are a number of reversible physiological situations, pathological processes, and pharmacologic interventions that can mimic autonomic dysfunction (see Table 2). However, there are other specific disease processes that are commonly associated with progressive neurologic impairment of the autonomic control system (Table 4). Whether these disease processes cause autonomic dysfunction because of afferent, central, or efferent lesions is not relevant to this discussion; however, their ability to compromise autonomic reflex mechanisms is extremely pertinent. I will briefly discuss one disease process, diabetes mellitus, and two clinical syndromes, chronic alcoholism and aging, that can lead to autonomic dysfunction.

Aging

A well-known phenomena associated with the aging process is an increased prevalence of postural hypotension. Epidemiologic studies reveal that approximately 20% of people over 65 years of age have postural hypotension (defined as a systolic blood pressure drop of at least 20 mm Hg or a diastolic blood pressure drop of greater than 10 mm Hg).[20] It is estimated that about one half of these patients are symptomatic; that is, experience dizziness, faintness, or loss of consciousness. Although there are clearly a number of reversible causes of orthostatic intolerance in the elderly such as prolonged bed rest, dehydration, varicose veins, anemia, arrhythmias, electrolyte imbalance, and a number of medications, some of the elderly have true neurologic degeneration of autonomic function.[32] It is well-known that the reflex regulation of heart rate, which is mediated primarily by parasympathetic mechanisms, declines progressively with age.[20–22] We have recently documented this phenomena in a group of 66

TABLE 4.
Pathological Impairment of the Autonomic Nervous System

Aging
Diabetes mellitus
Chronic alcoholism
Chronic renal failure
Hypertension
Idiopathic orthostatic hypotension
Spinal cord injury
Neurologic diseases
Tabes dorsalis
Syringomyelia,
Amyloidosis
Shy-Drager syndrome (multiple system atrophy)

healthy individuals ranging in age from 20 to 75 years (Fig 5). Interestingly, we found no significant age-related impairment of the reflex regulation of sympathetic outflow in the elderly. Additional support for a progressive age-related impairment of cardiac-vagal function has been provided by others who have shown that the degree of respiratory sinus arrhythmia progressively diminishes with increasing age.[20–22] These data suggest that there may be a selective or earlier impairment of parasympathetic function with aging with a minimal or a more gradual involvement of the sympathetic nervous system. The degree of autonomic impairment can be assessed by history and some simple bedside maneuvers previously described. Those with markedly impaired autonomic responses (see Table 3) should be given special attention.

Diabetes Mellitus

Diabetic autonomic neuropathy is a well-known clinical entity. Diabetic autonomic dysfunction may result from neuronal degeneration or metabolically related neuronal dysfunction.[23] The afferent, central, or efferent reflex pathways each can be involved. Diabetic autonomic neuropathy may increase in frequency with the duration of the disease.[23] The prevalence of diabetic autonomic neuropathy also appears to increase if other complications of diabetes mellitus are present, such as peripheral neuropathy and gastrointestinal dysfunction.[6, 23] Patients with nephropathy or proliferative retinopathy also have a higher incidence of reduced RSA than control subjects.[23] It has been suggested that the vagal neuropathy occurs earlier in the course of diabetes mellitus than the sympathetic neuropathy. For diagnostic purposes, it is useful to perform a number of bedside autonomic tests to better categorize the extent of autonomic dysfunction. The most sensitive test of cardiac parasympathetic impairment is that of determining the RSA during forceful breathing. Intolerance to the upright posture is often evident as well. Excessive decreases in systolic and diastolic blood

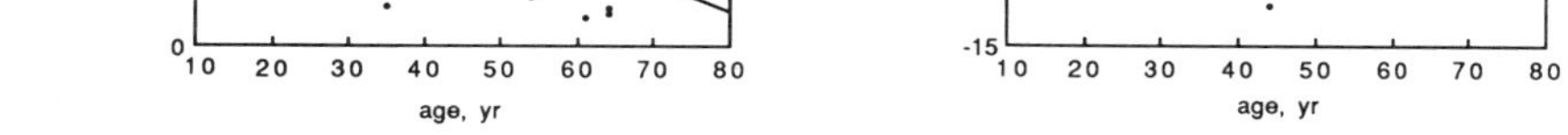

FIG 5.
The effects of aging on baroreflex sensitivity. The baroreceptor reflex control of heart rate (R-R interval), which is primarily due to parasympathetic mechanisms, declines linearly with increasing age. In contrast, the baroreflex regulation of peripheral sympathetic outflow does not show any consistent change with aging.

pressure with standing are strongly suggestive of failed peripheral sympathetic mechanisms. The presence of symptomatic postural hypotension is associated with a poor prognosis in the patient with diabetes mellitus.[33, 34] These patients are prone to sudden cardiac death. It has been reported that only 50% of diabetics who have abnormal autonomic function tests upon their first assessment will be alive after 3 to 5 years.[33, 34]

Autonomic neuropathy has been noted in 20% to 40% of all diabetics presenting to the hospital.[35] For those scheduled for surgery, there are several implications that are important to the anesthesiologist. Esophageal dysfunction and gastric hypotonia may be present, which increase the risk of regurgitation and aspiration in the perioperative period. Bradycardia, hypotension, and cardiopulmonary arrest have been reported among diabetics with autonomic neuropathy during the perioperative period.[36, 37] We have previously applied a number of routine autonomic stress tests to a group of 17 diabetics without renal disease and with minimal cardiac disease.[6] Almost all diabetics had retinopathy, and several were being treated for mild hypertension. We identified significant differences in the autonomic test results of these diabetics compared with those of 21 control patients. Moreover, the diabetics with the worst autonomic test results had the largest decrease in blood pressure after anesthetic induction and also had the highest requirement for intraoperative pressor agents to maintain stable hemodynamics (Fig 6). Undoubtedly, part of this morbidity is related to underlying cardiac disease in the patient with diabetes mellitus, although autonomic dysfunction appears to play an important role.

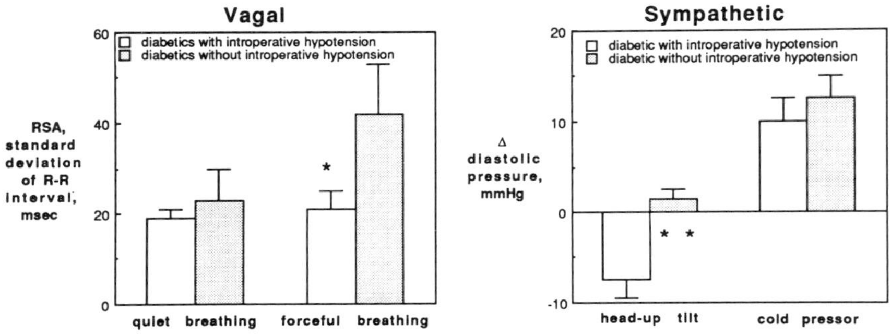

FIG 6.

Autonomic test results of diabetics who did and who did not develop hypotension during anesthesia and surgery. Autonomic tests were performed preoperatively during a separate testing session. Tests of vagal function included measuring the respiratory sinus arrhythmia. In this study, RSA was taken as the mathematical standard deviation of 256 consecutive R-R intervals. Tests of sympathetic function included the diastolic blood pressure response to 70-degree head-up tilt and a cold pressor test (hand in ice water for 1 minute). Diabetics who develop intraoperative hypotension had an impaired sympathetic vasoconstrictor response during head-up tilt testing as evidenced by the decline in diastolic blood pressure. (*, ** = $P < .05$ and $P < .01$ compared to diabetics without intraoperative hypotension.)

Alcoholism

Orthostatic intolerance and presumably autonomic dysfunction have been shown to occur not only in chronic alcoholics, but also after acute alcohol ingestion and during acute withdrawal of alcohol.[38] Although part of this response may be related to a direct effect of alcohol on the baroreceptors, it is clear that a combination of alcohol and poor nutrition impair the sympathetic nervous system at both central and peripheral levels. When Wernicke's encephalopathy and chronic liver disease are present, alcoholics frequently have orthostatic hypotension.[38] The Valsalva maneuver has been used to demonstrate the failure of sympathetic vasoconstrictor mechanisms (lack of blood pressure overshoot upon release) in a chronic alcoholic (Fig 7). There was a progressive improvement in the Valsalva response after 1 and 2 months of nutritional therapy in the patient. After treatment, orthostatic tolerance was restored. There is also evidence for impairment of parasympathetic function in alcoholics with polyneuropathy (i.e., peripheral and central neurologic damage). The Valsalva ratio, the cardiac slowing in response to baroreceptor stimulation, and the cardiac acceleration following intravenous atropine were all shown to be diminished in alcoholics with neurologic deficits.[38] Moreover, the 7-year survival rate of alcoholics with evidence of autonomic neuropathy was less than that of a normal population (Fig 8). Although one cannot be certain that survival is directly influenced by autonomic impairment, the presence of autonomic dysfunction clearly signals extensive systemic involvement from chronic alcoholism.

Autonomic Dysfunction: Why Should you be Concerned?

I have already cited evidence that life expectancy is reduced in diabetics and alcoholics with significant autonomic dysfunction (Fig 8). The impairment of the autonomic nervous system is coincident with severe systemic manifestations of these disease processes. However, it is conceivable that simple autonomic testing might identify individuals at risk of adverse perioperative events. Moreover, reduced autonomic function might even prove to be predictive of adverse outcome. I will cite several research reports in which pathophysiological alterations in autonomic function were shown to influence the morbidity and mortality in the perioperative and postoperative period.

First, we have carried out a prospective study that examined a diabetic population with reduced autonomic function and a control group of patients with normal autonomic function.[6] A battery of autonomic stress tests was given to each patient prior to their scheduled ophthalmologic surgery. All patients were induced with a standard anesthetic regimen by an investigator who was blinded to the patient groups. There were several interesting observations. Diabetics with autonomic dysfunction had greater reductions in blood pressure on anesthetic induction than the control group.

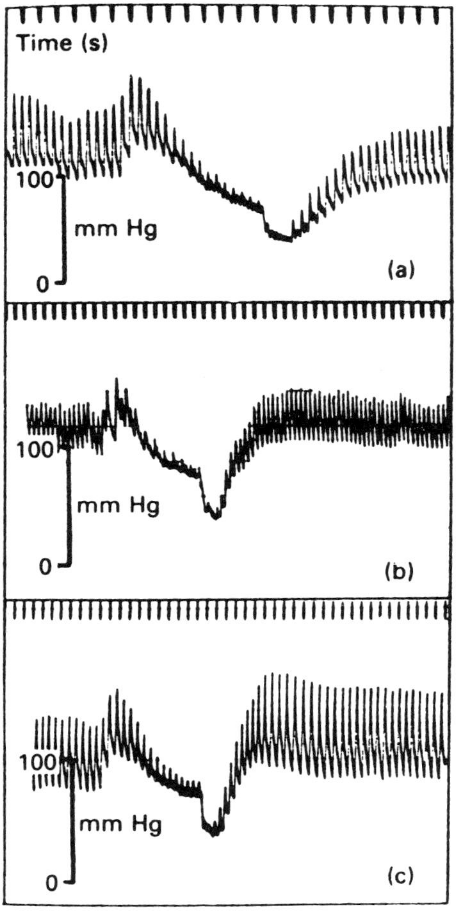

FIG 7.
The arterial blood pressure response to the Valsalva maneuver in one patient with chronic alcoholism and orthostatic hypotension. The top tracing was obtained upon hospital admission and syncope was noted to occur at the end of the period of raised intrathoracic pressure. The middle tracing was obtained 1 month and the bottom tracing obtained 2 months after treatment with vitamins and a normal diet. The recovery of autonomic reflex function is shown by the gradual restoration of the blood pressure overshoot upon release of the Valsalva strain. After treatment, this patient no longer had orthostatic hypotension. (From Barraclough and Sharpey-Schafer: *Lancet* 2:1121, 1963. Used by permission.)

Secondly, the diabetics with the most severe autonomic dysfunction had an increased requirement for intraoperative blood pressure support (see Fig 6). Recently, similar prognostic information has been derived from patients with cardiovascular diseases.[39] Autonomic reflex function was assessed with power spectral analysis of heart rate variability. Patients with

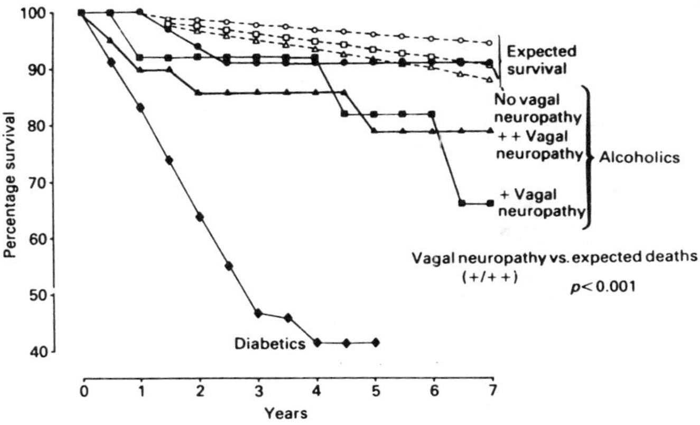

FIG 8.
Seven-year survival curves for alcoholics and diabetics who underwent autonomic function tests: *Solid circles* = 32 alcoholics with no evidence of parasympathetic neuropathy; *solid squares* = 25 alcoholics who had only one abnormal autonomic test; and *solid triangles* = 22 alcoholics who had two or more abnormal autonomic tests. Expected survival curves for the general population of New Zealand are shown by *broken lines* with age matching for each group *(open symbols)*. Survival curves for a diabetic population with autonomic neuropathy are also shown *(solid diamonds)*.[34, 35] The survival rates of alcoholics and diabetics were significantly decreased in the presence of parasympathetic neuropathy.

an impaired low-frequency (sympathetic peak) increase during head-up tilt testing had the greatest degree of hypotension after anesthetic induction. Thus, it appears that intact autonomic neural mechanisms are involved in maintaining cardiovascular stability during anesthetic induction and throughout the perioperative period.

In addition, impaired autonomic function may be predictive of adverse cardiac events following cardiac surgery. A high mortality rate following cardiac surgery has been correlated to several predisposing factors, which include recent myocardial infarction and preoperative dysrhythmias.[40] It is now well-established that a previous myocardial infarction imposes a significant risk to patients undergoing noncardiac surgery during the first 3 to 6 months following the infarction.[41] Recent work suggests that even the use of a pulmonary artery catheter to carefully monitor the cardiac and hemodynamic status during surgery may not improve outcome during this high-risk postinfarction period.[42] Could the presence of autonomic dysfunction be predictive of a poorer outcome after cardiac surgery? Clearly, heart rate variability (mediated primarily by cardiac-vagal activity) is reduced following myocardial infarction.[1–3] This low heart rate variability gradually improves over 3 to 12 months after the myocardial infarction.[28] Could this be related to the reduction in cardiac risk when surgery is performed more than 6 months after an infarction? Moreover, could the presence of preoperative dysrhythmias, which appear to be independent predictors of morbidity and mortality following surgery, be related to autonomic imbalances as well? It is now quite clear that infarction-related increases in cardiac sympathetic activity and/or reductions in cardiac-vagal activity increase the likelihood of new ischemia, reperfusion-induced arrhythmias, and sudden cardiac death.[1–3]

Finally, there are recent data in both animals and humans that suggest that the duration of myocardial ischemic episodes is attenuated in subjects with functional cardiac reflexes. For example, in dogs with myocardial infarctions, those who had preserved cardiac-vagal reflexes during ischemia had fewer episodes of malignant arrhythmias than dogs with impaired baroreflexes.[4] The activation of these vagal reflexes during ischemia are known to result in bradycardia and reduced myocardial oxygen demand and may counteract or lessen the likelihood of sympathetic hyperactivity. A human parallel has recently been published in which patients with ischemic heart disease and impaired cardiopulmonary reflex regulation of coronary vascular resistance had more prolonged spontaneous episodes of ischemia than a second group of patients with ischemia but normal cardiopulmonary reflex function.[5] These findings suggest that during ischemic episodes, activation of cardiac receptors may play an important role in terminating the ischemic event.

In summary, it appears that the autonomic nervous system plays an important role in maintaining hemodynamic stability and influencing outcome in patients undergoing anesthesia and surgery. Autonomic dysfunction is associated with reduced survival and predisposes to malignant arrhythmias and death. Moreover, intact autonomic reflexes are importantly involved in reducing the duration of spontaneous cardiac ischemic episodes. These favorable effects, mediated by preserved autonomic function, could be involved in reducing the incidence of cardiac morbidity and mortality in patients recovering from anesthesia and surgery. Thus, there is a need to evaluate the autonomic nervous system in the preoperative bedside visit. Normal reflex function suggests that patients will be at a lower risk of developing hemodynamic aberrations during the perioperative period. Moreover, the presence of intact cardiac-vagal reflexes may serve a protective role during the intraoperative and postoperative period, which may improve outcome.

References

1. Kleiger RE et al: Decreased heart rate variability and its association with increased mortality after acute myocardial infarction. *Am J Cardiol* 59:256–262, 1987.
2. Bigger JT et al: Components of heart rate variability measured during healing of acute myocardial infarction. *Am J Cardiol* 61:208–215, 1988.
3. Lombardi F et al: Heart rate variability as an index of sympathovagal interaction after acute myocardial infarction. *Am J Cardiol* 60:1239–1245, 1987.
4. DeFerrari GM et al: Vagal reflexes and survival during acute myocardial ischemia in conscious dogs with healed myocardial infarction. *Am J Physiol* 261:H63–H69, 1991.

5. Trimarco B et al: Prolonged duration of myocardial ischemia in patients with coronary heart disease and impaired cardiopulmonary baroreceptor sensitivity. *Circulation* 81:1792–1802, 1990.
6. Burgos LG et al: Increased intraoperative cardiovascular morbidity in diabetics with autonomic neuropathy. *Anesthesiology* 70:591–597, 1989.
7. Fleisher LA, Pincus SM, Rosenbaum SH: Approximate entropy (ApEn) as a correlate of postoperative cardiac dysfunction (abstract). *Proc Am Soc Crit Care Anesth* 1991, San Francisco.
8. Mancia G, Mark AL: Arterial baroreflexes in humans. In *Handbook of Physiology~The cardiovascular system III.* American Physiology Society, 1983, Bethesda, Md, pp 755–793.
9. Raczkowska M, Ebert TJ, Eckberg DL: Muscarinic cholinergic receptors modulate vagal cardiac responses in man. *J Auton Nerv Syst* 7:271–278, 1983.
10. Greene NM, Bachand RG: Vagal component of the chronotropic response to baroreceptor stimulation in man. *Am Heart J* 82:22–27, 1971.
11. Leon DF, Shaver JA, Leonard JJ: Reflex heart rate control in man. *Am Heart J* 80:729–739, 1970.
12. Sanders JS, Ferguson DW, Mark AL: Arterial baroreflex control of sympathetic nerve activity during elevation of blood pressure in normal man: Dominance of aortic baroreflexes. *Circulation* 77:279–288, 1988.
13. Mark AL, Giuseppe M: Cardiopulmonary baroreflexes in humans. In *Handbook of physiology~The cardiovascular system-peripheral circulation III,* section 2(2). American Physiology Society, 1983, Bethesda, Md, pp 795–813.
14. Ludbrook J: Cardiovascular reflexes from cardiac sensory receptors. *Aust NZ J Med* 20:597–606, 1990.
15. Bannister R, Mathias C: Testing autonomic reflexes. In Bannister R, editor: *Autonomic failure. A textbook of clinical disorders of the autonomic nervous system.* New York, Oxford University, 1988, pp 289–307.
16. Moore K, Newton K: Orthostatic heart rate and blood pressures in healthy young women and men. *Heart Lung* 15:611–617, 1986.
17. Ewing DJ et al: The value of cardiovascular autonomic function tests: 10 years experience in diabetes. *Diabetes Care* 8:491–498, 1985.
18. Dyrberg T et al: Prevalence of diabetic autonomic neuropathy measured by simple bedside tests. *Diabetologia* 20:190–194, 1981.
19. Robbins AS, Rubenstein LZ: Postural hypotension in the elderly. *J Am Geriatric Soc* 322:769–774, 1984.
20. Valvanne J et al: The occurrence of postural hypotension in age cohorts of 75, 80 and 85 years. A population study. *Arch Gerontol Geriatr* 2:421–424, 1991.
21. Wieling W et al: Reflex control of heart rate in normal subjects in relation to age: A data base for cardiac vagal neuropathy. *Diabetologia* 22:163–166, 1982.
22. Vita G et al: Cardiovascular reflex tests: assessment of age-adjusted normal range. *J Neurol Sci* 75:263–274, 1986.
23. Ewing DJ: Recent advances in the non-invasive investigation of diabetic autonomic neuropathy. In Bannister R, editor: *Autonomic failure. A textbook of clinical disorders of the autonomic nervous system.* New York, Oxford University, 1988, pp 667–689.
24. Malliani A et al: Cardiovascular neural regulation explored in the frequency domain. *Circulation* 84:482–492, 1991.

25. Inoue K et al: Power spectral analysis of blood pressure variability in traumatic quadriplegic humans. *Am J Physiol* 260:H842–H847, 1991.
26. Rimoldi O et al: Analysis of short-term oscillations of R-R and arterial pressure in conscious dogs. *Am J Physiol* 258:H967–H976, 1990.
27. Randall DC et al: SA nodal parasympathectomy delineates autonomic control of heart rate power spectrum. *Am J Physiol* 260:H985–H988, 1991.
28. Schwartz PJ et al: Baroreflex sensitivity and its evolution during the first year after myocardial infarction. *J Am Coll Cardiol* 12:629–636, 1988.
29. La Rovere MT et al: Baroreflex sensitivity, clinical correlates, and cardiovascular mortality among patients with a first myocardial infarction. *Circulation* 78:816–824, 1988.
30. Billman GE, Schwartz PJ, Stone HL: The effects of daily exercise on susceptibility to sudden cardiac death. *Circulation* 69:1182–1189, 1984.
31. Casadei B et al: Effects of vagal stimulation by transdermal scopolamine in patients post myocardial infarction. *Circulation* 84:II–555, 1991.
32. Schatz IJ: Orthostatic hypotension I. Functional and neurogenic causes. *Arch Intern Med* 144:773–777, 1984.
33. Bannister R. Clinical features of autonomic failure. Symptoms, signs, and special investigations. In Bannister R, editor: *Autonomic failure. A textbook of clinical disorders of the autonomic nervous system.* New York, Oxford University, 1988, pp 267–280.
34. Ewing DJ, Campbell IW, Clarke BF: Mortality in diabetic autonomic neuropathy. *Lancet* 1:601–603, 1976.
35. Ewing DJ, Campbell IW, Clarke BF: The natural history of diabetic autonomic neuropathy. *Q J Med* 49:95–108, 1980.
36. Ciccarelli LL, Ford CM, Tsueda K: Autonomic neuropathy in a diabetic patient with renal failure. *Anesthesiology* 64:283–287, 1986.
37. Page M Mcb, Watkins PJ: Cardiorespiratory arrest and diabetic autonomic neuropathy. *Lancet* 1:14–16, 1978.
38. Johnson RH: Autonomic failure in alcoholics. In Bannister R, editor: *Autonomic failure. A textbook of clinical disorders of the autonomic nervous system.* New York, Oxford University, 1988, pp 690–714.
39. Latson T, Sakai T, Whitten C: Autonomic reflex dysfunction in cardiac surgery patients may predict hypotension at induction. *Anesth Analg* 74:S174, 1992.
40. Tuman KJ et al: Does choice of anesthetic agent significantly affect outcome after coronary artery surgery? *Anesthesiology* 70:189–198, 1989.
41. Mangano DT: Perioperative cardiac morbidity. *Anesthesiology* 72:153–184, 1990.
42. Tuman KJ et al: Effect of pulmonary artery catheterization on outcome in patients undergoing coronary artery surgery. *Anesthesiology* 70:199–206, 1989.

Anesthetic Effects on Immune Function—Where Do We Stand?

A. Joseph Layon, M.D.

Associate Professor, Departments of Anesthesiology and Medicine, University of Florida, College of Medicine, Gainesville, Florida

Ammon B. Peck, Ph.D.

Professor, Department of Pathology and Laboratory Medicine, University of Florida, College of Medicine, Gainesville, Florida

An anaesthetic agent is not just a special poison of the nervous system; it anaesthetizes all elements, all tissues by numbing them temporarily blocking their irritability. (Claude Bernard, 1875.)

In the almost 125 years since Professor Bernard made the above observation, many groups have attempted to define the parameters of immune dysfunction caused, or worsened, by anesthetic agents.[1-8] Yet in spite of this work, serious questions remain regarding the exact nature of the immune modulation caused by anesthesia. Furthermore, as an anesthetic is not frequently delivered by itself, but as a means to a surgical end, the impact of surgical trauma on immune function in the same equation must be considered. The patient population involved in the operative intervention is another variable. While the use of anesthetic agents may influence in vitro immune function, in the healthy individual, this degree of dysfunction/modulation is unlikely to be clinically relevant.[1, 6-8] In a host already immunologically compromised, the same may not hold true. For example, whether the preexisting immune deficiency is mild, as in diabetes mellitus, or severe, as in the acquired immunodeficiency syndrome (AIDS) or trauma, anesthetic agents and/or surgical stress could further impair selected or global aspects of the immune system and thus result in a clinically relevant decrement in immune function that might be life-threatening.[9, 10]

The literature should allow us to resolve these issues; however, work in this area presents conflicting data. The major reasons for this are: (1) lack of correlation between in vitro studies and any measure of outcome; (2) difficulty in separating out the effects of anesthesia from those of the surgical procedure; and (3) limited preoperative immunological characterization in humans. Thus, 125 years after Claude Bernard's assertion, we remain limited in our ability to resolve the conflicting information and provide complete answers to the previous constructs. Outcome-based studies on either immunologically intact[9–12] or compromised animals are few and investigations in humans are quite difficult to interpret. In spite of these limitations, our intention is to review the current status of this area and delineate work that remains to be done. To accomplish this, we will first briefly summarize selective data, pro and con, suggesting that inducible defects of immune function are a consequence of anesthetic action. Thereafter, we will examine but a few of the latest relevant advances in the physiology of the immune system and examine in detail selected data in light of these findings. We will also summarize some of our own work in this area and conclude with the clinical implications of the data presented as well as suggestions for future work.

What are the Data Suggesting Potential Problems With Anesthesia?

Innate Immunity

Neutrophils

Neutrophils (polymorphonuclear leukocytes: PMNL) play a critical role in the host defense system. The response of the PMNL to invasion by extracellular microorganisms includes chemotaxis, phagocytosis, intracellular killing via both oxidative and hydrolytic systems, digestion, and release of lysosomal components.[13] This effector response is centrally regulated by the endotoxin-mediated stimulation of macrophages resulting in the production of cytokines. These macrophage-synthesized molecules, which include tumor necrosis factor (TNF), interleukin-1 (IL-1), IL-6, and members of the IL-8 family, induce adhesion of PMNLs to vascular endothelium followed by migration and accumulation at the site of infection.

The study of anesthetic effects on this cell system has yielded conflicting data. For example, Nunn and colleagues[14] studied the effect of the volatile potent inhaled anesthetic (PIA) agent halothane on PMNL random free movement on glass, chemotaxis through a 3-μm pore-size membrane against 0.5% casein, phagocytosis of polystyrene-latex particles (0.8 μm in diameter) opsonized with human IgG and evaluated by electron microscopy, and oxygen consumption as measured polarographically in a closed plastic chamber. Cells were obtained from healthy human volunteers, and the in vitro halothane concentration was carefully controlled during all stages of the experiments. Statistical methods were not described. No decrement in any of the measured parameters was found. Conversely, Edwards and colleagues[15] obtained cells from control subjects and healthy surgical patients preoperatively, immediately postoperatively, and for 5 days after the procedure. Each patient was exposed to multiple drugs in the perioperative period, making data interpretation difficult. Mitogen stimulation with polyclonal activators (phytohemagglutinin for T cell stimulation, pokeweed mitogen for T and B cell stimulation) and PMNL random migration assays were evaluated. Statistical analysis was well considered. While no differences in mitogen responses were observed, the authors reported a decrease in random migration of PMNLs when patients were compared to their own preoperative baseline. However, the authors did not report the raw data, and the figures used to show statistical significance proved unconvincing. This is especially disturbing because the variation in the normal control subjects, ranging from about 50% to 200% of baseline distance travelled, is not reported to be statistically different. Much less variation from baseline in the anesthetic groups is reported as significantly different from preoperative values.

Nakagawara and colleagues[13] studied the effects of the volatile anesthetic agents halothane, isoflurane, and enflurane on PMNL superoxide production, phagocytosis, and intracellular calcium mobilization in an in vitro assay with neutrophils obtained from healthy human volunteers. While the methods were elaborate, the statistical analysis was limited. For example, normality of distribution of the data was not evaluated, standard error of the mean rather than standard deviation was used, and it was extremely difficult, if not impossible, to determine the number of patients studied. Thus, it is possible that a nonparametric statistical analysis should have been used. Since it was not, and as we do not have the data to determine how the authors decided on the particular statistical method, it is possible that they have fallen into the quagmire of α-error (also called type I error[16]): detecting a difference where there was actually none. Nonetheless, these workers report some very interesting results, suggesting that the volatile agents caused a decrement in superoxide production that appeared to be partially a function of inhibited intracellular calcium mobilization. Phagocytic function did not appear to be adversely effected.

Welch[17] reported that, in clinically relevant concentrations, enflurane but not isoflurane reversibly inhibited killing and chemiluminescence of PMNLs obtained from healthy volunteers. This killing decrement was noted only if the neutrophils were stressed with a large bacterial challenge (i.e., bacteria to PMNL ratio of 100:1). The effect of enflurane on chemiluminescence was seen only at a concentration of 2% and resolved on exposure to air for 30 minutes. The mechanism(s) of these phenomena have not been worked out.

Perttila and colleagues,[18] studying granulocyte microbicidal function in 11 patients undergoing major abdominal surgery (7/11 for malignant diseases), obtained different results. The patients were anesthetized with balanced anesthetic technique, which included up to 1% enflurane. Blood was obtained preoperatively, immediately postoperatively, and daily for 3 days after the procedure. No decrement in the stimulated or unstimulated chemiluminescent response of granulocytes was found. Once again, however, there was no evaluation of the normality of distribution of the data collected prior to statistical analysis. In a small study, this could easily have influenced the results and conclusions.

In a well-designed study in humans, van Dijk and colleagues[19] found no adverse effects on PMNL chemiluminescence, phagocytosis, or stimulated chemotaxis after operative procedures for various, usually abdominal, disorders in 48 patients: 8 of these patients had underlying malignancies. The investigators found a decrement in the serum opsonic activity and about 30% of patients had depressed delayed hypersensitivity to recall antigens.

Similarly, ketamine has been shown, in an in vitro system, to impair the neutrophil cytotoxic myeloperoxidase-H_2O_2-Cl reaction as tested with the chemiluminescence assay.[20] The postulated mechanism is a scavenging effect of ketamine, related to its phenolic structure, of the cytotoxic free-radical intermediates generated by the reaction. However, statistical analysis and the data presentation make it unclear whether significance was ever reached.

Several obvious problems exist with these data in addition to those previously mentioned. While the methods are sophisticated, there have been no attempts to correlate the observed in vitro cellular defects with outcome changes. Furthermore, it is difficult to separate effects induced by the anesthetic agents from those resulting from the surgical procedure. Additionally, preoperative immunologic characterization of the patient is frequently lacking. Finally, we have suggested that issues of sample distribution and statistical analysis may be of significance in determining the validity of conclusions reached in some of the previous studies. This is of more than theoretical concern since the shape of the sampling distribution curve is a means to evaluate the precision of the statistic as an estimate of the population under study.[21] Utilization of parametric statistics to evaluate data when normality of distribution is not assured may result in *P* values that are of dubious value.[22]

It may well be that there are changes induced in neutrophil function by anesthetic agents and/or surgical intervention. These might include a decrement in the ability of the PMNL to either phagocytose or kill a previously phagocytosed bacterium. Indeed, resistance of bacteria to these important properties of PMNLs are recognized as important determinants of virulence. Almost 90 years ago, Snell,[2] in a remarkable series of experiments, alluded to precisely this effect of anesthetic agents on the immune system. Nonetheless, although the data presented are suggestive and interesting, they do not make a solid case for anesthetic-induced immunologic dysfunction due to methodologic failings.

Monocytes

The mononuclear phagocytic system comprises cells whose primary function, like the neutrophils, is phagocytosis. This system of phagocytic cells, initially termed the reticuloendothelial system (RES), includes the circulating monocyte, alveolar and peritoneal macrophage, hepatic Kupffer's cell, free and fixed macrophages of the bone marrow, the reticular cell of lymphatic tissue, and the microglial cell of the central nervous system. For many reasons, including recognition of differences that exist in the pinocytosis of the reticular and endothelial cells compared to phagocytosis of activated macrophages, the term RES has fallen from favor and it is now more appropriate to classify monocytes and macrophages as members of the mononuclear phagocyte system. A schematic of the development of this cell system is noted in Figure 1. These cells are important in both the nonspecific (natural) arm of the immune system as well as the specific (adaptive) arm. The most significant roles of the mononuclear phagocytic system include: (1) antigen presentation to antigen-specific T-lymphocytes; (2) expression of both cell-bound and secreted proteins that enhance T-cell activation; and (3) activation to more efficient killers through stimulation by cytokines (such as γ-interferon) secreted by helper T-cells, as well as by antibody-bound (opsonized) antigen that promotes more avid phagocytosis.

While anesthetic effects on monocyte function have not been evaluated in great detail, Everson,[23] using a ^{99}Tc-latex phagocytosis assay, found, in a group of surgical patients, that there was a statistically significant (P = .01) enhancement of monocyte function in the first 24 hours postoperatively in those with nonmalignant disease. In patients with malignant disease, there were no overall differences in preoperative and postoperative monocyte function. Interestingly, a control population consisting of ten individuals not undergoing any intervention appeared to have had a lower baseline level of monocytic function than did the study patients. This difference, which is not commented on by the authors, may have been due to variation in the assay used to evaluate monocyte function. In spite of minor shortcomings, this study is particularly interesting as there was an attempt to characterize the preoperative state of the monocytes as well as that existent after the operative intervention. Statistical analysis was well considered with nonparametric analysis for the most important comparison.

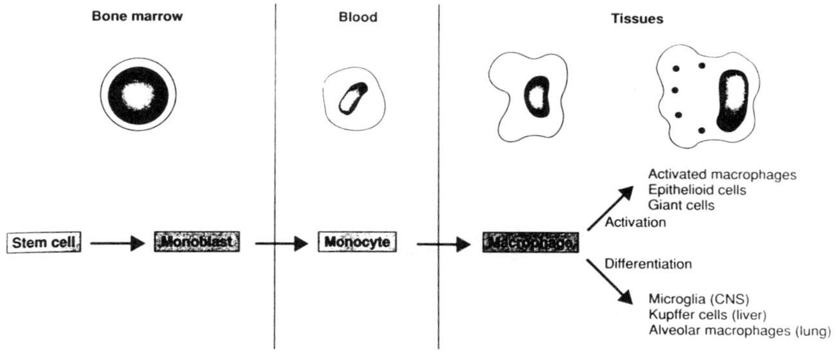

FIG 1.
Maturation of the mononuclear phagocyte from stem cell to monocyte to macrophage. The stem cell is acted on by granulocyte-monocyte CSF, monocyte-CSF, and IL-3 on its journey of differentiation. (From: Abbas AK, Lichtman AH, Pober JS: *Cellular and molecular immunology*. Philadelphia, 1991, Saunders, p 21. Used by permission.)

Adaptive Immunity

T and B Cells

Essentially, T cells are concerned with cell-mediated immunity. A T-cell subpopulation, the T-helper cell, serves as the focal point of the immune system and is intimately involved in providing the help that allows the B cell to transform into an antibody-producing cell. For example, when a protein antigen is introduced into an individual, the initial interaction (first signal) occurs primarily in the peripheral lymphoid tissue such as the spleen and lymph nodes. The initiating event in B-cell activation is the binding of antigen to membrane immunoglobulin (usually IgM or IgD, collectively termed SIg). The second signal, provided by the T-helper lymphocyte, comprises a variety of cytokines that assist the B cell in proliferation (IL-2, IL-4, IL-5) and isotype switching. Interestingly, the change in heavy chain class, also termed isotype switching, occurs with the secondary antibody response and the isotype produced is apparently determined (although the mechanism is not understood) by the combination of cytokines that stimulate the cell (Fig 2). For example, it appears that the combination of IL-4, IL-5, and IL-2 directs proliferating B cells to differentiate into plasma cells that produce pentamers of IgM. In a similar manner, the combination of IL-4, IL-6, IL-2, and interferon (IFN)-γ allow production of IgG by plasma cells. In a manner that is not understood, a portion of the antigen-stimulated B cells do not secrete antibody but, rather, become circulating long-term memory cells.

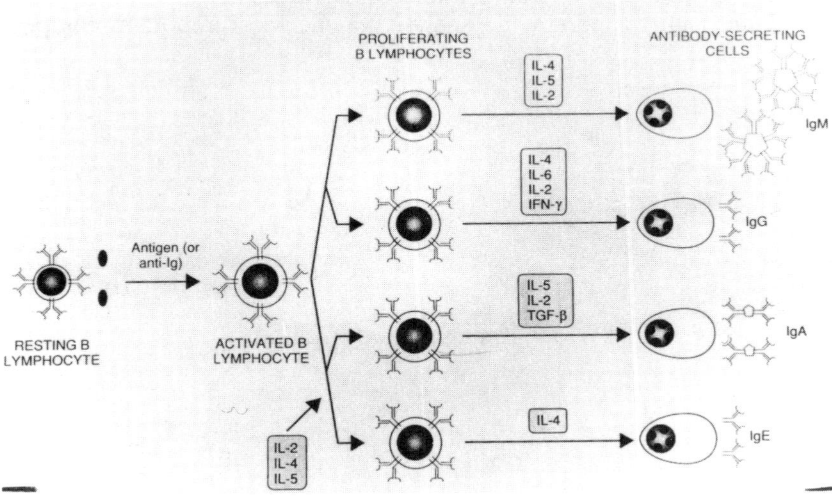

FIG 2.
Functions of cytokines in the proliferation and differentiation of B cells. Note the combinations of cytokines required for production of different isotypes (isotype switching). (From Abbas AK, Lichtman AH, Pober JS: *Cellular and molecular immunology.* Philadelphia, 1991, Saunders, p 196. Used by permission.)

B cells are not simply passively stimulated by the T-helper lymphocyte. The B cell can act as an antigen-presenting cell (APC). In this role, the B cell internalizes and processes the antigen bound to the SIg. This processed antigen is then presented, in conjunction with a bridge or carrier molecule termed the class II major histocompatibility complex (MHC) molecule, to the T-helper lymphocyte. The latter cell than secretes cytokines that assist in the proliferation and differentiation of the B cell. If there are very few B cells with SIg specific for a discrete antigen, the macrophage appears to be the APC of choice. This is also the case when particulate antigen, such as bacteria, must be presented to T-helper cells. In general, however, it appears that macrophages are the APC for induction of a primary antibody response, especially with particulate antigen. Once the B cell clones specific for the antigen are expanded, the B cell may well act as the APC.

Cytotoxic T cells develop from $CD3^+CD8^+$ precursors after activation by antigen-MHC class I receptor complex. These cells are expanded and mature by a combination of IL-2, IL-6, and IFN-γ produced by the helper T-cell ($CD4^+$). Cytotoxic lymphocytes (CTL) require at least two discrete signals for differentiation: class I MHC-associated antigen on a stimulator cell and cytokines secreted from stimulated T-helper cells. CTL killing is antigen-specific, requires that the target cell and the CTL have contact, and generally does not result in injury to the CTL itself. The method of killing appears to involve two specific mechanisms: exocytosis from the CTL of a pore-forming protein that polymerizes in the cell membrane of the target cell, resulting in cellular osmotic disruption, and secretion of a cell toxin related to lymphotoxin. Perhaps the most significant function of the CTL is the elimination of virus-infected cells.

The T-suppressor ($CD8^+$) cell, a fine-tuning controller, modulates the function of the immune system, at times even to the point of unresponsiveness. This cell can exercise inhibitory control over the B-cell as well as cytotoxic T-cells and macrophages. The mechanism of this control is unclear but may involve secretion of excess inhibitory cytokine secretion. For example, transforming growth factor (TGF)-β is a powerful inhibitor of T- and B-cell proliferation.

Eskola and colleagues[24] and Salo et al.,[25] using different models, found no decrement in either T-cell dependent or T-cell independent B-cell function after, respectively, high-dose fentanyl or "balanced" anesthesia, and a halothane anesthetic. The former study,[24] with human subjects, was small (N = ten patients per group) and appears to have used standard error of the mean where standard deviation was required for statistical analysis; no determination of normality of data distribution was performed. Otherwise, the experimental design is useful, involving a determination of polyclonal activation of peripheral blood lymphocytes and antibody secretion from the stimulated cells. Preoperative characterization of the immune response seems to have been carried out. The latter study[25] used a chicken model to evaluate the effect of differing concentrations of the PIA agent halothane on the antibody response to a protein antigen, bovine serum albumin, and a polysaccharide-type antigen, formalin-killed *Brucella abortus*. Antibody production to these antigens is, respectively, T-cell dependent and (relatively) T-cell independent. While the authors reported no significant differences between the anesthetic exposed and control animals, the number of animals studied was small, seven to eight chickens for each group, and statistical analysis seems not to have taken this into account. Nonetheless, this study may indicate that important T-cell, B-cell, and macrophage interactions are essentially intact after exposure to halothane. Unfortunately, there was no outcome arm of the study.

Robertson and colleagues[26] found no decrement in T- or B-cell function after either major or minor operative procedures under anesthesia that included halothane. Conversely, Khansari et al.,[27] in an in vitro system, studied the effect of phencyclidine (PCP) administration on uptake of ^{3}H-thymidine, ^{3}H-deoxyglucose, and immunoglobulin production in lymphocytes. They found that PCP, closely related to ketamine, significantly decreased lymphocyte DNA synthesis, immunologic activation (^{3}H-deoxyglucose uptake), and immunoglobulin production. The postulated mechanism(s) was potassium-channel blockade and/or reduction of monocyte IL-1 production. Slade and colleagues[28] and Whelan and Morris[29] described abnormalities in immune function after major and minor operative procedures in healthy subjects. Both T-cell[28, 29] and B-cell[29] abnormalities were noted in the general anesthesia group. A subgroup of patients undergoing a minor procedure and anesthetized with a regional technique had no depression of T- or B-cell mitogen responses. The authors suggested that a regional technique might be of use in patients at risk for perioperative immunodepression. However, no complications were reported in either group.[28, 29]

While we have been somewhat critical of these studies, perhaps the most serious problem remains the lack of evaluation of outcome in the series showing immunological dysfunction after anesthetic exposure. In the study by Salo and colleagues,[25] for example, it is unclear if minimum alveolar concentration (MAC) was achieved. In the study by Khansari et al.,[27] there was no in vivo exposure, and in the human studies,[28, 29] with the exception of that by Eskola et al.,[24] no attempt was made to separate out the differential effects of surgery and anesthesia. Furthermore, alterations in lymphocyte subsets, which may be of significance since one has access only to peripheral blood in humans, were not determined in these studies. Even the most interesting animal studies had significant flaws. Hansbrough et al.[10] attempted to show an outcome difference in a murine model after stress (burn, amputation, laparotomy) and anesthetic exposure. Unfortunately, the number of animals used was as small as five in some groups. This could have led to type I error, yet the data were not evaluated for normality nor were nonparametric statistics used to evaluate significance. Much the same problem seems to complicate a second work attempting to evaluate outcome.[9] Thus, these attempts to deal with issues previously raised have not been uniformly useful.

The recent exciting work by Knight and colleagues[30] shows that animals exposed to influenza virus during enflurane exposure have less pulmonary pathology and lower viral titers than animals exposed to halothane, pentobarbital, or diethyl ether. While evaluating the question of anesthetic-induced immune-modulation from an angle somewhat different than most have attempted, this work leaves little doubt about the significance of the area.

Natural Killer and Killer Cells

Natural killer (NK) lymphocytes, also termed large granular lymphocytes (LGLs), are a lymphocyte subset that share neither lineage nor phenotypic characteristics of T or B cells. These cells exhibit cytotoxicity to a variety of malignant, virus-infected, and normal cells, killing by mechanisms that are neither MHC restricted nor specific for a particular viral antigen. Thus, killing by NK cells remains part of the nonspecific arm of the immune system. NK cells require direct leukocyte-target cell interaction but do not need antibody or complement to kill the target. NK cells are responsive to cytokines, in as much as their ability to lyse target cells is enhanced by type I IFN, IFN-γ, TNF, or IL-2. While antibody is not required for killing by the NK cell, coating the target cell with IgG can enhance NK cell function, as the IgG is recognized by the NK F_c receptor (termed CD16). Cytolysis occurring in this manner is termed antibody-dependent cell-mediated cytotoxicity (ADCC), and NK cells are an important cellular mediator of this phenomenon. The mechanism used by NK cells to kill target cells are similar to those of cytotoxic lymphocytes, namely exocytosis of a pore-forming protein and secretion of a cell toxin. NK cells also produce and secrete IFN-γ and TNF; production appears to be enhanced when the CD16 receptor is stimulated by IgG.

Investigations of the effects of surgery and anesthesia on NK cell function have also yielded conflicting results. Pollock,[31] studying the effects of surgical stress on NK cell function in an acclimatized mouse model, found that surgery resulted in as much as a 59% decrease in NK cell-mediated cytotoxicity (NKCC). When NKCC was evaluated 24 hours after hindlimb amputation in mice who had been injected with Lewis lung carcinoma 7 days previously, a significant decrement in NK function was reported. Anesthesia (nembutal) was reported not to result in any decrement in NK function. However, when the tabular data are reevaluated, their conclusions appear less firm. In the experiment previously noted, in which the impact of tumor burden and surgery on NKCC were evaluated, only ten animals were used. This might have resulted in nonnormal distribution of data, but the appropriate statistical study to evaluate this possibility seems not to have been done. As we have mentioned several times, the statistical analysis of an experiment requires initial determination of the normality (or lack thereof) of data distribution, particularly when the sample size is small. From this analysis, one will then proceed to one of two general groups of statistical studies—parametric ones when the data are normally distributed and nonparametric ones for non-normally distributed data. In Pollock's study, there is some question as to whether this was done, so we question the statistical analysis, and logically, the inferences drawn from those analyses. Furthermore, the data are reported as mean ± standard error of the mean, and a *t*-test was performed to determine statistical significance. The *t*-test requires that we use standard deviation (SD), not the standard error of the mean (SEM)*; when we back-calculate and use SD instead of SEM in the *t*-test, statistical significance disappears. Nonetheless, the study by Pollock raises many excellent questions and provides some intriguing insights that demand follow-up.

Another group,[32] studying the effects of anesthesia on NK function in humans undergoing total hip arthroplasty, found an increase in activity after administration of preoperative oral benzodiazepine, a result maintained until the first postoperative day. The authors postulated the rapid rise in NK cell activity was due to mobilization of mature NK cells into the vascular space, but no data were given to support this hypothesis. The significance of the study is unclear. In a somewhat larger study, Tonnesen and colleagues[33] reported quite elaborately on the differential effects of epidural anesthesia vs. neuroleptanesthesia on NK activity, lymphocyte phenotype analysis, and stress hormone levels. Sixteen women scheduled to undergo abdominal hysterectomy for nonmalignant metrorrhagia were randomized to either epidural or neuroleptic techniques. With the blood draw always occurring between 0900 and 1100 hours, samples were removed for the previously mentioned analyses. The authors found no differences in the demographic or surgical data. NK function was significantly less between 1 and 3 days after surgery in the neuroleptanesthesia group when compared to preoperative NK function. There was a small but nonsignificant decrement in NK function in the epidural anesthesia group, but there were no significant differences when the two groups were compared. This held true for the phenotypic analyses as well: a significant decrement in pan–T cells, T-helper cells, B cells, and NK cells was seen 1 day after the procedure in the neuroleptanesthesia group compared to the preoperative period. No intergroup differences were noted. Serum cortisol levels were significantly different when compared between groups, with the neuroleptanesthesia group showing the higher values. No outcome data are reported in this paper.

Duncan et al.,[34] studying the effects of sodium thiopental on cell-mediated cytotoxicity (CMC) in a murine model, found that thiopental decreased cytotoxicity when the thiopental concentration was $\geq 5.7 \times 10^{-5}$ M. This effect was reversible with cell washing and was noted to be synergistic with the potent inhaled anesthetic agent, halothane. The proposed mechanism was impaired protein synthesis via disruption of microtubule/microfilament organization or a reduced cellular interaction between

*The mathematical formulation that describes these two methods of evaluation of variation around the mean value is:

$$\text{SEM} = \text{SD}\sqrt{n}$$

Where SEM = standard error of the mean; SD = standard deviation; and n = number of members of a sample group.

effector and target cells. There are several flaws with this study. Because of the cell preparation techniques used, it is likely that macrophages as well as NK cells were evaluated in this study. All analyses were carried out in vitro, so relevance to the intact animal is questionable. Finally, the statistical analysis is poorly done for the same reasons previously mentioned—small sample size, no evaluation of normality of distribution, and the possibility that the wrong studies were used to analyze the data. Yet again we are left with data that are suggestive and interesting, but incomplete.

McCredie[35] evaluated ADCC in a group of 70 critically ill patients. While we have no indicator of the severity of illness (i.e., APACHE II severity of illness score), the admission diagnoses suggest significant pathology. Peripheral blood was obtained from the patients on admission and at 3-day intervals until either discharge or death. Given the cell preparations used, it is likely that NK cells made up part, but not all, of the effector cells studied. ADCC was found to be significantly decreased in critically ill individuals as compared to healthy control subjects, those patients with benign diseases, and those with early—but not advanced—cancer. Those patients who went on to die in McCredie's series had lower initial and final levels of ADCC. Patients who became septic had decreased activity, but those who went on to die were noted to drop to even lower final values. The author suggests that ADCC activity might be used as a predictor of mortality in critically ill individuals. Statistical analysis is, in this study, problematic.

What is the Physiology of the Immune System?

In an area as extensive as this, we will only attempt to capture the spirit of the most recent significant advances to tie them into the issue at hand—the presence or absence of immune-modulating effects of anesthetic agents and their clinical relevance. Those areas of interest are as follows:

a. Ion-channel activation of lymphocytes[36–38] and the possible ion-channel blocking—either opened or closed—effects[39–42] or other transmembrane signaling alterations[43, 44] of the PIA or intravenous agents. This is of particular interest in the context of intracellular and intercellular communications requiring cytokines. The synthesis of these agents depends on ion-channel-mediated stimulation.

b. Complement protein C3 and complement receptor 2 (CR2) and their roles in antibody response.[45–49] This becomes even more interesting when data suggesting B-cell abnormalities after anesthesia[27, 29] are interpreted in the light of other work suggesting that anesthetic agents may compromise the quantity or quality of complement factor C3.[50]

c. Blood loss[51–56] as well as the utilization of transfused blood[57–59] in altering immune responsiveness. This, in the context of other possible immune modulation caused by anesthesia and surgery,[9] might be of significance.

Gardner[36] has reviewed in great detail the significant literature suggesting that activation of B- and T-lymphocytes requires functional ion channels. At least three ion channels are thought to take part in the activation process: a Ca^{2+} channel, a voltage-activated K^+ channel, and a Ca^{2+}-activated K^+ channel. DeCoursey and colleagues[37] reported, using whole cell and outside-out patch-clamp analyses, that the human T-lymphocyte has approximately 200 to 300 conducting K^+ channels per cell. Gating characteristics of the channels were altered within 1 minute of adding the polyclonal activator phytohemagglutinin (PHA) in concentrations known to produce mitosis. Specifically, the channels opened more rapidly and at more negative membrane potentials. PHA stimulation of T-lymphocytes was inhibited by adding the K^+ channel blockers tetraethylammonium and 4-aminopyridine (4AP). The authors suggest these results imply K^+ channels play a role in mitogenesis. Other cell types likely require ion channel function for activation as well. Sidell et al.,[38] using the whole-cell variation of the patch-clamp technique, found voltage-dependent K^+ current in human NK cells. This current was found to be reduced in a dose-dependent manner by the K^+-channel blockers 4AP and quinidine, as well as by the Ca^{2+}-channel blockers verapamil and cadmium. Verapamil and quinidine appear to block the K^+ channel after it has opened, resulting in a use- and time-dependent block that is only slowly reversible; 4AP and Ca^{2+} do not appear to block the K^+ channel in this manner. The K^+ channel appears to be required if the following are to occur: (1) binding of effector cell to target cell; (2) post-binding programming that precedes the release of cytotoxic factor; and (3) release of NK cytotoxic factor (NKCF). No killing will occur if NKCF is not released, and in these experiments, the ion channel blockers inhibited its release. As anticipated, addition of the K^+ channel blockers to the cell mixture after release of NKCF did not inhibit killing.

This work is important in our context because of data suggesting that the PIA agents have ion channel-blocking properties. Looking only at membrane fluidity changes in the presence and absence of halothane, Ueda and colleagues[39] found that halothane significantly increased monolayer membrane fluidity. While clearly not aimed at evaluating ion channels, this work suggests that cell membrane changes, and hence ion channels changes as well, might be seen with the PIA agents. Nelson and Sweo[40] evaluated the effects of PIA agents on Ca^{2+} uptake and Ca^{2+}-induced Ca^{2+} release in two separate sarcoplasmic reticulum membrane vesicle fractions obtained from the white muscle of rabbit back and hindlimb. It has been proposed that the Ca^{2+}-induced Ca^{2+} release is mediated by Ca^{2+} channels in the sarcoplasmic reticulum. Each of the PIA agents tested—enflurane, isoflurane, and halothane—tended to lower the threshold Ca^{2+} concentration at which Ca^{2+} release occurred (Fig 3). This was blocked by the Ca^{2+} channel-blocking agent ruthenium red (Fig 4). This suggests, minimally, that the PIA agents can influence membrane channels.

Brett and colleagues[41] used patch-clamp techniques to evaluate the effects of the PIA agent isoflurane on the acetylcholine receptor channel.

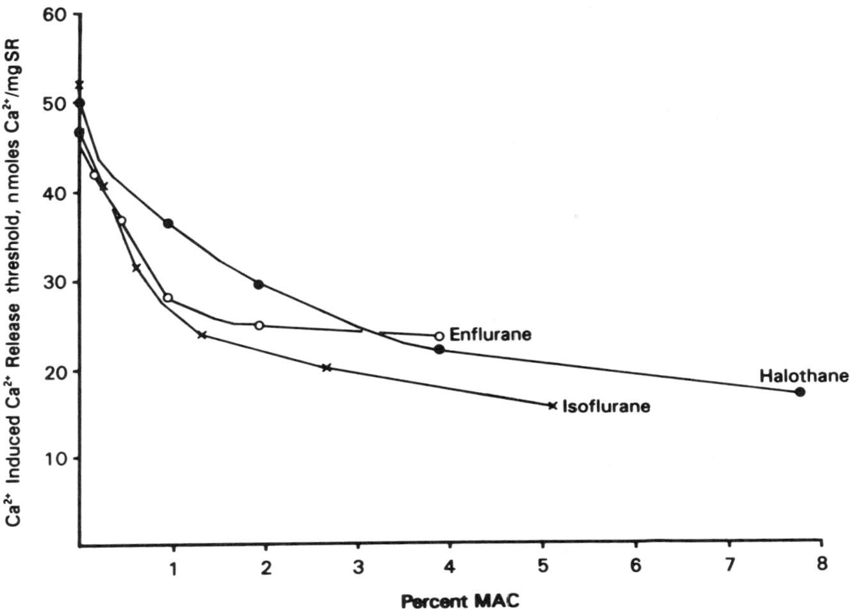

FIG 3.
Plot of the effect of three potent inhaled anesthetic agents on the threshold for Ca^{2+} release from isolated skeletal muscle sarcoplasmic reticulum membrane vesicles. The Ca^{2+} load needed for Ca^{2+}-induced Ca^{2+} release is decreased by each of the anesthetic agents. (From Nelson TE, Sweo T: *Anesthesiology* 69:571–577, 1988. Used by permission.)

The technique, quite intriguing in itself, involved utilization of a glass micropipette. The polished tip was placed in contact with the surface of a cell membrane. Gentle suction was then applied and the patch of membrane covered by the pipette tip pulled slightly into the opening of the micropipette. In this way, a high resistance seal was formed (Fig 5). It was the high resistance seal as well as the small area of the patch being studied that allowed the resolution of microcurrents associated with activation of the ion channels. The major components for the patch clamp technique are presented in Figure 6. In the series of experiments by these authors, a second micropipette was used to deliver or remove isoflurane from the area of the membrane being studied (Fig 7). Data obtained from this type of experiment are shown in Figure 8. Channel openings are shown by a downward threshold crossing, while closings are designated by upward threshold crossings. Any individual opening may actually be made up of several opening/closing events that are occurring too fast to be resolved. When the authors exposed their membrane patches to 5mM (9.7 volumes percent) isoflurane, the duration of brief closures increased, open and burst durations decreased in length, the duration of brief closures as a percentage of

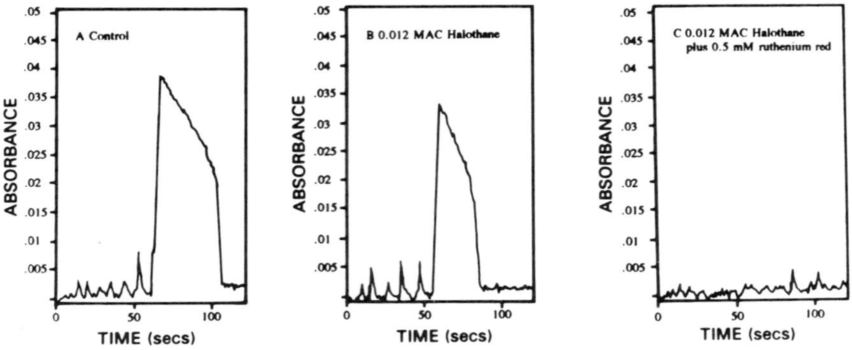

FIG 4.
A series of plots showing the consequence of the Ca^{2+} channel blocker ruthenium red on halothane's lowering of the Ca^{2+} threshold for Ca^{2+}-induced Ca^{2+} release in rabbit heavy sarcoplasmic reticulum (SR) fraction. Block A is the control and shows that a total of 40 nmol Ca^{2+}/mg SR is required to reach threshold. Block B shows that in the presence of 0.012 MAC halothane, the threshold (Ca^{2+}) is decreased to 30 nmol Ca^{2+}/mg SR. Block C shows that, after the addition of 0.5 mM ruthenium red to the mixture containing 0.012 MAC halothane, even adding up to 85 nmol Ca^{2+}/mg SR does not result in any Ca^{2+} release. (From Nelson TE, Sweo T: Anesthesiology 69:571–577, 1988. Used by permission.)

control increased, and the duration of long closures as a percentage of control decreased (Fig 9[9]). The flickering nature of the channel when exposed to isoflurane resembles the effect of local anesthetics on the same channel. While the clinical significance of these data are not entirely clear, it does appear that the PIA agents affect channel function. These data also

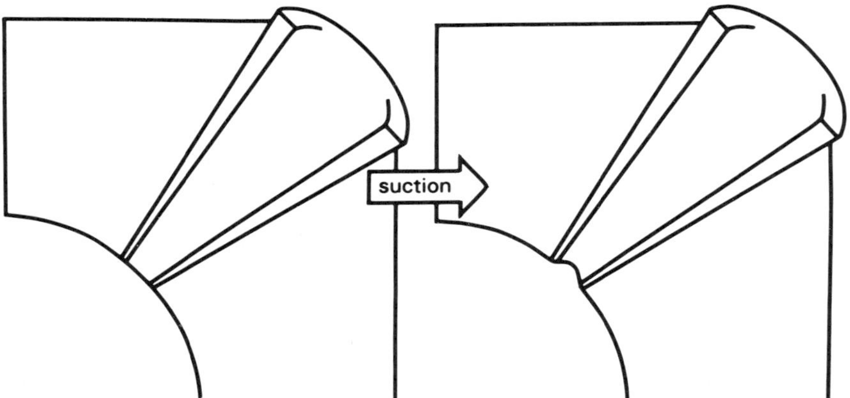

FIG 5.
A schematic representation of the seal formed between the polished tip of the micropipette and the patch of cell membrane under it when gentle suction is applied to the pipette. (From Brett RS, Dilger JP, Yland KF: *Anesthesiology* 69:161–170, 1988. Used by permission.)

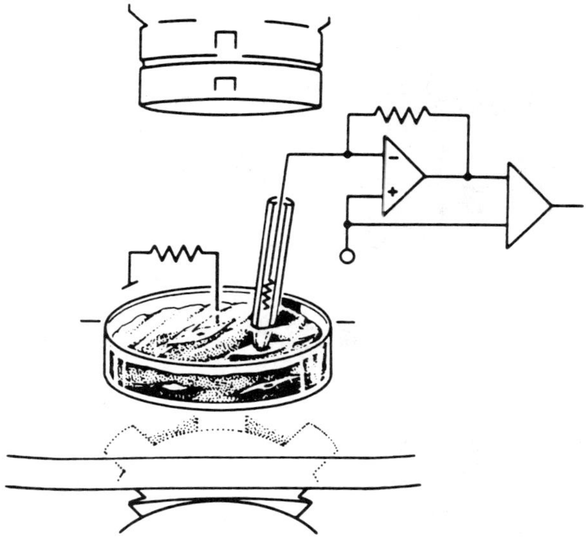

FIG 6.
A diagrammatic representation of the major components of the apparatus required to perform the patch clamp experiments. Cells grown in culture are viewed through an inverted microscope. The micropipette, attached to a micromanipulator (not shown), has been placed onto a segment of cell as shown in Figure 5. A silver chloride wire is used to provide electrical continuity between the saline solution inside the pipette and a current-voltage converter/amplifier. (From Brett RS, Dilger JP, Yland KF: *Anesthesiology* 69:161–170, 1988. Used by permission.)

raise questions about the possible effects of the PIA agents on other channels in other cell types, for example the K^+ channel of the T-lymphocyte and NK cell.

Furthermore, the interesting data of Robinson-White et al.,[43] using a different cell system, provide additional hints that anesthetic agents might influence membrane function. This group looked at cell signal transduction after exposure to one of several barbiturates. They hypothesized that barbiturates exerted their effect through inhibition of guanosine triphosphate (GTP)-binding proteins that are required to couple the signal produced after receptor stimulation by agonist. Successful coupling (as when barbiturates are not present) results in hydrolysis of inositol phospholipids, which subsequently leads to the generation of two synergistic signals: release of intracellular Ca^{2+} from the endoplasmic reticulum by inositol 1,4,5 triphosphate, and the activation of protein kinase C by 1,2-diacylglycerol (Fig 10). The interaction of these two signals results in a cellular response. Thus, the authors looked for agonist-stimulated release of ^{3}H-inositol phospholipids with and without pentobarbital present. They found that the presence of pentobarbital caused a significant decrement in the hydrolysis of inositol phospholipids (Figs 11, 12). The effects of pentobarbital were hypothesized to be the result of G-protein or phospholipase C inhibition. Once

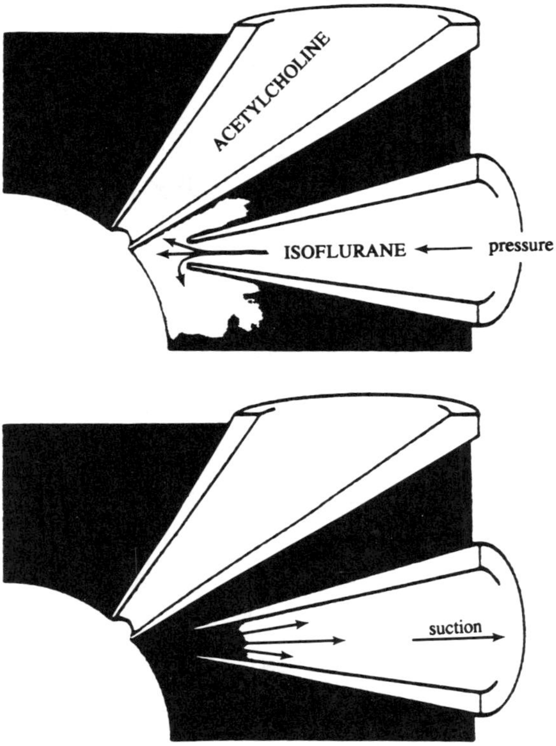

FIG 7.
Diagrammatic representation of the apparatus used for the local microperfusion technique of applying and removing isoflurane. The patch of membrane under study has been isolated in the upper pipette; the lower pipette contains a solution of isoflurane in saline. (From Brett RS, Dilger JP, Yland KF: *Anesthesiology* 69:161–170, 1988. Used by permission.)

again, the significance of these data are the hints they give as to the cell membrane effects of anesthetic agents. At present, these studies raise more questions than answers. Furthermore, while the clinical relevance of these data may be questionable, this area is one of potential fruitful collaboration between basic scientists and clinicians that will yield, in the near future, a good deal of basic scientific data about both drug and cellular mechanisms. This work, in sum, requires aggressive follow-up and expansion.

A second major area of interest involves the complement system. Recent data suggest that complement protein C3 and CR2 play a role in antibody responses.[45–49] For example, Böttger and Bitter-Suermann[45] have shown that guinea pigs genetically deficient in C3 have an impaired antibody response to the T-cell dependent antigen bacteriophage ϕX 174. Interestingly, this decrement in antibody response was strictly dose-dependent.

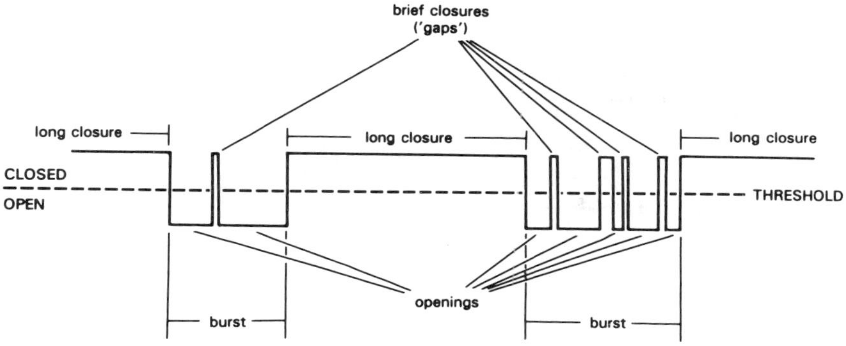

FIG 8.
A schematic representation of the acetylcholine receptor channel currents. The terminology is discussed in the text. (From Brett RS, Dilger JP, Yland KF: *Anesthesiology* 69:161–170, 1988. Used by permission.)

When the antigen dose was increased, the immune response returned to normal. Heyman[46] reviewed data suggesting that stimulation of the B-cell complement receptor by IgM enhances production of both IgM and IgG and potentiates induction of memory cells. The degree of stimulation varies with concentration of antigen and antibody, is antigen- but not epitope-

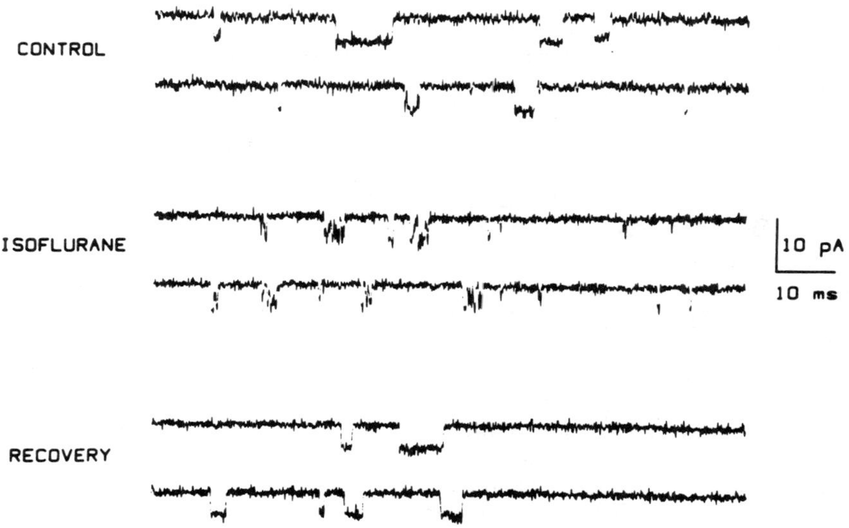

FIG 9.
Examples of unitary acetylcholine receptor channel currents before, during, and after perfusion with 5 mM isoflurane. Channel openings are noted by the downward deflection of the current trace. See text for more detail. (From Brett RS, Dilger JP, Yland KF: Anesthesiology 69:161–170, 1988. Used by permission.)

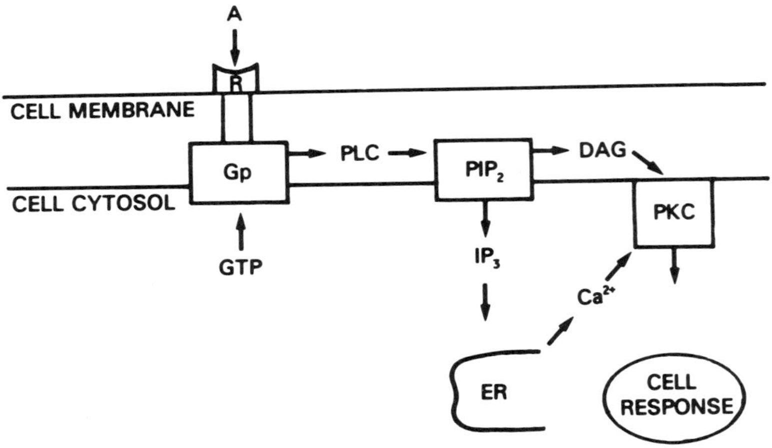

FIG 10.
Schematic representation of the G-protein regulated inositol phospholipid hydrolysis and signal transduction. Activation of receptor (R) by agonist (A) causes phospholipase C (PLC) to hydrolyze phosphatidylinositol biphosphate (PIP_2) through the intervention of the putative GTP binding protein (G_p). The rest of the schema is as described in the text. *ER* = endoplasmic reticulum, IP_3 = inositol triphosphate, *PKC* = protein kinase C, *DAG* = 1,2-diacylglycerol. (From Robinson-White AJ et al: *Anesthesiology* 72:996–1004, 1990. Used by permission.)

specific, and will not occur if the IgM is injected after the antigen. The humoral response to both particulate and soluble antigen- is enhanced by IgM. The importance of the complement system in this phenomenon has been suggested by two lines of evidence: First, mutant IgM unable to activate complement cannot enhance the humoral response of normal mice. Second, normal IgM cannot induce augmentation in complement-depleted mice. One proposed mechanism for this phenomenon is that triggering of the B cell occurs following cross-linking of surface Ig and complement receptors. Calcium influx has been shown to occur after cross-linking. It has been reported that IgG can also enhance antibody production to soluble, but not particulate, antigen. The proposed mechanism involves complement activation by the IgG. The importance of complement receptor 1 (CR1) and CR2 in immunoregulation has been reviewed recently.[47, 48] Finally, Matsumoto and colleagues[49] have recently presented data suggesting that the B cell has on its membrane surface a signal transduction complex, separate from the antigen receptor complex, composed of B-cell-restricted proteins, CR2, CD19 (a member of the Ig superfamily), as well as other components that are still ill-defined. These data may lead to an understanding of the molecular mechanism involved in the complement-mediated augmentation of Ig production. These data become even more interesting for the clinician when considered with reports suggesting B cell abnormalities after anesthesia,[27, 29] and work suggesting that anesthetic

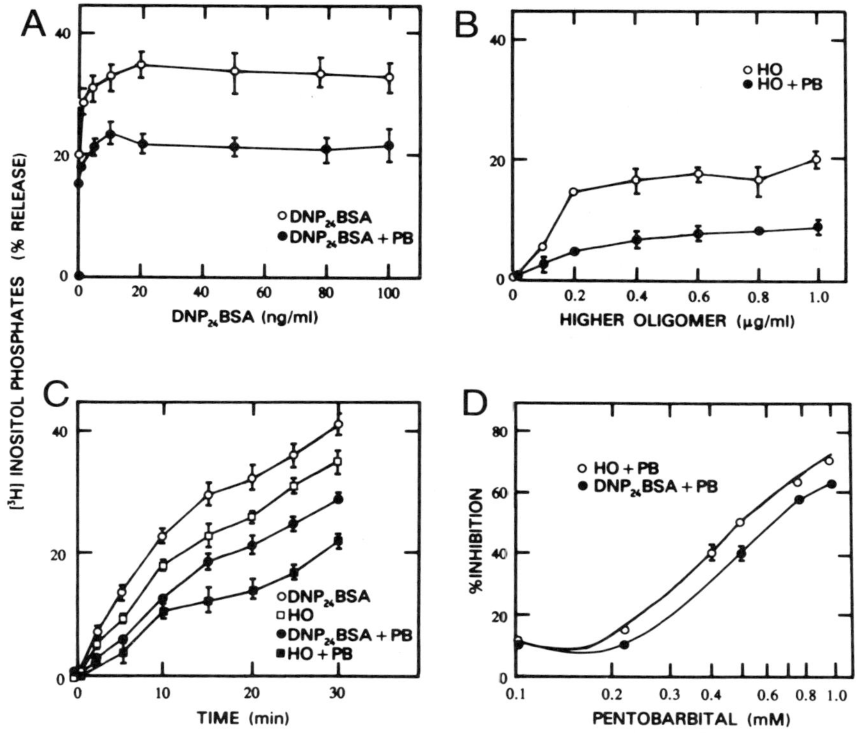

FIG 11.
Time and dose-response curves of antigen and oligomer-induced (tetrameres of IgE) ^{3}H-inositol phospholipid hydrolysis in intact RBL-2H3 cells. **A,** the effect of pentobarbital on hydrolysis as induced by increasing concentrations of dinitrophenol-conjugated bovine serum albumin ($DNP_{24}BSA$) or, **B,** oligomers of IgE. **C,** time course of the inhibition by pentobarbital of $DNP_{24}BSA$ (10 ng/mL) and oligomers of IgE (1 mcg/mL)-induced hydrolysis. **D,** concentration curves of the inhibition by pentobarbital of $DNP_{24}BSA$ (10 ng/mL) and oligomers of IgE (1 mcg/mL)-induced hydrolysis. Response to stimulants in the presence of pentobarbital was significantly different from controls, $P < .01$ for panels **A, B,** and **C,** $P < .03$ for panel **D.** (From Robinson-White AJ et al: *Anesthesiology* 72:996–1004, 1990. Used by permission.)

agents may compromise the quantity or quality of complement factor C3.[50] This latter work involved the study of 98 patients who were exposed to anesthetic agents and underwent operative intervention. In 33 of 98 patients, the hemolytic compliment (CH_{50}) was decreased, so individual component levels were assayed. The authors reported that CH_{50} levels were significantly decreased 15 minutes after anesthetic induction (10% decrease), and 120 minutes after anesthetic induction (i.e., during surgery, 25% decrease). C3 was found to be decreased in approximately 63% of the individuals in whom it was measured. While there are the usual prob-

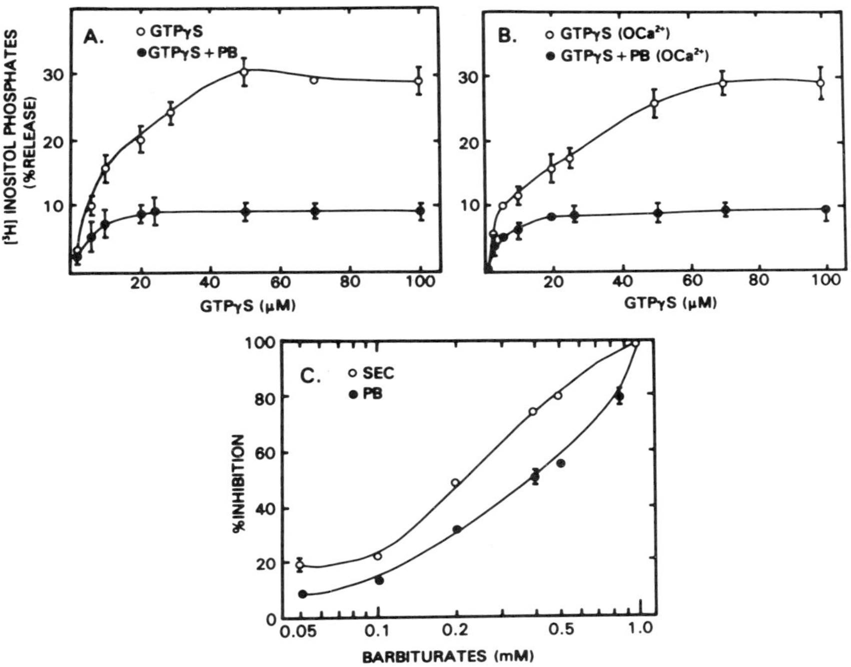

FIG 12.
Inhibition of GTPγS (a nonhydrolyzable analog of GTP)-induced ^3H-inositol phospholipid release in permeabilized RBL-2H3 cells by pentobarbital and secobarbital. In panel **B,** 0 Ca^{2+} signifies incubation without calcium. In panel **C,** *SEC* = secobarbital and PB = pentobarbital. Statistical values: $P < 0.01$ for panels **A** and **B,** $P < 0.05$ for panel **C.** (From Robinson-White AJ et al: *Anesthesiology* 72:996–1004, 1990. Used by permission.)

lems with patient selection and statistical analysis, we are once again presented with very interesting and potentially significant findings that demand follow-up and expansion.

Finally, there is a significant body of data suggesting that blood loss[51–56] as well as the utilization of transfused blood[57–59] may alter immune responsiveness. Jubert and colleagues[51] found that the anesthetic agents halothane and ether, and blood loss greater than 500 mL decreased responsiveness of lymphocytes to polyclonal activators. The data are of interest although there were only 18 patients studied. Esrig et al.[52] evaluated the effects of hemorrhagic shock on neutrophil function and animal survival in a rat model. After blood pressure was held at 30 mm Hg for 30 minutes, the animals were resuscitated with Ringer's lactate solution and then injected intraperitoneally with either 1 mL lysed sheep red blood cells (RBCs) or sheep RBCs plus 3×10^9 colony-forming units (cfu) of *Escherichia coli.* Neutrophil phagocytosis and killing were also evaluated. Although the animals injected with sheep RBCs and *E. coli* suffered a 90%

mortality rate, neutrophil function appeared to be unchanged. While the study is limited by its small size—four groups of ten animals—and lack of statistical analysis, the results presented are quite intriguing. The pathophysiology of hemorrhage-induced immune dysfunction has been evaluated in some detail by Abraham and colleagues in a series of studies.[53, 54, 56] In these experiments, both human and animal, several points are clarified: (1) PHA lymphocyte stimulation is decreased by almost 50% within 2 hours after a 30% total blood volume hemorrhage; (2) a dialyzable molecule of between 13,000 and 23,000 molecular weight appears to be responsible for the decreased PHA response; (3) IL-2 production, as measured with bioassay, is decreased from 56% to 85% in humans who have suffered moderate-to-severe injury (trauma and hemorrhage); and (4) in a murine model, 30% total blood volume hemorrhage resulted in decreased IL-2, IL-3, and IL-5, a significant decrement in IL-2R expression, and decreased proliferative response to concanavalin A (Con A). Similarly, Stephan et al.[55] used a C3H/HeJ mouse model to evaluate mortality and lymphocyte responsiveness to Con A after the animals were bled to a mean blood pressure of 35 mm Hg and held at that level for 1 hour. This group found Con A responsiveness had decreased significantly beginning 1 day after the bleed, then slowly began to recover, returning to normal 10 days after the insult. Three days following the bleed, animals were subjected to cecal ligation and puncture as a model of sepsis; mortality was followed for an additional 3 days. All of the experimental animals ($N = 10$) died as compared to 58% (11/20) of the control subjects. While these data are interesting, the reader is not told if the data were normally distributed, and why the only statistical analysis performed on the nonproportional data was the paired *t*-test.

A related line of study involves the immunosuppressive effects of transfused blood.[57–59] In a recent review, Schriemer and colleagues[57] point out that NK function may be altered by transfusion and in this way transfusion may thus be involved in tumor progression and metastases. Waymack and colleagues[58] found that rats exposed to an unknown concentration of methoxyflurane (i.e., methoxyflurane-soaked gauze sponges until the animals were asleep) for 2 to 3 minutes and then, over a period of 7 days, challenged intravenously with 1×10^8 cfu/mL *E. coli* did not have an increase in mortality compared with control rats. This also held for animals given an autologous transfusion of 0.5 mL and then exposed intravenously to *E. coli* as described. Interestingly, when the bacterial challenge was administered intraperitoneally, there was a significant decrease in survival in both the anesthetic and transfused animals when compared to that in control animals. It is unclear why differences in survival between animals injected with the bacterial challenge intravenously vs. intraperitoneally were seen. In a more recent paper, Waymack and colleagues[59] found that intravenous transfusion of autologous blood 7 days before challenge by *E. coli* resulted in enhanced survival when compared to control animals. These data, when placed in the context of other possible immune modulation caused by anesthesia and surgery,[9] suggest that this is a fertile area for further work. For example, we[11, 12] have not found an increase in mortality over control nor a change in responsiveness to polyclonal activators when healthy BALB/c mice were injected intraperitoneally with 4.5×10^7 *E. coli* after exposure to 1.3 MAC of either isoflurane or halothane for 1½ hours. Whether this will hold true when animals are subjected to an intravenous *E. coli* exposure, a 30% total blood volume hemorrhage prior to anesthetic exposure, or to a 30% hemorrhage after a 25% total body surface area full-thickness burn is presently being evaluated.

Summary

For the past century, a great many studies have attempted to evaluate the issues raised by Claude Bernard in 1875. In reviewing these data, we have attempted to make sense of the direction in which this work has led. Unfortunately, we must frankly state that there is a significant portion of the literature that brings us no closer to answering Professors Bernard's question. What is to be done? Studies providing suggestive, but unclear results must be repeated. The rush to utilize molecular and other high-technology techniques must not blind us to the importance of determining, in the first instance, whether or not there is a whole-animal phenomenon that should be studied in molecular detail. Carefully thought-out experiments that build on previous work must be designed and carried out by collaborators in the clinical and basic sciences. This point cannot be overemphasized; collaborative work is the order of the day. Clinicians know what happens in the operating room, in the intensive care unit, and on the hospital ward. Thus the physician, knowing what is clinically relevant, can pose the question to the basic scientist and together they can develop a relevant, well-controlled animal model. In the area of anesthetic-induced immune-dysfunction/modulation, this is what we should aim for at present.

References

1. Salo M: Effects of anaesthesia and surgery on the immune response. In Watkins J, Salo M, editors: *Trauma, stress and immunity in anaesthesia and surgery.* London, 1982, Butterworth Scientific, pp 211–253.
2. Snel JJ: Immunität und Narkose. *Berl Klin Wochenschr* 40:212–214, 1903.
3. Rubin G: The influence of alcohol, ether, and chloroform on natural immunity in its relation to leukocytosis and phagocytosis. *J Infect Dis* 1:425–444, 1904.
4. Graham EA: The influence of ether and ether anesthesia on bacteriolysis, agglutination, and phagocytosis. *J Infect Dis* 8:147–175, 1911.
5. Kolmer JA, Pearce RM: Studies in non-specific complement fixation. III. The influence of splenectomy and anesthetics on the non-specific complement fixation sometimes shown by normal rabbit and dog sera. *J Infect Dis* 18:32–45, 1916.
6. Moudgil GC: Update on anaesthesia and the immune system. *Can Anaesth Soc J* 33:54–60, 1986.

7. Lee Y-T N: Effect of anesthesia and surgery on immunity. *J Surg Oncol* 9:425–430, 1977.
8. Bruce DL, Wingard DW: Anesthesia and the immune response. *Anesthesiology* 34:271–282, 1971.
9. Lundy J, Ford CM: Surgery, trauma and immune suppression: Evolving the mechanism. *Ann Surg* 197:434–438, 1983.
10. Hansbrough JF et al: Alterations in splenic lymphocyte subpopulations and increased mortality from sepsis following anesthesia in mice. *Anesthesiology* 63:267–273, 1985.
11. Layon AJ et al: Cellular and nonspecific immune function and outcome after anesthesia with isoflurane in mice (abstract). *Anesth Analg* 74:S178, 1992.
12. Aleixo L et al: Effects of halothane anesthesia on immune function and outcome from a septic challenge in healthy mice (abstract). *Crit Care Med* 20:S77, 1992.
13. Nakagawara M et al: Inhibition of superoxide production and Ca^{2+} mobilization in human neutrophils by halothane, enflurane, and isoflurane. *Anesthesiology* 64:4–12, 1986.
14. Moore DS: *Statistics: Concepts and controversies.* San Francisco, 1979, Freeman, pp 295–299.
15. Nunn JF et al: Halothane does not inhibit human neutrophil function *in vitro*. *Br J Anaesth* 51:1101–1108, 1979.
16. Edwards AE et al: The effects of three differing anaesthetics on the immune response. *Anaesthesia* 39:1071–1078, 1984.
17. Welch WD: Effect of Enflurane, isoflurane, and nitrous oxide on the microbicidal activity of human polymorphonuclear leukocytes. *Anesthesiology* 61:188–192, 1984.
18. Perttila J, Salo M, Rajamäki A: Granulocyte microbicidal function in patients undergoing major abdominal surgery under balanced anaesthesia. *Acta Anaesthesiol Scand* 31:100–103, 1987.
19. van Dijk WC et al: Neutrophil function, serum opsonic activity, and delayed hypersensitivity in surgical patients. *Surgery* 92:21–29, 1982.
20. Pekoe GM, Peden D, Van Dyke K: Impairment of leukocyte myeloperoxidase bactericidal mechanisms with ketamine (Ketalar). *Agents Actions* 13:59–62, 1983.
21. Moore DS: *Statistics: Concepts and controversies.* San Francisco, 1979, Freeman, pp 146–150.
22. McClave JT, Dietrich FH II: *Statistics,* ed 2. Santa Clara, Calif, 1982, Dellen, pp 436–437.
23. Everson NW et al: The effect of surgical operation upon monocytes. *Br J Surg* 68:257–260, 1981.
24. Eskola J et al: Impaired B-lymphocyte function during open-heart surgery: Effects of anaesthesia and surgery. *Br J Anaesth* 56:333–338, 1984.
25. Salo M et al: Effect of halothane anaesthesia on primary antibody response in the chicken. *Acta Anaesth Scand* 23:344–348, 1979.
26. Robertson AJ et al: Effect of anaesthesia and surgery on the pre-S-phase cell cycle kinetics of mitogen-stimulated lymphocytes of previously healthy people. *Br J Anaesth* 55:339–347, 1983.
27. Khansari N, Whitten HD, Fudenberg HH: Phencyclidine-induced immunodepression. *Science* 225:76–78, 1984.
28. Slade MS et al: Immunodepression after major surgery in normal patients. *Surgery* 78:363–372, 1975.
29. Whelan P, Morris PJ: Immunological responsiveness after transurethral resec-

tion of the prostate: General versus spinal anaesthetic. *Clin Exp Immunol* 48:611–618, 1982.
30. Knight Pr et al: Alterations in influenza virus pulmonary pathology induced by diethyl ether, halothane, enflurane, and pentobarbital anesthesia in mice. *Anesthesiology* 58:209–215, 1983.
31. Pollock RE et al: Surgical stress-mediated suppression of murine natural killer cell cytotoxicity. *Cancer Res* 44:3888–3891, 1984.
32. Tonnesen E, Mickley H, Grunnet N: Natural killer cell activity during premedication, anaesthesia and surgery. *Acta Anaesthesiol Scand* 27:238–241, 1983.
33. Tonnesen E, Wahlgreen C: Influence of extradural and general anaesthesia on natural killer cell activity and lymphocyte subpopulations in patients undergoing hysterectomy. *Br J Anaesth* 60:500–507, 1988.
34. Duncan PG, Cullen BF, Ray-Keil L: Thiopental inhibition of tumor immunity. *Anesthesiology* 46:97–101, 1977.
35. McCredie JA: Antibody-dependent cellular cytotoxicity in critically ill surgical patients. *Surgery* 88:544–550, 1980.
36. Gardner P: Patch clamp studies of lymphocyte activation. *Annu Rev Immunol* 8:231–252, 1990.
37. DeCoursey TE et al: Voltage-gated K^+ channels in human T lymphocytes: A role in Mitogenesis? *Nature* 307:465–468, 1984.
38. Sidell N et al: Potassium channels in human NK cells are involved in discrete stages of the killing process. *J Immunol* 137:1650–1658, 1986.
39. Ueda I et al: Do anesthetics fluidize membranes? *Anesthesiology* 64:67–71, 1986.
40. Nelsen TE, Sweo T: Ca^{2+} uptake and Ca^{2+} release by skeletal muscle sarcoplasmic reticulum: Differing sensitivity to inhalational anesthetics. *Anesthesiology* 69:571–577, 1988.
41. Brett RS, Dilger JP, Yland KF: Isoflurane causes flickering of the acetylcholine receptor channel: Observations using the patch clamp. *Anesthesiology* 69:161–170, 1988.
42. Strichartz GR: Through the eye of the channel: Considerations of a reductionist view of general anesthesia (editorial). *Anesthesiology* 69:155–156, 1988.
43. Robinson-White AJ et al: Evidence that barbiturates inhibit antigen-induced responses through interactions with a GTP-binding protein in rat basophilic leukemia (RBL-2H3) cells. *Anesthesiology* 72:996–1004, 1990.
44. Maze M: Transmembrane signalling and the holy grail of anesthesia (editorial). *Anesthesiology* 72:959–961, 1990.
45. Böttger EC, Bitter-Suermann D: Complement and the regulation of humoral immune responses. *Immunol Today* 8:261–264, 1987.
46. Heyman B: The immune complex: Possible ways of regulating the antibody response. *Immunol Today* 11:310–313, 1990.
47. Ahearn JM, Fearon DT: Structure and function of the complement receptors, CR1 (CD35) and CR2 (CD21). *Adv Immunol* 46:183–219, 1989.
48. Cooper NR, Moore MD, Nemerow GR: Immunology of CR2, the B lymphocyte receptor for Epstein-Barr virus and the C3d complement fragment. *Annu Rev Immunol* 6:85–113, 1988.
49. Matsumoto AK et al: Intersection of the complement and immune systems: A signal transduction complex of the B lymphocyte-containing complement receptor type 2 and CD19. *J Exp Med* 173:55–64, 1991.
50. Lewis RE Jr, Cruse JM, Richey JV: Effects of anesthesia and operation on the classical pathway of complement activation. *Clin Immunol Immunopathol* 23:666–671, 1982.

51. Jubert AV et al: Effects of surgery, anesthesia and intraoperative blood loss on immunocompetence. *J Surg Res* 15:399–403, 1973.
52. Esrig BC et al: Predisposition to infection and neutrophil function following hemorrhagic shock. *Rev Surg* Nov–Dec:431–433, 1976.
53. Abraham E, Regan RF: The effects of hemorrhage and trauma on interleukin 2 production. *Arch Surg* 120:1341–1344, 1985.
54. Abraham E, Chang Y-H: Cellular and humoral bases of hemorrhage-induced depression of lymphocyte function. *Crit Care Med* 14:81–86, 1986.
55. Stephan RN et al: Hemorrhage without tissue trauma produces immunosuppression and enhances susceptibility to sepsis. *Arch Surg* 122:62–68, 1987.
56. Abraham E, Freitas AA: Hemorrhage produces abnormalities in lymphocyte function and lymphokine generation. *J Immunol* 142:899–906, 1989.
57. Schriemer PA, Longnecker DE, Mintz PD: The possible immunosuppressive effects of perioperative blood transfusion in cancer patients. *Anesthesiology* 68:422–428, 1988.
58. Waymack JP, Miskell P, Gonce S: Alterations in host defense associated with inhalation anesthesia and blood transfusion. *Anesth Analg* 69:163–168, 1989.
59. Waymack JP et al: Alterations in host defense associated with anesthesia and blood transfusions: Effect on response to endotoxin. *Arch Surg* 126:59–62, 1991.

Update on Anesthesia for Intracranial Aneurysm Surgery

Michael E. Mahla, M.D.

University of Florida College of Medicine, Department of Anesthesiology, Gainesville, Florida

Approximately 20% of individuals reading this page have or will develop an intracranial aneurysm during their lifetime. Fortunately, most of these people will never experience a subarachnoid hemorrhage (SAH) and will remain totally asymptomatic. An intracranial aneurysm is produced by a weakening in the wall of a blood vessel, usually at a bifurcation (Fig 1, A). Turbulent flow of blood at the bifurcation predisposes that area to formation of aneurysms. As the aneurysm enlarges, the compliance of the aneurysm wall decreases. Wall tension rises, and the risk of rupture increases (Fig 1, B). If the aneurysm does not rupture, it may continue to grow becoming a giant aneurysm (>2 cm diameter) (Fig 1, C).

Most aneurysms remain small and do not rupture. Nonetheless, SAH from intracranial aneurysm is a major health concern in the United States. Approximately 11 of 100,000 patients can be expected to experience an SAH during their lifetime. About 28,000 aneurysmal hemorrhages occur annually in the United States.[1] Despite improvements in surgical, anesthetic, and medical treatment of these patients, the overall mortality rate of

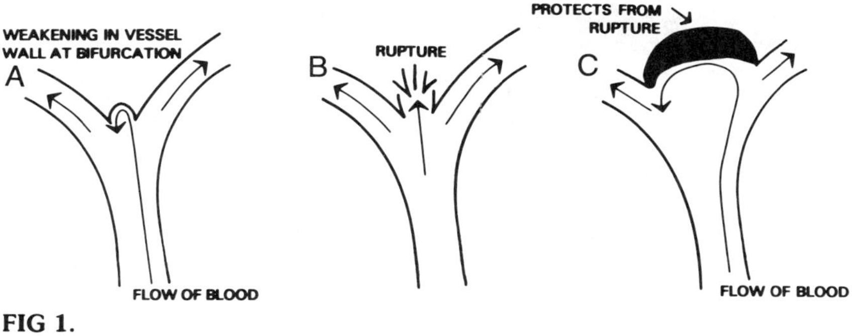

FIG 1.
Schematic representation of aneurysm development. **A,** asymptomatic small intracranial aneurysm; **B,** aneurysmal rupture; **C,** formation of giant aneurysm with wall reinforced by clot that may be calcified.

aneurysmal SAH remains at about 50%. The most common causes of mortality include rebleeding and vasospasm (delayed ischemic encephalopathy). Of those who survive the initial hemorrhage, 20% of patients with SAH whose aneurysms are not surgically clipped will experience rebleeding in the first 2 weeks, and half of the patients who experience rebleeding will die.[1] Roughly 40% of patients with SAH, clipped or unclipped, will develop vasospasm. Approximately half of these patients will have symptoms ranging from focal neurologic deficit to massive stroke and death.[2]

SAH from an aneurysm is a medical condition that requires urgent surgical repair to prevent rebleeding. There is no reliably effective medical management. Timing of aneurysm surgery after SAH is controversial. Because SAH may produce cerebral swelling, aneurysm exposure immediately after SAH may be technically more difficult and associated with increased brain retraction to expose the aneurysm. This retraction will subject the neural tissue to increased retractor pressures at a time when the brain may already be ischemic. On the other hand, early surgery prevents further morbidity and mortality from aneurysm rebleeding. Finally, early clipping of the aneurysm increases the safety of hypervolemic, hypertensive therapy, a promising approach to the treatment and prevention of vasospasm. During the mid-1980s, a multicenter prospective International Cooperative Study on the Timing of Aneurysm Surgery[3–5] was undertaken. This study demonstrated that many patients for whom surgery was delayed had major complications or died prior to surgery. However, patients who survived until surgery had better postoperative results if surgery was delayed until the second week after SAH. The overall morbidity and mortality was nearly identical for both the early and delayed surgery groups. I will discuss the perioperative treatment of the patient with aneurysmal SAH, emphasizing how the pathophysiology of each individual aneurysm guides anesthetic management.

Preoperative Evaluation: Neurologic System

The major factors determining anesthetic management during aneurysm clipping are aneurysm location, size, whether it has ruptured, presence of vasospasm, preoperative neurologic grade, non-central nervous system (CNS) systemic manifestations of SAH, and preexisting medical illnesses (Table 1). The location of the aneurysm will determine the positioning of the patient. In general, anterior circulation aneurysms may be approached with the patient supine and the head slightly turned. A roll under the shoulder will prevent stretch of the brachial plexus (Fig 2). Basilar aneurysms may be approached either with the patient in the full lateral position or supine with the head turned to a greater extent. Posterior fossa aneurysms are usually approached in the three-quarter prone or prone positions.

TABLE 1.
Schematic for Preoperative Evaluation

Location
Size
Ruptured?
Vasospasm?
Systemic manifestations of subarachnoid hemorrhage
Preexisting medical illness

Aneurysms are surrounded by brain tissue and can be exposed by spreading anatomic fissures or by retraction on a lobe of the brain (Fig 3). Anterior circulation aneurysms are usually approached via the Sylvian fissure with retraction on the frontal and temporal lobes. Basilar apex aneurysms are usually approached by retracting the temporal lobe superiorly. Therapy directed at decreasing brain bulk is useful in decreasing the amount of retractor pressure necessary to expose the aneurysm (Table 2). Retractor pressure reduces perfusion to the underlying brain tissue and may produce neurologic damage particularly if blood flow is already reduced by vasospasm or induced hypotension.

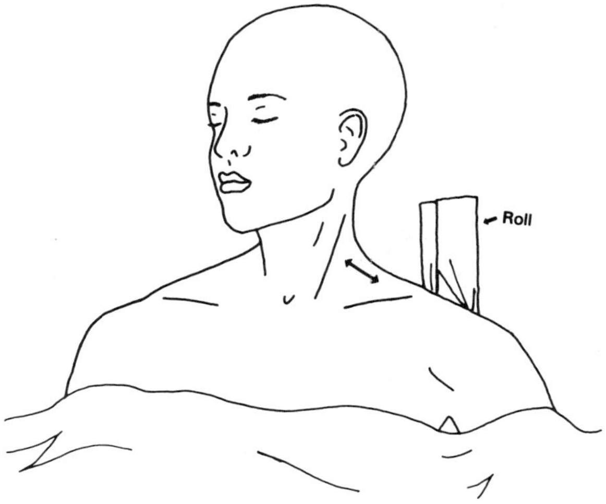

FIG 2.
A roll under the shoulder *(arrow)* prevents stretch of the brachial plexus *(double arrow)*, which could be produced by excessive lateral rotation and extension of the neck.

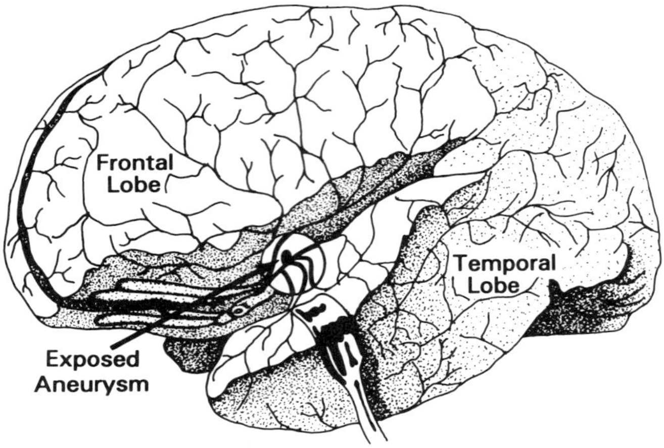

FIG 3.
Aneurysms are generally accessible only by retracting brain tissue. In this case, the Sylvian fissure is split and retracted, revealing a middle cerebral artery aneurysm.

The location of the aneurysm also affects planning for intraoperative catastrophic rupture. Hemorrhage from aneurysms located at birfurcations of terminal arteries (such as the middle cerebral artery) may be readily controlled with a temporary clip on the parent vessel (Fig 4). Aneurysms located on vessels with multiple inflow and outflow vessels are more problematic. For example, an aneurysm on the anterior communicating artery may require temporary clips on both anterior cerebral arteries to control intraoperative hemorrhage. While intravenous (IV) access is needed in all cases, greater access is needed in cases in which hemorrhage cannot be easily controlled.

TABLE 2.
Methods to Minimize Retractor Pressure Needed for Exposure

Hyperventilation
Mannitol
Cerebrospinal fluid drainage
Lumbar drain
Ventriculostomy
Pharmacologic (e.g., barbiturates, etomidate)
Lower cerebral metabolic rate
Lower cerebral blood volume

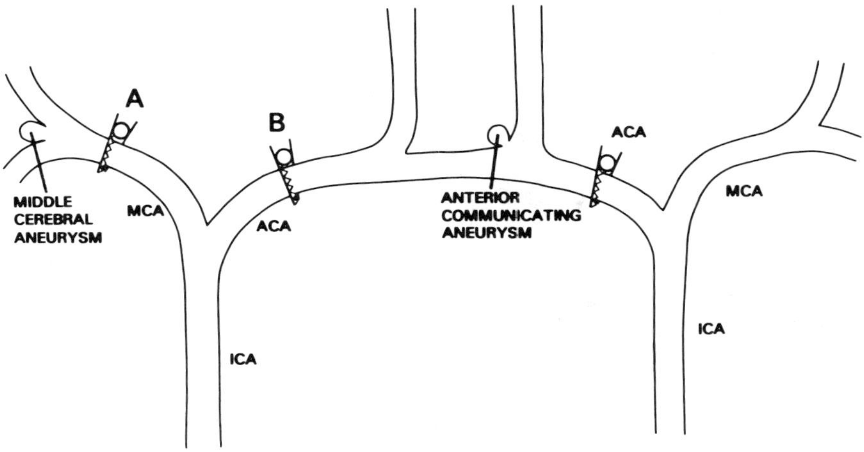

FIG 4.
Planning for rupture. *A* indicates a temporary clip on the middle cerebral artery *(MCA)* that stops most bleeding from a ruptured MCA aneurysm. *B* indicates a ruptured anterior communicating artery aneurysm that may require clips on both anterior cerebral arteries *(ACA)* to control intraoperative hemorrhage. *ICA* = internal carotid artery.

The size of the aneurysm may create special problems. Aneurysms greater than 2 cm are called giant aneurysms. As aneurysms enlarge, it becomes more likely that major outflow vessels and perforating vessels will be involved in the dome of the aneurysm (Fig 5, A). Blood may become relatively stagnant inside larger aneurysms (see Fig 1, C), resulting in clot formation. This clot subsequently organizes and may become calcified, thus reinforcing the aneurysm wall. Patients with giant aneurysms may present with rupture, but often they present with mass effect (such as a focal neurologic deficit or elevated intracranial pressure), convulsions, or stroke from particulate emboli arising from the intraluminal clot. Repair of these large aneurysms will sometimes involve temporary occlusion of the vessels supplying the aneurysm (Fig 5, B). In these cases, cerebral metabolic rate may be decreased by the administration of barbiturates and decreasing the patient's temperature, thereby increasing the time arterial occlusion can be tolerated without neurologic damage. Review of the angiogram and preoperative discussion with the surgeon can help anticipate the need for hypothermia or for pharmacologic reduction of the cerebral metabolic requirement for oxygen ($CMRO_2$). Poor intracranial compliance or frankly elevated intracranial pressure (ICP), caused by the aneurysmal mass, may require the use of the head-elevated position and hyperventilation during surgery to facilitate exposure of the aneurysm.

Aneurysms that have ruptured are at high risk for rebleeding. Risk of rebleeding may be minimized by carefully controlling blood pressure. Preoperative insertion of invasive arterial monitoring facilitates this control, but

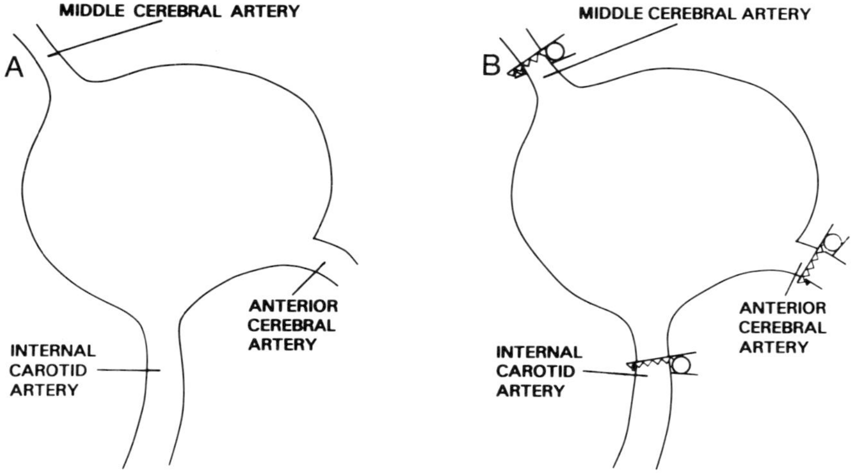

FIG 5.
Giant aneurysms. **A,** as aneurysms enlarge, they may involve other vessels in addition to the parent vessel. Shown here, an internal carotid artery bifurcation aneurysm enlarges to involve both the middle and anterior cerebral arteries. **B,** operative repair (if possible) may involve temporary occlusion of major cerebral vessels.

insertion of this line must be as painless as possible since noxious stimuli may cause hypertension. Patients with preoperative hypertension who need sodium nitroprusside for control of blood pressure require invasive monitoring. Patients who are normotensive and stable may have the arterial catheter placed after induction but preferably before laryngoscopy. Aneurysmal wall tension is directly related to the radius of the aneurysm, which in turn is related to the pressure inside the aneurysmal lumen (Fig 6). It is important to remember that sudden increases or decreases in blood pressure, unless the aneurysm is partially thrombosed, are fully transmitted to the aneurysm wall, alter wall tension, and may result in rupture. A study conducted in humans undergoing aneurysm clipping showed that the pressure inside the aneurysm lumen and the artery supplying it are equal unless the aneurysm is thrombosed.[6]

Aneurysmal rupture causes a rapid increase in ICP. Classically, ICP rises immediately after SAH. This increase in ICP helps to tamponade the aneurysm and bleeding stops. ICP usually returns to normal over a period of hours. However, blood in the cerebrospinal fluid (CSF) interferes with CSF reabsorption and may cause hydrocephalus. In addition, hemorrhage into the parenchyma of the brain may produce an intracerebral hematoma. In either of these cases, ICP may be elevated when the patient arrives in the operating room. In patients with altered mental status and hydrocephalus, a ventriculostomy may be inserted preoperatively. CSF pressure is then gradually reduced over several hours to improve cerebral perfusion but is generally not reduced below 20 mm Hg. Sometimes dramatic improve-

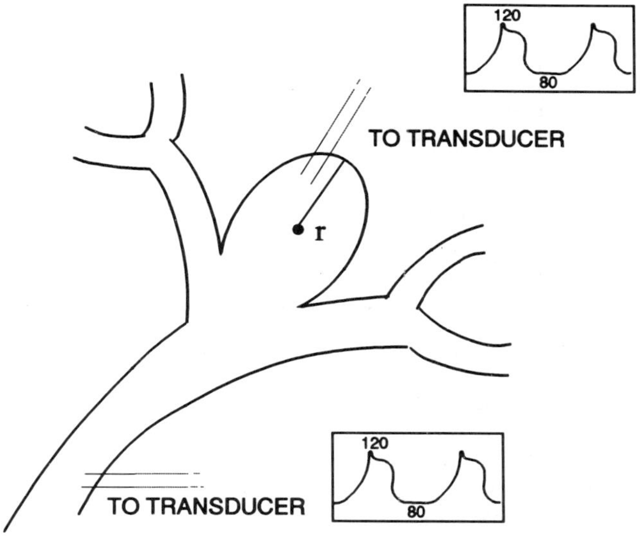

FIG 6.
Changes in systemic pressure are transmitted directly to a cerebral aneurysm. Increases in pressure will increase the radius and wall tension of the aneurysm. Decreases in pressure will likewise decrease radius and wall tension.

ments in neurologic status may be seen after this intervention. While decreasing ICP will improve cerebral perfusion and cerebral blood flow, aneurysmal transmural wall pressure will increase and make rebleeding more likely. When ICP is elevated and hyperventilation or spinal fluid drainage is needed to facilitate exposure of the aneurysm, they should be instituted gradually just before or at opening of the dura mater. Rapid institution of hyperventilation or spinal fluid drainage may decrease ICP too quickly and produce rebleeding. In patients with giant aneurysms, large intracerebral hematomas, or massive hydrocephalus, hyperventilation may be necessary at the beginning of the operation to control intracranial hypertension.

Aneurysmal rupture can cause loss of autoregulation, which may be diffuse or restricted mainly to the vascular bed involved with the SAH. Reductions in blood pressure, which normally do not cause a decrease in cerebral blood flow (CBF), may cause marked decreases in CBF (Fig 7). Reduction in brain bulk to avoid excess retractor pressure and maintenance of adequate cerebral perfusion are particularly important in patients with loss of autoregulation. When hypotension is necessary in these patients, the adequacy of cerebral perfusion may be monitored with electroencephalography (EEG) or somatosensory-evoked potentials (SEPs), if available.[7, 8]

Vasospasm is a potentially devastating complication occurring the first 72 hours following SAH. Manifestations of vasospasm are highly variable, ranging from asymptomatic vasospasm seen only with angiography to se-

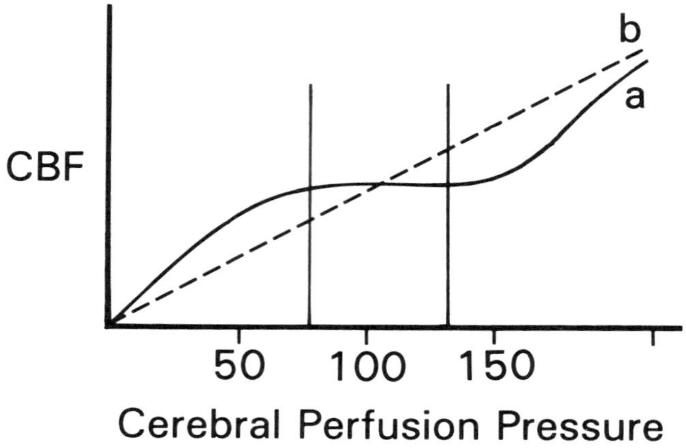

FIG 7.
Schematic of cerebral autoregulation. *a*, With normal autoregulation, no significant blood flow changes with blood pressure changes would be expected during anesthesia and surgery. *b*, When autoregulation is lost, large changes in blood flow can occur with similar changes in blood pressure.

vere cerebral ischemia with focal or global neurologic deficit and massive stroke. A recent review suggests that vasospasm may cause more morbidity and mortality following SAH than rebleeding.[9] Vasospasm is thought to be caused by the breakdown of blood in cerebrospinal fluid. Risk of vasospasm increases with an increased amount of blood in the CSF.[10] Vasospasm is initially diagnosed clinically by a typical gradual deterioration in the level of consciousness and the development of focal neurologic findings. Headache is common, and blood pressure frequently increases. These clinical findings could also be caused by other treatable lesions such as rebleeding, hematoma, hydrocephalus, or metabolic abnormalties (commonly hyponatremia). Once these other lesions are ruled out, the diagnosis of vasospasm can be confirmed with angiography. Recently, studies have demonstrated that noninvasive transcranial doppler (TCD) measurements of blood flow velocities in the basal arteries of the brain can depict and document the severity of vasospasm.[11–14] The TCD uses sound waves to measure the velocity of blood flowing in the basal arteries of the brain. Sound waves are transmitted through the relatively thin temporal bone (Fig 8). When these sound waves come in contact with blood, they are reflected off the red blood cells back through the brain and skull to a detector. The velocity of the sound waves reflected back to the surface will be changed since the blood cells themselves are in motion either toward or away from the sound wave detector. This phenomenon is known as the Doppler shift and is directly related to the velocity and flow direction of the blood cells. The velocity of the blood cells will be faster during systole and slower during diastole. The blood in the center of the lumen will move faster than the blood near the vessel wall. Thus, a spectrum of flow veloc-

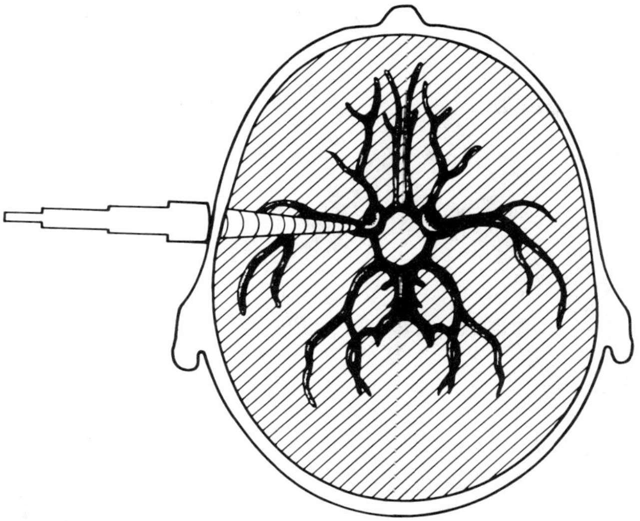

FIG 8.
Schematic of transcranial Doppler. Sound waves penetrate the relatively thin temporal bone and are reflected by red blood cells in the basal arteries of the brain back to a detector.

ities is produced. This spectrum resembles the shape of the waveform produced by the pulse oximeter or an arterial pressure transducer (Fig 9). As the diameter of the arterial lumen decreases with vasospasm, the velocity of blood flowing through the narrowed vessel must increase if flow is to be maintained (Fig 10). If studies involving greater numbers of patients confirm reasonable sensitivity and specificity for TCD diagnosis of vasospasm, TCD may greatly facilitate the detection of vasospasm in patients who are still asymptomatic.

Detection of vasospasm is very important since patients with vasospasm are at particular risk during hypotension. Vessels involved or distal to vasospasm are no longer able to dilate or constrict according to metabolic needs or inflow pressure, and reductions in cerebral blood flow may occur with decreases in blood pressure even within the normal range (see Fig 7). Decreases in blood pressure that would normally not be treated may produce critical decreases in cerebral blood flow. In the awake patient, such a reduction in blood flow would be detected because of the onset of a focal or global neurologic deficit. While the patient is anesthetized, the neurologic examination is unavailable, and electrophysiologic brain monitoring may be used to determine lower limits of blood pressure tolerated by the brain supplied by the vasospastic vessels.[7, 8] With monitoring, the clinician may properly balance the need for decreased blood pressure to prevent aneurysm rupture and facilitate clipping against the need for higher blood pressure to assure adequate perfusion of brain supplied by vasospastic vessels.

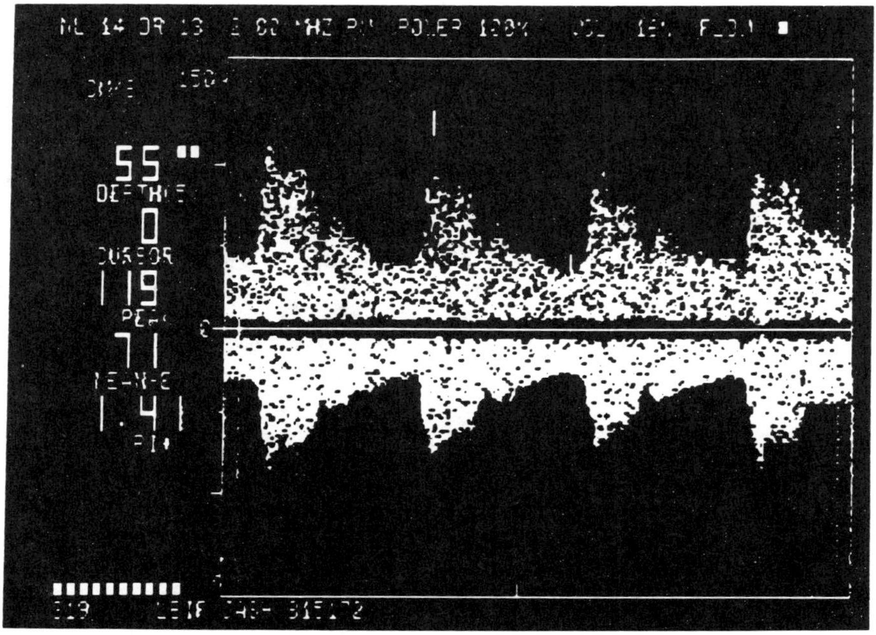

FIG 9.
Normal transcranial Doppler tracing – transtemporal scan. This tracing shows a blood flow velocity spectrum at the carotid bifurcation. Blood is flowing both toward the probe (middle cerebral artery) and away from the probe (anterior cerebral artery).

There is no reliably effective treatment for vasospasm. It has been postulated that increasing cardiac output and mean arterial pressure can overcome the vessel narrowing produced by vasospasm and restore normal blood flow. A prospective study examining the effects of prophylactic hypervolemic, hypertensive therapy (HHT) (Table 3) demonstrated a marked reduction in morbidity and mortality in patients with post-SAH vasospasm.[15] In this study, 87% of 56 patients had normal neurologic examinations or had only minor deficits following SAH. Treatment of established vasospasm with HHT was also shown to be effective in a series of 188 consecutive patients with SAH.[16] Forty-two of these patients developed vasospasm. All were treated with HHT. Overall, the rate of death and major neurologic deficit in this series was an impressively low 7%.

Further studies involving larger numbers of patients are needed before this therapy becomes standard care. Early results, however, are promising, and this treatment regimen has already found widespread clinical use. When this treatment is used preoperatively, the patient must be examined carefully for evidence of pulmonary edema. Increased concentration of oxygen and continuous positive airway pressure may be necessary intraoperatively in these patients to attain adequate oxygenation. HHT produces a

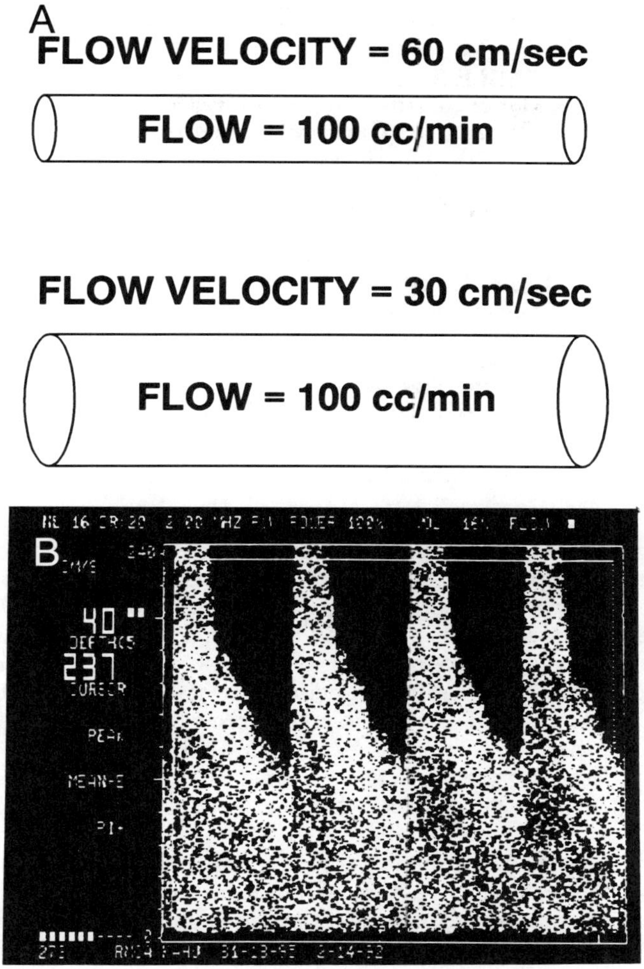

FIG 10.
A, schematic of blood flow velocity changes during vasospasm. When narrowing occurs as in vasospasm, if constant flow is to be maintained, flow velocity must increase. **B,** transcranial Doppler tracing in a patient with severe vasospasm. Peak flow velocities exceed the maximum scale of the measurement device.

hyperdynamic circulation and may increase the risk of rupture if initiated prior to the clipping of the aneurysm. Thus, early aneurysm clipping allows this treatment of vasospasm to be undertaken with less risk. Treatment of vasospasm by increasing blood pressure and cardiac output with vasopressors and IV fluids may be undertaken without fear of either rupturing the aneurysm or causing cerebral swelling, which would impede surgical aneurysm exposure.

TABLE 3.
Hypervolemic Hypertensive Therapy for Cerebral Vasospasm

Systolic arterial pressure >10 mm Hg higher than premorbid state
Cerebral venous pressure, 10–12 cm H_2O
Pulmonary capillary wedge pressure, 12–16 cm H_2O
Hematocrit, 30%–33%
Cardiac index >3.0
Use vasopressors if increased filling pressures are not enough to accomplish this.

Calcium channel blockers used for prophylaxis against and treatment of established vasospasm appear promising and can be used safely whether or not the aneurysm is clipped.[17, 18] Nimodipine has been shown in several trials to reduce the incidence and severity of post-SAH vasospasm. The mechanism for improvement in outcome is unclear. Reduced vessel caliber seen with vasospasm on angiography is not improved by nimodipine. Calcium channel blockers may help prevent influxes of calcium at a cellular level that occur during ischemia, thus helping maintain cellular integrity and lessening the impact of ischemia. In addition, calcium channel blockers may improve collateral circulation to areas affected by vasospasm.[19]

One common effect of many calcium channel antagonists is the reduction of peripheral vascular resistance. If calcium channel blockers are used preoperatively, greater amounts of intravenous fluids or vasopressors may be needed to maintain an adequate blood pressure while the patient is anesthetized.

Since the risk of cerebral vasospasm increases with the amount of blood in the subarachnoid space, removal of the clot could theoretically lessen vasospasm. Early trials with surgical irrigation to remove blood had promising results,[20] but clot removal takes time, may be difficult, and may itself produce brain damage. Recently, a phase 1 trial with recombinant tissue plasminogen activator instilled via ventriculostomy to facilitate clot removal was completed.[21] Ten patients with grade 3 or 4 SAH were enrolled in the study. Sixty percent of these patients showed good outcome 3 months after SAH. These results, though promising, must be duplicated with larger numbers of patients.

Patients who fail medical treatment of vasospasm may respond to cerebral angioplasty. A small number of patients have been reported to have good results following forced balloon dilation of vasospastic vessels.[22] There is a risk of arterial rupture or dissection following this procedure; therefore, this treatment is used only on patients with severely narrowed vessels not responsive to medical management.

Finally, it is important to gauge the severity of neurologic dysfunction (neurologic grade) that is present preoperatively to plan for postoperative respiratory care. Patients with higher grade SAH or symptomatic vasospasm may have large areas of brain either irreversibly damaged or ischemic but still viable. These patients should retain their endotrachial tube at the conclusion of surgery. Even transient hypoxemia or hypercarbia may produce irreversible damage to ischemic but still viable brain. Continued intubation will allow careful control of arterial oxygen and carbon dioxide levels during this critical period and will facilitate hypervolemic therapy of vasospasm with its attendant risk of pulmonary edema.

Preoperative Evaluation: Non-CNS Manifestations of SAH

SAH may produce marked abnormalities in organ systems that have no intrinsic disease or exacerbate problems in already diseased systems. The most overt SAH-induced problems occur in the cardiovascular and pulmonary systems. New onset hypertension or exacerbation of previously existing hypertension is common and frequently requires intravenous antihypertensive agents such as nitroprusside, nitroglycerin, esmolol, or labetalol for control. Cardiac ischemia may also be produced. There are many descriptions of electrocardiogram (ECG) changes with SAH.

Early articles suggested that ECG changes did not correlate with significant myocardial damage or dysfunction.[23–25] More recently, evidence has suggested that patients with ECG changes consistent with myocardial damage may have subendocardial ischemia and areas of focal necrosis, and may be at increased risk for serious dysrhythmias.[26] A recent study suggests that serious myocardial dysfunction following SAH may occur and should be considered in patients with SAH who also show significant ECG abnormalities.[27] This study of 13 patients with SAH documented marked myocardial dysfunction including myocardial infarction with severe wall motion abnormalities in four patients. None of the patients with evidence of myocardial infarction (MI) who subsequently died showed any evidence of coronary artery disease on postmortem examination. The exact mechanism producing cardiac damage is not clear. It is also unclear how often cardiac dysfunction occurs after SAH or what implications such myocardial dysfunction has in management. Because some patients with ECG changes apparently do have significant myocardial dysfunction, a work-up of ECG abnormalities suggestive of ischemia or MI should be performed if time and clinical circumstance permits. Usually, both ECG changes and functional changes such as wall motion abnormalities will resolve within a few days following SAH.

Pulmonary edema has also been reported after SAH. Pulmonary edema may be cardiogenic or noncardiogenic, and treatment with increased inspired oxygen, positive pressure ventilation, and continuous positive airway pressure may be required in the perioperative period.

Preexisting cardiac disease may present problems in patients sustaining SAH. As already discussed, SAH has the potential to cause ischemic myocardial damage in patients without coronary disease. The impact of this damage may be greater on patients with preexisting coronary artery disease (CAD). Reductions in diastolic blood pressure and increases in heart rate accompanying induced hypotension needed for aneurysm clipping may not be tolerated by the patient with CAD. Thus, when induced hypotension is used, careful monitoring of ST segments should be performed in every case. Patients with significant symptomatic coronary artery disease may benefit from pulmonary artery pressure monitoring or two-dimensional echocardiography to improve detection of myocardial ischemia.

Patients with preexisting pulmonary disease may experience marked decreases in $Pa{O_2}$ if induced hypotension is required. In patients with areas of atelectasis, inhibition of hypoxic pulmonary vasoconstriction by vasodilators[28] will lead to worsening of shunt and decreases in $Pa{O_2}$. Continuous pulse oximetry will aid the clinician in detecting this problem.

Patients with preexisting renal disease also may suffer worsening of renal function if induced hypotension is utilized. Careful monitoring of urine output may help in detection of worsening renal function, but administration of mannitol may obscure decreases in urine output that would otherwise occur.

Preparation for Surgery

Patients undergoing cerebral aneurysm clipping are often heavily premedicated to prevent anxiety and pain-induced fluctuations in blood pressure. The preoperative neurologic condition of the patient may, however, make the unmonitored use of premedicants dangerous. Patients with elevated ICP from hydrocephalus or intracranial hematoma may have further increases in ICP if premedication causes hypoventilation. Patients with global depression of mental status caused by the SAH itself or by subsequent vasospasm should be given premedications only with close monitoring since they may be inordinately sensitive to the premedication. Heavy premedication resulting in somnolence may simulate neurologic changes that could occur with rebleeding or worsening vasospasm. Both rebleeding and vasospasm may preclude surgery, and it is therefore important to be able to distinguish between premedication effects and rebleeding.

Patients with subarachnoid hemorrhage are at high risk for seizures. They are usually given diphenylhydantoin (Dilantin) or phenobarbital on admission to the hospital. Anticonvulsant levels should be checked if possible, and the anticonvulsant agent should be continued throughout surgery into the postoperative period.

Invasive arterial blood pressure monitoring should be started if possible before induction for any patient with SAH and hypertension. Many of these patients require intravenous antihypertensive agents and will already have such monitoring. Normotensive otherwise healthy patients may have the arterial line started after induction. Preoperative arterial blood gas measurement with baseline $Paco_2$ measurement is particularly useful in avoiding hyperventilation and undesired decreases in ICP. Some patients with SAH who are thought to be at high risk for vasospasm may already have a pulmonary artery catheter in place to help monitor HHT prior to surgery. These patients are sometimes markedly hypervolemic and will show arterial hypoxemia if allowed to breathe room air. Oxygen saturation should be monitored closely.

Induction and Maintenance of Anesthesia

There are multiple anesthetic regimens that could be used in the patient with intracranial aneurysm. The common goals of any of these techniques are listed in Table 4. After induction of anesthesia, IV access should be attained. A central line is useful for the administration of vasoactive drugs and for measurement of central pressures. Patients with preoperative symptomatic vasospasm may benefit from pulmonary artery pressure monitoring with continuous mixed venous saturation measurements. This monitor will help the clinician maintain adequate filling pressures and cardiac output. The mixed venous oxygen saturation will provide early warning of decreasing cardiac output.

TABLE 4.
Anesthetic Goals During Aneurysm Surgery

Prevention of rapid increases or decreases in blood pressure
Prevention of rapid increases or decreases in intracranial pressure
Reduction of brain oxygen consumption
Maintenance of adequate cerebral blood flow
Just before removal of bone flap, reduction in brain bulk to minimize retraction
Minimal suppression of evoked potentials or electroencephalogram if employed
Rapid return of normal neurologic function at the conclusion of surgery

Particular care should be taken with positioning as these operations are frequently very long. Padding of pressure points is even more important if induced hypotension is planned since perfusion of compressed skin can be further reduced by hypotension.

Patients with SAH rarely have increased ICP. Normocapnia based on preoperative blood gas measurements (if available) should be maintained throughout surgery. Hyperventilation may lower ICP and increase transmural aneurysmal pressure. Hyperventilation may, however, be necessary to reduce brain bulk and retractor pressure if other methods such as spinal fluid drainage or mannitol diuresis are inadequate. Mannitol should be withheld until just before the removal of the bone flap. This regimen will produce the maximum decrease in brain bulk at a time when the aneurysm is being exposed. Spinal fluid drainage via a ventriculostomy or by a spinal drain may be used during some aneurysm clippings. If this technique is used, no more than 25 mL of fluid should be drained at one time, and this fluid should be allowed to drain slowly over 10 to 20 minutes by gravity (never aspirated). Rapid drainage of CSF may produce both hypertension and a decrease in ICP and therefore increase the risk for rupture of the aneurysm.

The patient should be kept normovolemic during surgery to maintain adequate blood pressure and cardiac output. This therapy will help minimize the effects of preexisting vasospasm. After the aneurysm is clipped, particularly if the patient is at risk for vasospasm, the patient should be kept moderately hypervolemic. The type of IV fluid that is used for this therapy is somewhat controversial. Most clinicians would use a mixture of crystalloid, colloid, and blood to produce the hypervolemia.[15, 16]

Evoked Potential Monitoring During Aneurysm Surgery

Cortical SEPs may be used to monitor cerebral function during aneurysm clippings.[7, 8, 28–33] These evoked potentials are the summation of excitatory and inhibitory postsynaptic potentials produced in response to stimuli applied to either the median or posterior tibial nerve. The electrical stimulus produces an action potential in the nerve that is conducted centrally. The response passes through the dorsal root ganglion and is conducted rostrally in the posterior columns. The posterior columns terminate in nucleus gracilis (information from the leg and trunk) or nucleus cuneatus (information from the arm) in the medulla. There, the response is conducted across a synapse and crosses to the opposite side. The response ascends in the medial lemniscus, which then terminates in the ventral posterolateral nucleus of the thalamus. The response is then conducted rostrally to the somatosensory cortex via the thalamocortical radiations, which pass through the anterior limb of the internal capsule.[34] Sites where the evoked potential may be recorded and a typical somatosensory-evoked potential are shown in Figure 11.

SEPs are useful during aneursym surgery if the vessel involved with the

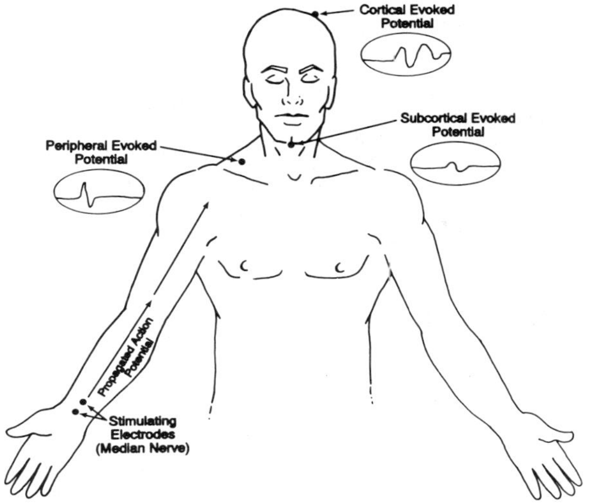

FIG 11.
Schematic of a medial nerve SEP recording. Evoked potentials may be recorded over the peripheral nerve, near the brain stem, and at cortical levels. Similar recording sites are used for posterior tibial nerve SEPs except the peripheral recordings are made over the tibial nerve at the knee.

aneurysm supplies blood to either the cortex generating the SEP or to the subcortical SEP pathway. Figure 12 shows the areas of the cortex responsible for generating cortical somatosensory-evoked responses. Figure 13 shows the cerebral cortex divided into regions according to its blood supply. As one can see from these two figures, the somatosensory cortex producing the response generated by median nerve stimulation is supplied by the middle cerebral artery. The somatosensory cortex producing the response generated by posterior tibial nerve stimulation is supplied by the anterior cerebal artery. The thalamocortical radiations are supplied by the

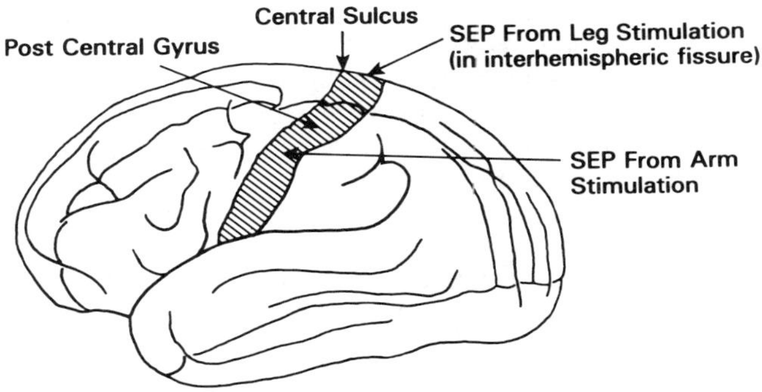

FIG 12.
Schematic of cortical generating sites for SEPs.

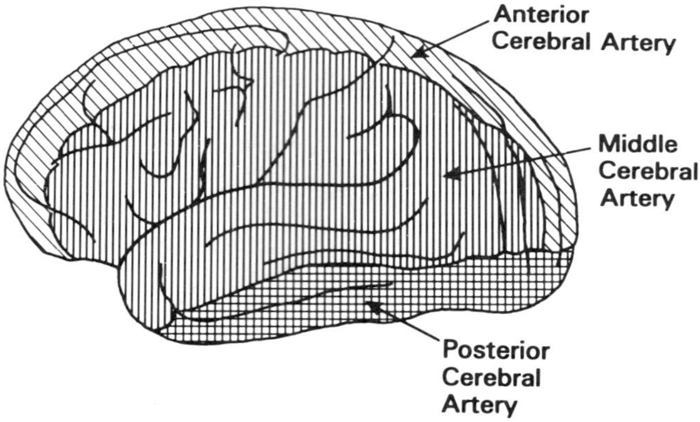

FIG 13.
Schematic of the distribution of the blood supply to the cerebral cortex.

lenticulostriate arteries arising from the proximal middle cerebral artery. The relationship between cerebral blood flow and the cortical SEP has been studied in animals.[35–37] In a primate study,[38] the amplitude of the cortical SEP was found to be well maintained until cortical blood flow decreased to below 16 mL/100 g/min. There was a steep decline in amplitude until flow reached 12 mL/100 g/min, at which point the SEP was lost.

Clinical studies, involving large numbers of patients, used EEG during carotid endarterectomy[39, 40] and established a similar relationship between the EEG and cerebral blood flow in humans. The threshold at which EEG changes were consistent with ischemia was anesthetic-dependent and occurred at 20 mL/100 g/min with halothane, 15 mL/100 g/min with enflurane, and 10 mL/100 g/min with isoflurane. Unfortunately, a study with EEG, SEPs, and cerebral blood flow measurements to establish a similar relationship for SEPs in humans does not exist. However, clinical experience during cerebral aneurysm clippings[7, 8, 28–33] and limited experience during carotid endarterectomy[41–45] suggest that a threshold relationship does exist and that cortical SEPs become abnormal at a slightly lower cortical blood flow than the level at which EEG changes occur.[46] SEPs are most useful and correlate best with outcome during anterior circulation aneurysm clippings. If blood flow to the cerebral cortex supplied by either the anterior or middle cerebral arteries is reduced, the SEP will be attenuated or lost. Since most aneurysms are relatively proximally located, all sections of cortex supplied by the artery will be equally affected, and loss of SEP will correlate with loss of motor function as well. Figures 14 and 15 demonstrate two examples of changes in SEP during aneurysm clippings at my institution. Figure 14 shows SEP changes that occurred when the retractors were removed following an uneventful middle cerebral aneurysm clipping. Removal of retraction apparently allowed the brain to displace the aneurysm clip and caused kinking of the middle cerebral artery. Replacement of retraction and clip adjustment resulted in restoration of the SEP. Figure 15

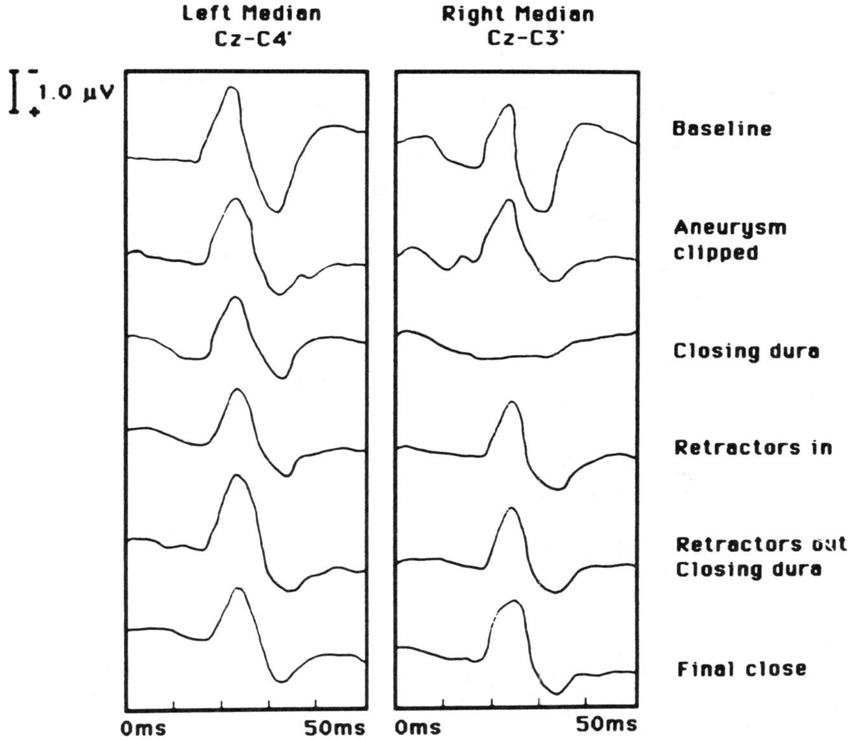

FIG 14.
SEP changes during aneurysm surgery. Removal of retraction on the frontal and temporal lobes allowed brain tissue to move and cause kinking of the left middle cerebral artery during dural closure. Note, there were no changes in simultaneously monitored right cortical SEPs, thus ruling out anesthetic changes as a cause of SEP loss. Readjustment of the clip solved the problem, and the patient awakened without neurologic compromise.

shows an example of a clip on a middle cerebral artery aneurysm that inadvertently included a lenticulostriate perforating artery, which supplies blood to part of the subcortical somatosensory pathway. Adjustment of the clip again resulted in restoration of SEP and good outcome.

Correlation with outcome is not as good during posterior circulation aneurysm clippings. The posterior circulation does provide blood via perforating vessels to the somatosensory pathway as it ascends through the brain stem to the thalamus. However, this same circulation also supplies blood via perforating vessels to large portions of the brain stem not involved with the somatosensory pathway. Thus damage may occur to motor pathways and to the reticular formation, resulting in motor deficits or global depression of consciousness without any change in SEP.[47]

Anesthetic technique may profoundly influence the usefulness of cortical

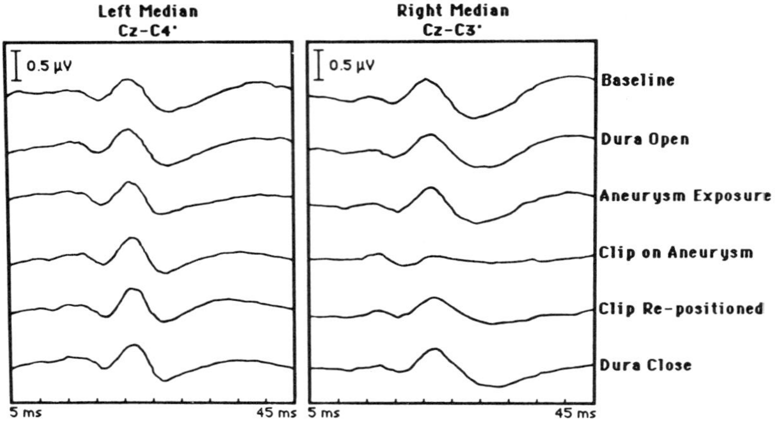

FIG 15.
SEP changes during aneurysm surgery. Placement of a clip on a proximal left middle cerebral artery inadvertently included a small perforating artery supplying blood to the internal capsule. Note again, there were no changes in simultaneously monitored right cortical SEPs, thus ruling out an anesthetic cause of the SEP change. Clip readjustment resulted in restoration of SEP, and the patient awakened without neurologic compromise.

SEP monitoring. High doses of potent inhaled agents may profoundly depress the cortical SEP, rendering it useless for monitoring cortical function. Generally, intravenous agents have much less effect on cortical-evoked potentials. For example, if two minimum alveolar concentration (MAC) or greater concentrations of isoflurane are used to suppress the EEG and produce cerebral protection, the cortical SEP will also be profoundly depressed. If thiopental is used, however, for the same purpose, the cortical SEP is preserved much better and remains useful for monitoring.[48]

In summary, anterior circulation aneurysm clippings may benefit from somatosensory-evoked potential monitoring if available. Evoked potentials are particularly useful for determining adequacy of cerebral blood flow during vasospasm, during induced hypotension or hyperventilation, after placement of aneurysm clip, and during temporary occlusion of major cerebral vessels. Evoked potentials may also be useful for monitoring the brain during clipping of posterior circulation aneurysms. Correlation with outcome is not as good, however, as when evoked potentials are used to monitor anterior circulation aneurysm clippings.

Induced Hypotension

The lumina of most intracranial aneurysms are in direct contact with the arterial lumina. The pressure inside the aneurysm is therefore about the same as arterial pressure.[6] The radius of the aneurysm changes in direct proportion to arterial pressure, and aneurysmal wall tension changes proportionately to the fourth power of the aneurysmal radius (Laplace's law). Deliberate hypotension can therefore greatly decrease wall tension and the risk of intraoperative rupture. Induced hypotension may also be used to decrease the bulk of the aneurysm, thereby facilitating placement of a clip on the neck of the aneurysm that otherwise would be obscured by the dome of the aneurysm. Induced hypotension is not without risk. Cerebral blood flow may be reduced below critical levels, producing ischemia. This problem is most likely when the patient has preexisting vasospasm and/or long-standing arterial hypertension. Hypotension should be used only with caution in these patients, and EEG or cortical SEPs may be very helpful in determining limits of hypotension when it is needed. Certain hypotensive agents preserve cerebral blood flow better than others in the face of hypotension. At this time, sodium nitroprusside (SNP) and/or isoflurane appear to be the agents of choice for hypotension. Nitroprusside is very easy to titrate and preserves adequate cerebral blood flow even in the face of severe hypotension (mean arterial pressure, 40 mm Hg).[49] This ability to preserve blood flow even at very low mean arterial pressures makes nitroprusside very useful if intraoperative rupture of the aneurysm occurs. Reductions in mean arterial pressure to 30 to 40 mm Hg will greatly reduce bleeding and allow the surgeon to see the aneurysm or parent vessel to place a clip and stop the hemorrhage. Rapid adjustments of blood pressure are more difficult with isoflurane. Isoflurane has a potential advantage over nitroprusside because it maintains cerebral blood flow and reduces brain oxygen consumption. Isoflurane in high concentrations necessary for hypotension, however, suppresses both the EEG and cortical-evoked potentials. Thus, during isoflurane-induced hypotension, although CBF may be adequate to supply the brain with oxygen, there is no way to monitor the adequacy of CBF.

Hyperventilation reduces CBF and should be used with caution when induced hypotension is used. One study in dogs[50] demonstrated that hypocarbia (Pa_{CO_2} = 22 mm Hg) and induced hypotension within the autoregulatory range (mean arterial pressure $>$ 50 mm Hg) will usually maintain adequate CBF.

Cerebral Protection

When a major conducting vessel to the brain must be occluded temporarily during aneurysm surgery, the brain may be relatively protected from ischemic damage by reducing $CMRO_2$. This reduction in oxygen demand may be accomplished by two mechanisms. First, the temperature of the patient may be actively reduced or allowed to passively fall. Cerebral oxygen demand is reduced approximately 5% to 10% per degree celsius fall in temperature.[51, 52] The patient's temperature should be kept above 33° C, however, since the incidence of serious ventricular arrhythmias begins to increase at that level. Second, the oxygen consumed by the generation of spontaneous EEG activity may be reduced by the administration of a barbiturate or isoflurane. These drugs are administered until spontaneous EEG activity is lost. With complete suppression of spontaneous EEG activity, the oxygen requirement of the brain is reduced about 50%.[53, 54] Such EEG suppression may require large doses of barbiturate (e.g., loading dose of 15 mg/kg of thiopental followed by an infusion of up to 20 to 30 mg/kg/hour or two MAC or more of isoflurane). Additional barbiturate or isoflurane will not produce any more reductions in cerebral oxygen demand once EEG activity is suppressed. Since high-dose barbiturate administration is accompanied by marked cardiovascular depression, inotropic support of the circulation usually is required. Many different vasopressors including phenylephrine, dopamine, dobutamine, epinephrine, and others have been successfully used in this setting. If barbiturate suppression is planned, the EEG should be monitored so that the minimum dose of barbiturate needed to produce EEG suppression can be used.

Emergence From Anesthesia

Quick emergence from anesthesia at the conclusion of the operation is necessary to allow for assessment of neurologic status. If the patient does not promptly return to baseline status, a computed tomography scan will be needed to rule out a postoperative hematoma, and an angiogram may be needed to rule out inadvertent occlusion of cerebral vessels. Patients who were obtunded preoperatively will usually not improve in the immediate postoperative period. They should not be extubated until mental status has improved. In addition, patients with vasospasm who are undergoing vigorous hydrotherapy may need continued postoperative positive pressure ventilation to treat pulmonary edema and to improve oxygenation. Even in cases in which postoperative intubation is planned, it is important to be able to frequently assess the patient's neurologic status. After initial neurologic assessment, careful sedation may be useful in these patients to help them tolerate prolonged intubation. After sedation is discontinued, a rapid return to normal mental status is very important.

Conclusion

In summary, providing anesthesia for the patient with aneurysmal SAH is one of the most difficult challenges an anesthesiologist can face. Careful preoperative evaluation of the patient can help the clinician plan for special techniques (such as induced hypotension, cerebral protection with barbiturates, spinal drainage, or temporary vessel occlusion with induced hypertension and barbiturates) that may be needed during surgery. Clearly, careful control of blood pressure is important, but how the patient is ventilated and oxygenated as well as the anesthetic that is used can also profoundly affect the functioning of the brain. Evoked potential and EEG monitoring can help the anesthesiologist to ascertain the impact of hyperventilation, induced hypotension or hypertension, pharmacologic reductions in $CMRO_2$, temporary clipping of major vessels, and permanent clipping of the aneurysm on cerebral function. Communication between the surgeon, anesthesiologist, and electrophysiologist will enable the patient to attain the best possible outcome.

Acknowledgements

The editorial assistance of Anita Yeager and the artistic talents of Maggie Hope, Diane Pettey, and Kendra Kuck are gratefully acknowledged.

References

1. Philips LH et al: The unchanging pattern of subarachnoid hemorrhage in a community. *Neurology* 30:1034–1039, 1980.
2. Weir B: Medical aspects of the preoperative management of aneurysms: A review. *Can J Neurol Sci* 8:21–26, 1981.
3. Flamm ES: The timing of aneurysm surgery. *Clin Neurosurg* 33:147–158, 1986.
4. Adams HP: Early management of the patient with recent aneurysmal subarachnoid hemorrhage. *Stroke* 17:1068–1070, 1986.
5. Disney L, Weir B, Petruk K: Effect on management mortality of a deliberate policy of early operation on supratentorial aneurysms. *Neurosurgery* 20:695–701, 1987.
6. Ferguson GG: Direct measurement of mean and pulsatile blood pressure at operation in human intracranial saccular aneurysms. *J Neurosurg* 36:560–568, 1972.
7. Yamada S et al: Safety limits of controlled hypotension in humans. *Acta Neurochir* 42:14–17, 1988.
8. Symon L, Momma F, Murota T: Assessment of reversible cerebral ischaemia in man: Intraoperative monitoring of the somatosensory evoked response. *Acta Neurochir* 42:3–7, 1988.
9. Kassell NF et al: Cerebral vasospasm following aneurysmal subarachnoid hemorrhage. *Stroke* 16:562–572, 1985.
10. Fisher CM, Kistler JP, Davis JM: Relation of cerebral vasospasm to subarachnoid hemorrhage visualized by computerized tomographic scanning. *Neurosurgery* 6:1–8, 1980.
11. Seiler RW et al: Cerebral vasospam evaluated by transcranial ultrasound correlated with clinical grade and CT-visualized subarachnoid hemorrhage. *J Neurosurg* 64:594–600, 1986.
12. Harders AG, Gilsbach JM: Time course of blood velocity changes related to vasospasm in the circle of Willis measured by transcranial Doppler ultrasound. *J Neurosurg* 66:718–728, 1987.
13. Sekhar LN et al: Value of transcranial Doppler ultrasound examination in the diagnosis of cerebral vasospasm after subarachnoid hemorrhage. *Neurosurg* 22:813–821, 1988.
14. Klingelhöfer J et al: Cerebral vasospasm evaluated by transcranial Doppler ultrasonography at different intracranial pressures. *J Neurosurg* 75:752–758, 1991.

15. Solomon RA, Fink M, Lennihan L: Early aneurysm surgery and prophylactic hypervolemic hypertensive therapy for the treatment of subarachnoid hemorrhage. *Neurosurgery* 23:699–704, 1988.
16. Awad IA et al: Clinical vasospam after subarachnoid hemorrhage: Response to hypervolemic hemodiluton and arterial hypertension. *Stroke* 18:365–372, 1987.
17. Tettenborn D et al: Survey of clinical experience with nimodipine in patients with subarachnoid hemorrhage. *Neurosurg Rev* 10:77–84, 1987
18. Allen GS et al: Cerebral arterial spasm - a controlled trial of nimodipine in patients with subarachnoid hemorrhage. *N Engl J Med* 309:308–310, 1983.
19. Hubschmann OR, Natnanson DC: The role of calcium and cellular membrane dysfunction in experimental trauma and subarachnoid hemorrhage. *J Neurosurg* 62:698–703, 1985.
20. Saito I, Sano K: Early operation and washout of blood clots for prevention of cerebral vasospasm. From Wilkins RH, editor: *Cerebral arterial spasm: Proceedings of the second international workshop.* Baltimore, 1980, Williams and Wilkins, pp 510–513.
21. Zabramski JM et al: Phase I trial of tissue plasminogen activator for the prevention of vasospasm in patients with subarachnoid hemorrhage. *J Neurosurg* 75:189–196, 1991.
22. Zubrov YLN, Nikiforov BM, Shustin VA: Balloon catheter techniques for dilation of constricted cerebral arteries after aneurysmal subarachnoid hemorrhage. *Acta Neurochir* 70:65–79, 1984.
23. Beard EF, Robertson JW, Robertson RCL: Spontaneous subarachnoid hemorrhage simulating acute myocardial infarction. *Am Heart J* 58:755–759, 1959.
24. Cropp GJ, Manning GW: Electrocardiographic changes simulating myocardial ischemia and infarction associated with spontaneous intracranial hemorrhage. *Circulation* 22:25–38, 1960.
25. Diamond T, Segal F: Subarachnoid hemorrhage masquerading electrocardiographically as acute myocardial infarction. *Heart Lung* 13:451–453, 1984.
26. Marion DW, Segal R, Thompson M: Subarachnoid hemorrhage and the heart (review). *Neurosurgery* 18:101–106, 1986.
27. Pollick C et al: Left ventricular wall motion abnormalities in subarachnoid hemorrhage: An echocardiographic study. *J Am Coll Cardiol* 12:600–605, 1988.
28. Friedman WA et al: Monitoring of somatosensory evoked potentials during surgery for middle cerebral artery aneurysms. *Neurosurgery* 29:83–88, 1991.
29. Buchthal A, Belopavlovic M: Somatosensory evoked potential in cerebral aneurysm surgery. *Klin Wochenschr* 66:27–34, 1988.
30. Carter LP et al: Somatosensory evoked potentials and cortical blood flow during craniotomy for vascular disease. *Neurosurgery* 15:22–28, 1984.
31. Schramm J et al: Surgical and electrophysiological observations during clipping of 134 aneurysms with evoked potential monitoring. *Neurosurgery* 26:61–70, 1990.
32. Symon I et al: Perioperative use of somatosensory evoked responses in aneurysm surgery. *J Neurosurg* 60:269–275, 1984.
33. Friedman WA et al: Evoked potential monitoring during aneurysm operation Observations after fifty cases. *Neurosurgery* 20:678–687, 1987.
34. Grundy BL: Monitoring of sensory evoked potentials during neurosurgical operations: Methods and applications. *Neurosurgery* 11:556–575, 1982.
35. Lessick JE, Michele JJ, Simeone FA: Alteration of somatosensory evoked potentials in response to global ischemia. *J Neurosurg* 60:490–494, 1984.

36. Branaston NM, Symon L, Crockard HA: Recovery of the cortical evoked response following temporary middle cerebral artery occlusion in baboons: Relation to local blood flow and Po_2. *Stroke* 7:151–157, 1976.
37. Hargadine JR, Branston NM, Symon L: Central conduction time in primate brain ischemia — a study in baboons. *Stroke* 11:637–641, 1980.
38. Branston NM et al: Relationship between the cortical evoked potential and local cortical blood flow following acute middle cerebral artery occlusion in the baboon. *Exp Neurol* 45:195–208, 1974.
39. Sharbrough FW, Messick JM, Sundt TM: Correlation of continuous electroencephalograms with cerebral blood flow measurements during carotid endarterectomy. *Stroke* 4:674–683, 1973.
40. Messick JM et al: Correlation of regional cerebral blood flow (rCBF) with EEG changes during isoflurane anesthesia for carotid endarterectomy: Critical rCBF. *Anesthesiology* 66:344–349, 1987.
41. McPherson RW, Johnson RM, Graf M: Intraoperative neurologic monitoring during carotid endarterectomy: Electroencephalogram versus somatosensory evoked potential (abstract). *Anesthesiology* 59:368, 1983.
42. Lam AM et al: Monitoring electrophysiologic function during carotid endarterectomy: A comparison of somatosensory evoked potentials and conventional electroencephalogram. *Anesthesiology* 75:15–21, 1991.
43. Markand ON et al: Monitoring of somatosensory evoked responses during carotid endarterectomy. *Arch Neurol* 41:375–378, 1984.
44. Gigli GL et al: Monitoring of subcortical and cortical somatosensory evoked potentials during carotid endarterectomy: Comparison with stump pressure levels. *Electroencephalogr Clin Neurophysiol* 68:424–432, 1987.
45. De Vleeschauwer P, Horsch S, Matamoros R: Monitoring of somatosensory evoked potentials in carotid surgery: Results, usefulness and limitations of the method. *Ann Vasc Surg* 2:63–68, 1988.
46. Nuwer MR: Use of somatosensory evoked potentials for intraoperative monitoring of cerebral and spinal cord function. *Neurol Clin* 6:881–897, 1988.
47. Little JR, Lesser RP, Luders H: Electrophysiologic monitoring during basilar aneurysm operation. *Neurosurgery* 20:421–426, 1987.
48. Drummond JC, Todd MM, U HS: The effect of high dose sodium thiopental on brain stem auditory and median nerve somatosensory evoked responses in humans. *Anesthesiology* 63:249–254, 1985.
49. Pinaud M et al: Cerebral blood flow and oxygen consumption during nitroprusside-induced hypotension to less than 50 mm Hg. *Anesthesiology* 70:255–260, 1989.
50. Artru AA, Katz RA, Colley PS: Autoregulation of cerebral blood flow during normocapnia and hypocapnia in dogs. *Anesthesiology* 70:288–292, 1989.
51. Michenfelder JD, Theye RA: Hypothermia: Effect of canine brain and whole body metabolism. *Anesthesiology* 29:1107–1111, 1968.
52. Bering EA Jr: Effect of body temperature change on cerebral oxygen consumption in the intact monkey. *Am J Physiol* 200:417–421, 1961.
53. Michenfelder JD: The in vivo effects of massive concentrations of anesthetics on canine cerebral metabolism. *In Fink BR, editor: Molecular mechanisms of anesthesia.* New York, 1975, Raven, p 537.
54. Newberg LA, Milde JH, Michenfelder JD: The cerebral metabolic effects of isoflurane at and above concentrations that suppress cortical electrical activity. *Anesthesiology* 59:23–29, 1983.

An Update on the Perioperative Management of the Patient With Peripheral Vascular Disease

John A. Youngberg, M.D.

Associate Professor of Anesthesiology, The Department of Anesthesiology, Tulane University School of Medicine, New Orleans, Louisiana

Donald Lea Akers, Jr., M.D.

Assistant Professor of Surgery, The Department of Surgery, Tulane University School of Medicine, New Orleans, Louisiana

This chapter will address the preoperative evaluation and intraoperative management of patients scheduled for surgery involving the abdominal aorta and peripheral vasculature. In addition, the issues of risk assessment and the role of endovascular procedures will be discussed.

Preanesthetic Evaluation

Patients undergoing peripheral vascular surgery often have significant cardiac, pulmonary, renal, and/or endocrine disease. A detailed medical history is imperative in this patient population.[1–4] The majority of postoperative deaths following major vascular surgery are secondary to myocardial infarctions (Table 1).[5] Myocardial infarctions account for approximately 55% of the postoperative deaths and a perioperative myocardial infarction is associated with a mortality rate of approximately 70%.[6, 7] Major risk factors include a family history of heart disease, a history of smoking, hyperlipidemia, hypercholesterolemia, obesity, hypertension, left ventricular hypertrophy on the electrocardiogram and, in some studies, a history of diabetes mellitus requiring medical treatment. A history of typical or atypical chest pain; nocturnal dyspnea; dyspnea on exertion, exposure to cold, or during defecation; a history of congestive heart failure or pulmonary edema; and a history of dysrythmias or previous myocardial infarction should be elicited.

TABLE 1.
Mortality Related to Cardiac Dysfunction*

Aortic Reconstructive Series	Deaths/Total Number of Patients	Mortality Caused by Cardiac Dysfunction, %
Szilagi et al. (1966)	59/401	48
Young et al. (1977)	7/144	100
Hicks et al. (1975)	19/225	53
Thompson et al. (1975)	6/108	83
Mulcare et al. (1978)	14/140	79
Whitemore et al. (1980)	1/110	100
Crawford et al. (1981)	1/860	54
Hertzer (1983)	22/523	64

*From Roizen MF et al: *Vascular surgery: Principals and practice.* New York, 1987, McGraw-Hill, pp 312–321. Used by permission.

Hypertension is often a common finding in patients who have peripheral vascular disease, although hypertension has not been reported to be a consistent independent predictor of perioperative cardiac events in patients undergoing noncardiac surgery.[1, 8–10] Gotto and Farmer reported that systolic hypertension has been a more powerful predictor of coronary artery disease than has diastolic hypertension.[11] Patients with a history of hypertension are understandably more likely to experience perioperative hypertensive episodes than are normotensive patients. Interestingly, Bedford et al. reported that patients who had an abnormal blood pressure on admission to the hospital and who were not under medical treatment for hypertension were often the patients who experienced the highest blood pressures during laryngoscopy and intubation, were more likely to require vasodilator therapy, and were more likely to develop periods of myocardial ischemia.[12] The concurrent presence of other conditions in patients with hypertension may cloud the issue of the importance of adequately controlling hypertension preoperatively. Hartford et al. have reported the beneficial physiologic effects of adequate control of hypertension, and Stone et al. have demonstrated the beneficial effects of a single dose of a beta-adrenergic blocker administered 90 minutes prior to the induction of anesthesia in patients with untreated hypertension.[13, 14]

A history of primary cardiac disease is a definitive and independent predictor of perioperative cardiac events. Of the approximately 24.5 million noncardiac surgeries performed each year, there are approximately one million surgeries performed in patients with known coronary artery disease, two to three million performed in patients who are at risk for coronary artery disease, and an additional four million procedures performed on patients over the age of 65.[15] On physical examination, the patient should be

TABLE 2.
Previous MI and Risk of Reinfarction

Study	Months Since MI	Reinfarction Rate, %
Tarhan et al.[18]	<3	37
Steen et al.[17]	<3	27
Rao et al.[10]	<3	5.8
Shah et al.[21]	<3	4.3
Tarhan et al.[18]	3–6	16
Steen et al.[17]	3–6	11
Rao et al.[10]	3–6	2.3
Shah et al.[21]	3–6	0
Tarhan et al.[18]	>6	6
Steen et al.[17]	>6	4.1
Rao et al.[10]	>6	1.7
Shah et al.[21]	>6	5.7

evaluated for cardiac murmurs, hepatojugular reflux, hepatic distention, peripheral edema, and the presence of third or fourth heart sounds. The presence of a third heart sound often signifies left ventricular dysfunction while the presence of a fourth heart sound is often present in patients who have a poorly distensible or low compliance ventricle such as is found in patients with hypertension or those who have ischemic heart disease.

The history of a previous myocardial infarction (MI) is a consistently reported major risk factor for perioperative cardiovascular complications.[1, 16–19] A myocardial infarction that occurred less than 6 months previous to the proposed surgery imports a greater degree of risk while the risk of a recurrent myocardial infarction remains relatively constant after a period of 6 months.[1, 16–19] More recent studies have indicated that the rate of reinfarction may be lessened if invasive monitoring is used, the anesthetic management is judicious, and postoperative care is excellent.[10, 20, 21] These differences in reinfarction rate are summarized in Table 2.

Interestingly, the Shah et al. study reported a reinfarction rate in the group with previous myocardial infarctions greater than 6 months old to be 5.7%, which is considerably higher than the 1.7% reported by Rao et al.[10, 21] The authors explain that this apparent difference in recurrence rate of myocardial infarctions is secondary to the surgical procedures the patient underwent. In the Shah study, 36 of the 55 patients in the MI older than 6 months group underwent aortic or peripheral vascular surgery, and the reinfarction rate was 17% in these 36 patients. If only nonaortic/nonvascular operations were considered, the reinfarction rate was 2.9%—a significant difference. These findings are in agreement with those of Jeffrey et al. and Domaingue et al., who have reported that patients undergoing aortic surgery are at greater risk for cardiac complications than if they were undergoing nonaortic operations.[7, 22]

A history of congestive heart failure (CHF) is also a major determinant of perioperative risk. Over two million Americans have CHF, and the mortality rate of patients with CHF is reported to be 15% to 60%. The incidence of CHF has been reported to double with each decade between ages 45 to 75 years. Goldman et al. have reported that the risk of perioperative pulmonary edema following major surgery in patients over the age of 40 is 23% in patients with a history of pulmonary edema, 25% in patients who are New York Heart Association functional class IV, 30% in patients with jugular vein distention and signs of left heart failure, and 35% in patients with an S3 gallop.[16] The physiologic picture of CHF often includes: (1) acidosis, (2) increased ventricular filling pressures, (3) increased systemic vascular resistance, and (4) decreased cardiac output. Therapy is directed toward decreasing ventricular filling pressures (preload), decreasing systemic vascular resistance (afterload), and increasing cardiac output. Dysrhythmias are often present in patients with CHF and their presence may increase morbidity.[23]

The presence of dysrhythmias may primarily be an indicator of the severity of underlying cardiac disease rather than an independent variable in the prediction of perioperative morbidity.[1, 16, 24, 25] The logical approach would be to search for the underlying cause of the dysrhythmias rather than focusing on treating the manifested dysrhythmias.

The presence of ischemic heart disease is of paramount concern in patients undergoing vascular surgery. Pasternack et al. reported that the incidence of perioperative myocardial infarctions was directly related to the total duration of ischemia in patients undergoing peripheral vascular surgery.[26] Angina can be divided into a variety of types: (1) stable angina is usually consistent and fairly well reproduced at a given level of stress or activity, (2) unstable angina is myocardial ischemia that occurs at a new lower level of stress or activity or is present at rest for the first time, (3) new angina is self-explanatory, and (4) Prinzmetal's angina is angina that occurs at rest and may occur at night. This form of angina is associated with coronary artery spasm, and patients may not experience angina during exercise. Detsky et al. have suggested that patients undergoing noncardiac surgery are more at risk for perioperative cardiac events if they have unstable angina vs. stable angina.[27]

There are a great number of methods available to the clinician to evaluate patients suspected of having coronary artery disease (Table 3). When determining which test or tests of the cardiovascular system to employ, it is important to be cognizant of the sensitivity and specificity of a given test. Sensitivity is defined as: Total positive (TP) results divided by total positive results plus false-positive (FP) results (sensitivity $= TP \div TP + FP$). Specificity is defined as total negative results divided by total negative (TN) re-

TABLE 3.
Tests for Ischemic Coronary Disease

Electrocardiogram
24-hour Holter monitoring
Stress test
Bicycle ergometer
Radionuclide angiography
Echocardiography
Dipyridamole-thallium scintigraphy
Coronary angiography

sults plus false-negative (FN) results (specificity = TN ÷ TN + FN). A standard electrocardiogram is indicated for all patients scheduled for major vascular surgery. Special attention should be given to evidence of a previous myocardial infarction, evidence of left ventricular strain or hypertrophy, electrolyte or conduction abnormalities, the presence of ischemia, and the existence of dysrhythmias. The resting 12-lead electrocardiogram (ECG) may be normal in 25% to 50% of patients with coronary artery disease and only represents a window in time and is therefore somewhat limited as a diagnostic tool. The sensitivity (80%) and specificity (53%) of the ergometric bicycle test when the patient is unable to raise his heart rate above 90 beats/min after supine exercise for 2 minutes at 50 revolutions per minute compares favorably with the sensitivity of 60% and specificity of 64% for the Goldman Risk Index. Exercise stress testing is commonly used to evaluate patients with suspected coronary disease. False-positive results are more common in women, digoxin therapy is often a cause of false-positive tests, and exercise stress tests are often difficult to interpret in the presence of left bundle branch block or Wolf-Parkinson-White syndrome. By contrast, 24- to 48-hour Holter monitoring with ST segment analysis has a reported sensitivity of 92% and a specificity of 88%. Positive predictive value is reported to be 38% while negative predictive value is reported to be 99%. Limitations of this test include the presence of left bundle branch block, left ventricular hypertrophy with strain, and medications such as minoxidil and digoxin. Dipyridamole thallium scintigraphy has been reported by Boucher et al. to have a sensitivity of 100%; however, Mangano et al. recently reported a much lower specificity and sensitivity with use of dipyridamole thallium scintigraphy.[28, 29]

The stress test is a fairly standardized test that is used to evaluate patients for the manifestation of ischemia during a period of exercise. Exercise can be tested on treadmills, bicycles, or during the performance of isometric exercises. A variety of protocols including the familiar Bruce protocol and others such as the Balhe, Ellestad, Sheffield, Naughton, and Astrand are used. The overall sensitivity is approximately 70% and the specificity is approximately 90% in patients who have coronary artery disease risk factors. The patient's electrocardiogram is observed for the development of ST segment depression, which is an indication of subendocardial ischemia. The evidence for ischemia is more reliable if the ST segment depression is present in more than one lead and the appearance of the depression is either flat or downward sloping. The depression should be at least 0.5 to 2.0 mm (0.05 to 0.2 mV) on a standardized strip or recorder, depending on which protocol is being used. ST depression that worsens during the recovery period is often associated with a worse prognosis. As with the standard electrocardiogram and 24-hour Holter monitor, female gender, drugs such as minoxidil or digoxin, and cardiac conditions such as Wolf-Parkinson-White syndrome are all associated with a greater incidence of false-positive readings. The presence of bundle branch blocks also makes the test difficult to interpret.

Other findings associated with an exercise stress test may be the occurrence of dysrhythmias, conduction abnormalities, or ST segment elevation. In the setting of exercise stress testing, ST segment elevation (usually 1.5 mm or more) is more likely to represent transmural myocardial ischemia or a greater degree of dyskinesis in the area of a previous myocardial infarction rather than the coronary spasm that produces Prinzmetal's angina, which is more commonly experienced at rest.

In addition to observation and recording of the electrocardiogram, the patient is observed for changes in blood pressure and heart rate in response to exercise. If systolic blood pressure does not rise or paradoxically decreases during a period of exercise, the patient may have moderate-to-severe cardiac dysfunction. Clearly, there are marked limitations to the use of exercise stress testing in patients who have moderate-to-severe major vascular disease. These patients may be unable to perform the test secondary to claudication or increases in blood pressure may result in unacceptable pressures on the wall of an aortic aneurysm. Patients with aneurysms are often best evaluated with some other means. Patients with claudication may be more suitable for arm crank ergometric evaluation. Cutler et al. reported the use of arm ergometry and found that only about 9% of patients with peripheral vascular disease were unable to complete the protocol.[30]

The predictive capability of exercise stress testing has been evaluated by a number of investigators. McPhail et al. reported that patients who were not able to achieve at least 85% of their predicted maximal heart rate during either arm crank or treadmill exercise testing experienced a 25% perioperative cardiac complication rate in contrast to a 6% complication rate in patients who achieved greater than 85% of their predicted maximum heart rate. The addition of ST depression of greater than 1 mm to an inability to achieve 85% of predicted maximum heart rate increased the risk to 33%.[31] Gerson et al. reported that the inability to increase the heart rate above 90 beats per minute after supine bicycle exercise for 2 minutes was predictive of a perioperative myocardial infarction with a sensitivity of 80%.[32]

Twenty-four hour Holter monitoring with ST segment analysis is also an effective method for evaluating patients at potential risk for perioperative myocardial events. Raby et al. reported a study of 176 patients scheduled for major vascular surgery. Thirty-two patients had 75 episodes of ST segment depression. Interestingly, 73 of the 75 episodes were asymptomatic or "silent." Twelve of these 32 patients suffered perioperative events compared to only 1 of 144 patients who did not have episodes of ST segment depression.[9] In 10% of the cases, the ST segment data were difficult to interpret. This study supports previous studies, which have reported that 80% or more of ischemic episodes are asymptomatic or silent even in patients who do not have diabetes mellitus. The sensitivity of this test is therefore 92% with a specificity of 88% and a negative predictive value of 99% but a positive predictive value of only 38%.

Echocardiography is an excellent tool that can be used to evaluate wall motion abnormalities, wall thickening, valve function, ventricular function, and ejection fraction. M mode echocardiography records only structures that lie parallel to the beam whereas two-dimensional echocardiography simultaneously has the capability of scanning an entire sector of a field rather than the ice-pick view of M mode.

Dipyridamole thallium scintigraphy (DTS) is receiving a great deal of scrutiny as a diagnostic tool in evaluating patients at risk for perioperative myocardial events. The nonexercise DTS test is performed by administering dipyridamole followed by thallium (which is taken up by viable myocardial tissue) and an initial scan is obtained. The myocardium will either present a picture of relative homogeneous uptake (white on a black-and-white scan) or there will be one or more areas of decreased or lack of uptake (dark areas on a black-and-white scan). The patient is then scanned a second time approximately 3 to 4 hours after the first scan if areas of decreased or no uptake were present on the initial scan. If the darker areas appear to have filled in on the second scan, the patient is termed to have evidence of redistribution. Patients who exhibit redistribution have been reported to be at greater risk for developing a perioperative myocardial infarction than patients who had a normal initial scan or who had persistent defects (reflecting old stable scars or injury) on the subsequent scan.[3, 28, 33, 34] However, a number of investigators have recently questioned the utility of the DTS as a screening test.[29, 35–37] Younis et al. have reported that patients with a positive DTS appear to have a poorer prognosis.[38] Cambria et al. recently reported that although selective use of DTS based on certain clinical markers of coronary artery disease will identify the approximately 10% of patients undergoing major vascular surgery who are at an increased risk of a significant perioperative myocardial event, the significant predictors of postoperative death were more than 5 hours of operative time, operation for aortoiliac disease, and a history of ventricular ectopy.[37] A persistent defect may also represent an area of protracted ischemia rather than an old scar.

Dipyridamole thallium scintigraphy is not without real and potential risks. Dipyridamole is a coronary artery dilator and a "steal" may be produced.

Patients may develop angina, dysrhythmias or infarctions. Drug reactions are also a potential source of sequelae. The "gold standard" for evaluating the severity of coronary artery disease is coronary angiography. Some authors have recommended the routine use of coronary angiography prior to aortic surgery.[39, 40] Leppo et al. reported that exercise thallium scanning was not predictive of evidence of ischemia in 9 of 30 patients who had angiographically documented triple vessel disease.[41] Like DTS, however, angiography is not without risk and when used as a routine diagnostic tool angiography may yield a positive indication for angioplasty or coronary artery bypass grafting in less than 40 percent of the cases.[31] Selective use of coronary angiography would appear to be appropriate. A possible evaluation scheme to identify the patient at risk for a perioperative myocardial event is presented in Figure 1.

Organ Protection

Renal

One of the major organs at risk during major vascular surgery is the kidney. The kidney is at risk from a variety of causes, including ischemia from aortic cross-clamping, direct manipulation, embolization of debris or air, drug effects, and hypotension. The renal arteries usually arise from the aorta at a level of T10 to L1 but may come off as high as T8. The kidneys normally receive 20% to 25% of the cardiac output. Renal blood flow then is in the range of 1250 mL/min based on a cardiac output of 5.0 L/min, renal plasma flow would be approximately 750 mL/min, glomerular filtration rate would be approximately 50% of renal plasma flow (125 mL/min), and urine output normally is 1 to 2 mL/kg/min.

When the aorta is cross-clamped at the level of the thoracic aorta, the reported incidence of acute renal failure is 2.7% to 13.8%.[42–44] Although renal dysfunction is far less frequent when the aorta is cross-clamped at an infrarenal level, the serum creatinine level has been reported to increase by 0.5 mg/dL or more in 15% of patients.[45] Indeed, cardiovascular surgery is emerging as the primary cause of acute renal failure.[46] Cross-clamping the aorta in the thoracic region has been reported to decrease renal blood flow by 85% to 94%, whereas infrarenal cross-clamping of the aorta decreases renal blood flow by 40%.[47, 48] The mortality rate in patients who develop acute renal failure following aortic aneurysm surgery may be as high as 40%. Both preexisting cardiac disease and renal ischemic time that exceeds 30 minutes have been identified as factors that increase the risk of renal failure.[49]

Anesthesia and the type of anesthetics used produce effects on normal renal function. Mechanical ventilation and the use of positive end expiratory pressure (PEEP) both may be associated with a reduction in renal function.[50] PEEP can be associated with a reduction in plasma levels of atrial natiuretic factor and a decrease in the excretion of sodium in the urine. Atrial natiuretic factor is a peptide hormone in the atrial cardiocyte

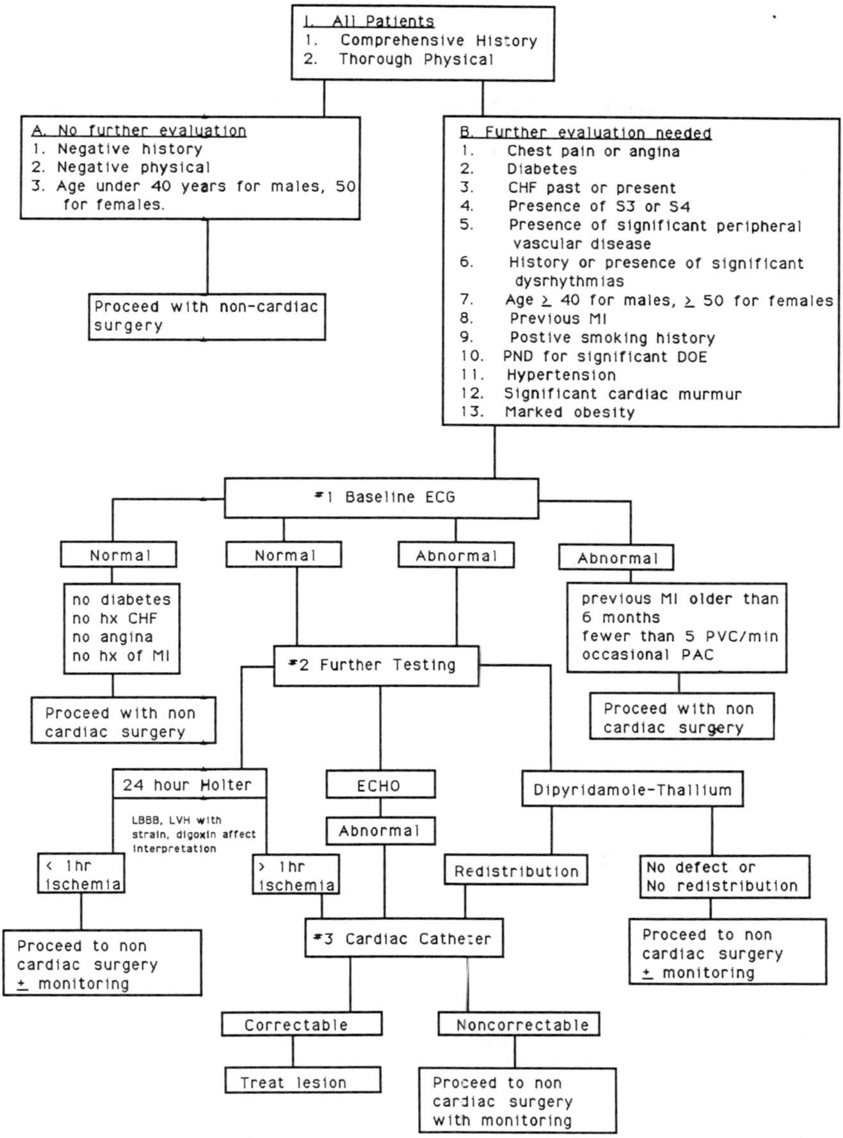

FIG 1.
Algorithm for preoperative evaluation of patient undergoing vascular surgery.

that produces natiuresis and diuresis with only a moderate kaliuresis. Atrial natiuretic factor increases glomerular filtration rate while renal blood flow is only minimally affected.

Both isoflurane and enflurane have been reported to decrease glomerular filtration rate; however, isoflurane may produce less of an alteration in

TABLE 4.
Preserving Renal Function

Volume loading
Maintain urine output greater than ½ to 1 mL/kg/hr
Mannitol 20–30 min prior to aortic cross-clamping
Retrograde femoral-femoral bypass in special circumstances
Local renal cooling
Use of renin antagonists
Use of calcium channel blockers
Low dose dopamine
Loop diuretics
Maintain adequate potassium and magnesium levels
Prevent debris from embolizing to the renal arteries
Oxygen free radical scavengers

renal blood flow at equipotent doses than enflurane.[51, 52] The alterations in glomerular filtration rate may result in a lower urine output with both agents. Fentanyl has also been reported to produce a decrease in the glomerular filtration rate while the effects on renal blood flow appear to be somewhat less consistent.[53, 54] Merin et al. have reported that desflurane produces similar effects on renal blood flow as those produced by isoflurane.[55] The effects of major regional anesthetics such as spinal or epidural anesthesia are largely secondary to the production of a sympathectomy and the resultant decreases in arterial pressures.

The primary key to the preservation of renal function is the prevention of injury. A variety of modalities have been presented in the literature as methods to preserve renal well-being (Table 4). Potassium depletion prior to renal ischemia has been reported to accentuate renal injury.[56] Loop diuretics inhibit tubule salt reabsorption, produce a vasodilator effect, and inhibit tubuloglomerular feedback. Mannitol is an impermeant solute and limits osmotic cell swelling in addition to being a potential scavenger of oxygen free radicals. Mannitol possesses vasodilator actions, may increase renal prostaglandin, may decrease renal renin, and has been reported to shift blood flow to the cortex of the kidney. Dopamine is a natiuretic hormone, which in low doses increases renal plasma flow resulting in an increase in glomerular filtration rate. Dopamine also inhibits the tubular transport of sodium and may produce a redistribution of intrarenal blood flow. A new dopamine-receptor agonist, fenoldopam, has been evaluated as an agent for renal preservation. Fenoldopam appears to possess properties in common with both mannitol and dopamine: systemic vascular resistance is reported to decrease while sodium excretion, creatinine clearance, and urine flow are all reported to increase.[57, 58]

There is a developing body of knowledge primarily in animal models that suggests that pretreatment with calcium entry blockers may be beneficial, depending on the resultant effects on perfusion pressure to the kidney and the cause of renal hypotension.[59, 60]

Ischemic damage to the kidneys may in part be a result of less well-understood and investigated factors such as the role of neutrophils, leukotrienes, oxygen free radicals, and arachidonate metabolites. In animals, superoxide dismutase, an oxygen free radical scavenger, may provide some degree of protection if administered prophylactically prior to renal ischemia.[61] Free radical scavengers may also decrease the production of thromboxane A2, which is a renal vasoconstrictor, and produce a resultant preservation in renal perfusion.[62] I am not aware of data or literature that have indicated that free radical scavengers per se are approved for use in humans or that superoxide dismutase is available or recommended for use in humans for the purposes of renal or spinal cord protection. Other areas of investigation include phosphodiesterase inhibitors, angiotensin-converting enzyme inhibitors, and the use of epidermal growth factor.

Spinal Cord

Although the risk of injury to the spinal cord is less than that of injury to the kidneys, the spinal cord is another vulnerable organ that may require protection during major vascular surgery. The spinal cord receives its blood supply from three primary arteries: two posterior spinal arteries and a single anterior spinal artery. The anterior spinal artery is usually the major blood supply to the spinal cord and perfuses all areas except the posterior columns and the tips of the posterior horns. The posterior spinal arteries arise from the posterior cerebellar arteries, while the anterior spinal artery is formed by the union of the two vertebral arteries, which are branches of subclavian arteries.

The spinal arteries' blood supply is reinforced by spinal branches of the deep cervical, ascending cervical, vertabral, posterior intercostal, lumbar, and lateral sacral arteries. The largest radicular artery supplying the anterior spinal artery is often called the artery of Adamkiewicz. The artery of Adamkiewicz can arise from the aorta anywhere from T5 to L3 but comes off at a level of T9 to T12 in 75% of cases. Like the brain, the spinal cord has both a forward perfusion pressure and a pressure that retards perfusion (equation I).

Equation I:

$$SCPP = MAP - CSFP$$

where SCPP = spinal cord perfusion pressure, MAP = mean arterial pressure, and CSFP = central spinal fluid pressure.

TABLE 5.
Spinal Cord Preservation

Hypothermia
CSF drainage
Shunts
Retrograde bypass
Steroids
Opiate antagonists
Intrathecal papaverine
Intrathecal local anesthetics
Superoxide dismutase
Calcium channel blockers
Magnesium

A net driving pressure (SCPP) of at least 30 mm Hg has been reported in dogs and spinal cord perfusion has been reported to be adequately maintained in dogs with a distal mean aortic pressure as low as 50 mm-Hg.[63] The incidence of paraplegia depends on factors such as preexisting aortic disease, level of aortic cross-clamping, duration of clamping, central spinal fluid pressure, collateral circulation, and prophylactic measures instituted. The reported incidence of spinal cord injury associated with major vascular surgery varies from 24% following acute rupture of the aorta to 0.19% following repair of nonruptured aneurysms.[64, 65] In a series of 1,188 patients undergoing surgery for aortoiliac occlusive disease, there were no patients who suffered spinal cord injury.[64] Cross-clamping the aorta at the level of the subclavian artery in dogs resulted in a 94% decrease in spinal artery blood flow.[47] The warm ischemic time to the spinal cord has been reported to be 20 to 30 minutes.[64, 66]

The key to preservation of spinal cord function is the prevention of injury by maintaining an adequate perfusion pressure and/or limiting the period of ischemia. A variety of procedures and techniques have been presented in the literature as methods to preserve spinal cord integrity (Table 5). Drainage of spinal fluid to increase spinal cord perfusion pressure was proposed by McCullough et al. in 1988.[67] Both Svensson and Grum have published reports combining the drainage of cerebrospinal fluid with the addition of intrathecal papaverine.[68–71] In these various studies, the authors use an indwelling continuous spinal catheter for removal of cerebrospinal fluid (CSF). Twenty milliliters of CSF is removed prior to aortic cross-clamping and 3 mL of 1% papaverine is injected 10 minutes prior to aortic cross-clamping. During the period of aortic cross-clamping, 15 to 20 mL of CSF is drained every 15 minutes to maintain cerebrospinal fluid pressure between 5 and 15 mm Hg. An upper limit of 50 to 75 mL of CSF is drained off depending on the study (Grum et al., personal communication, 1988). Svensson et al. recommend an upper limit of 50 mL of CSF drainage secondary to a potential risk of herniation. They also reported that papaverine injected at room temperature produced hypotension and recommended warming the papaverine to 37°C.[71] Papaverine is a smooth muscle relaxant, an arteriolar dilator, blocks calcium entry into cells, and also is reported to be an indirect oxygen free radical scavenger. Studies in both primates and humans have led Svensson and Grum to conclude that the combination of CSF drainage coupled with the use of intrathecally administered papaverine may offer protection to the spinal cord. The numbers of patients (11 total) in these studies are small; and for that reason, these reports should be considered preliminary.

A variety of other techniques of prophylaxis against cord injury have also been investigated. Hill et al. reported that the use of a calcium channel blocker may offer some protection against reperfusion injury in dogs.[72] Laschinger et al. reported that in a dog model the use of corticosteroids may also lessen the risk of spinal cord injury following aortic cross-clamping.[73] Magnesium has also been reported to offer protection against spinal cord or central nervous system injury.[74, 75] Vacanti et al. demonstrated that rabbits cooled to 3°C and administered 5 mmol/kg of magnesium experienced a threefold increase in ischemic time when compared to control animals.[74] Magnesium activates alkaline phosphates and pyrophosphates, affects calcium uptake, affects adenyl cyclase generation of cyclic adenosine monophosphate, affects membrane sodium-potassium adenosine triphosphatase, and produces vasodilation and the familiar curariform activity at the neuromuscular junction. It has been reported that magnesium sulfate can be given intravenously at a rate of 40 mmol (10 g) in 24 hours followed by 24 mmol per day for 2 to 5 days for slow replacement, or magnesium sulfate may be administered on an emergent basis as 8 mmol (2 g) in 10 mL of 5% dextrose in water solution (D5W) over 10 minutes followed by 20 mmol (5 g) in 500 mL D5W over 3 to 12 hours (Table 6).[76] More recently the use of superoxide dismutase, an oxygen free radical scavenger, has been reported to offer some degree of cardiovascular stability and spinal cord protection in dogs following cross-clamping of the aorta.[77, 78] Breckwoldt et al. reported that 0.3 mL of 1% tetracaine administered subarachoid in rabbits was protective against ischemia to the spinal cord for 30 minutes. No mechanism was proposed.[79]

There is little evidence in the literature to recommend one anesthetic or an anesthetic technique as being superior with respect to spinal cord protection. There are questions raised in the literature, however, concerning the potential for deleterious effects of various agents at least on a theoretical basis. Nitroprusside has been reported to produce an increase in central spinal fluid pressure and a lowering of spinal cord perfusion pressure while other investigators have not demonstrated an increase in central spinal fluid pressure.[70, 80, 81] Isoflurane has been reported to decrease spinal cord perfusion pressure primarily by decreasing diastolic arterial pressure.[70]

Monitoring the spinal cord with somatosensory-evoked potentials does not guarantee against spinal cord injury in that only the posterior and lat-

TABLE 6.
Magnesium Requirements and Replacement

Serum level 0.7–1.05 mmol/L
Daily intake approximately 12.5 mmol
Slow replacement: intravenous 40 mmol (10 g) of magnesium sulfate in 24 h followed by 24 mmol (6 g) per day for 2–5 days
Emergent replacement: 8 mmol (2 g) in 10 mL of D5W over 10 min followed by 20 mmol in 500 mL D5W in not less than 3 hr but usually over 8–12 hr

eral columns of the spinal cord are monitored. Motor deficits can occur despite normal recordings. Laschinger et al. have reported the use of motor-evoked potentials in dogs to obviate this limitation.[82]

The Bowel

The incidence of gastrointestinal complications following aortic surgery and/or reconstruction has been reported to range from 1.5% to 7.3% with a mortality rate of up to 24% in patients who develop gastrointestinal complications.[83, 84] The inferior mesenteric artery arises from the aorta at the level of L1 to L5. Although infrarenal cross-clamping of the aorta may produce little effect on splanchnic flow, suprarenal cross-clamping of the aorta may markedly decrease flow. Use of vasodilators such as nitroprusside or nitroglycerin may increase arteriovenous shunting in the splanchnic bed. Manipulation of the bowel can result in a mesenteric traction response, which is often initially associated with hypotension and tachycardia and is mediated by release of prostacyclin. This process is usually self-limiting, lasting less than 20 to 30 minutes, but a period of hypertension mediated by increased levels of thromboxane may follow. Pretreatment with ibuprofen 12 mg/kg given orally 1 to 1½ hours preoperatively or 800 mg given in three divided doses 6 hours apart have both been reported as successful therapies to decrease the levels of 6-keto-$PGF_{1\ alpha}$, which is a metabolite of prostacyclin.[85, 86] Ibuprofen is a cyclooxygenase inhibitor and therefore reduces the formation of prostacyclin. Aspirin therapy also reduces the formation of prostacyclin. Although not yet reported in a prospective randomized study, it would appear that keroralac, another cyclooxygenase inhibitor, should have similar protective effects. The treatment for the mesenteric traction syndrome once it occurs is symptomatic and includes the administration of fluids, the use of vasoconstrictors, and potentially the use of diphenhydramine, etc. The potential drawback to the routine administration of ibuprofen is the reported increase in blood loss secondary to alterations in platelet function. In a recent study by Hudson et al., however, there was no reported significant difference in blood loss between control patients and patients treated with ibuprofen who were undergoing aortic surgery.[86]

The Heart

As previously described, the greatest incidence of morbidity and mortality following major vascular surgery is cardiac in origin. There are a variety of factors involved including events in both the intraoperative and postoperative periods. Some of these factors include the effects of anesthetics on the coronary circulation and vascular system, the general stress response to surgery, hemodynamic consequences of aortic cross-clamping and unclamping, fluid shifts associated with major vascular surgery, altered states of coagulation postoperatively, changes in pulmonary function and oxygenation postoperatively, and the management of pain postoperatively.

Coronary ischemia has been reported in the presence of abnormal hemodynamics, normal hemodynamics, secondary to coronary vasospasm, and as a result of intracoronary steal. In patients undergoing major vascular surgery, the ECG is routinely monitored with many authors recommending the monitoring of both leads II and V_5 simultaneously. When both leads are monitored simultaneously, 85% to 90% of the episodes of ischemia may be manifest.[87] Many authors also recommend the use of a pulmonary artery catheter and/or transesophageal echocardiography (TEE). Although Tuman et al. reported that pulmonary artery catheters (PAC) did not play a significant role in influencing outcome after cardiac surgery, Ansley et al. reported no consistent relationship between the central venous pressure (CVP) and pulmonary capillary wedge pressure (PCWP) during aortic surgery in patients with either good or poor left ventricular function.[88, 89] Indeed, in the study by Ansley et al., the CVP and PCWP were reported on occasion to move in opposite directions. More recently, Berlauk et al. reported that when a PAC was used to optimize patients hemodynamically 3 to 12 hours preoperatively, the perioperative mortality rate was 1.5% compared to 9.5% in patients who did not receive PAC monitoring.[90]

The use of TEE has proven to be beneficial in identifying wall motion abnormalities, which may indicate ischemia and can help evaluate valve function, identify intracardiac air and structural abnormalities, and assess volume status at the end of both systole and diastole, which enables the clinician to determine stroke volume and calculate cardiac output. By combining the volume data from the TEE and the pressure data from the PAC, an estimation of ventricular compliance can be made. The use of TEE may be beneficial in the assessment of volume status prior to aortic cross-clamping and unclamping and in the evaluation of ventricular performance and valve function during aortic cross-clamping.

TABLE 7.
Percent Change in Variable if Aorta Occluded at Various Levels*

Variable	Supraceliac Level	Infraceliac-Suprarenal Level	Infrarenal Level
Mean arterial blood pressure	54	5	2a
Pulmonary capillary wedge pressure	38	10a	0a
End-diastolic area	28	2a	9a
End-systolic area	69	10a	11a
Ejection fraction	−38	−10a	−3a
Abdominal wall motion (% of patients)	92	33	0
New myocardial infarctions	8	0	0

*From Roizen MF et al: *J Vasc Surg* 1:300–305, 1984. Used by permission.

An intraarterial catheter is used almost routinely in patients undergoing major vascular surgery. In patients with peripheral vascular disease (PVD), the right and left arm blood pressures may not be similar. In a study reported by Frank et al., systolic blood pressure was found to vary by 20 mm Hg or more in one arm vs. the other arm in 21% of 58 patients with PVD and in 3% of 38 patients with coronary artery disease (CAD) whereas the pressures were often the same in patients without PVD or CAD.[91] The higher pressure was in the right arm 60% of the time. In patients with PVD, it would appear to be important to know which arm was used to obtain baseline blood pressures on the ward and to note any differences between the arm pressures prior to surgery.

Roizen et al. reported cardiovascular changes observed when the aorta was cross-clamped at the supraceliac, infraceliac/suprarenal, and at the infrarenal level (Table 7).[92] Although Roizen et al. found limited changes in cardiovascular parameters associated with infrarenal aortic cross-clamping, Attia et al. reported a 30% incidence of myocardial ischemia following infrarenal aortic cross-clamping in patients with known coronary artery disease.[92, 93] Kouchoukas et al. have reported 35%, 56%, 43%, and 90% increases in mean arterial pressure, CVP, mean pulmonary artery pressure, and PCWP, respectively, when the descending thoracic aorta was cross-clamped.[94] In this study of eight patients, the authors also reported a 29% decrease in cardiac index.

Myocardial ischemia intraoperatively may or may not be related to hemodynamic changes such as hypotension, hypertension, tachycardia, or changes in filling pressures. Additionally, the anesthesiologist may need to be able to differentiate supply ischemia from demand ischemia. Factors that may produce a decrease in coronary blood flow include tachycardia, diastolic hypotension, increased preload, hypocarbia, and coronary spasm. Coronary artery perfusion pressure (CAPP) is directly related to diastolic blood pressure (DBP) and inversely related to left ventricular end diastolic pressure (LVEDP) so that CAPP = DBP − LVEDP. Any significant degree of coronary stenosis may produce a significant decrease in diastolic pressure distal to the stenosis. Decreased oxygen delivery to the myocardium may also be produced by alkalosis, anemia, hypoxia, decreased 2,3-diphosphoglycerate levels, and a decrease in cardiac index. An increase in myocardial oxygen demand can be produced by tachycardia, increased preload, increased afterload, and increased contractility.

It is apparent that both tachycardia and an increased preload may have adverse effects on both the supply and demand sides of the myocardial oxygen supply/demand balance and should be avoided. Tachycardia decreases diastolic filling time, thereby decreasing coronary perfusion, while at the same time the increased heart rate increases myocardial work and oxygen demand. An increase in preload produces an increase in myocardial cell fiber length, which increases oxygen demand, while at the same time CAPP may be adversely affected secondary to the relationship CAPP = DBP − LVEDP. The myocardium potentially at the greatest risk is the subendocardium.

In 1988, Buffington et al. presented data concerning patients with steal-prone coronary anatomy.[95] In this study, the authors reviewed the angiograms from 16,249 patients with coronary artery disease who had been part of the Coronary Artery Surgery Study (CASS). From their analysis, Buffington et al. concluded that 23% of these patients fulfilled the anatomic requirements for the potential of the development of coronary steal.[95] Steal-prone anatomy is defined as a combination of three factors: (1) total occlusion of a coronary vessel, (2) presence of intercoronary collateral vessels from a second coronary vessel supplying blood to the occluded vessel beyond the area of total occlusion, and (3) a 50% or greater stenosis of the coronary vessel supplying the collateral vessels. Any agent that produces significant epicardial vasodilation of the coronary vasculature could have the potential for producing a coronary steal by shunting blood away from the collateral system.

A number of investigators have reported that isoflurane has the potential for producing coronary steal and in selected cases has been associated with myocardial lactate production as evidence of myocardial ischemia.[96–98] Conversely, although desflurane is reported to be associated with many of the same cardiovascular effects as isoflurane including tachycardia, desflurane has not been found to produce effects on the coronary circulation that would produce a steal.[99, 100] Hartman et al. have also questioned the potential for isoflurane producing steal effects in vivo.[100] Both sodium nitroprusside and adenosine can produce an intracardiac steal effect in coronary blood flow whereas nitroglycerine does not appear to produce a steal.[100–102]

Just as cross-clamping the aorta may be associated with hemodynamic instability, unclamping the aorta may also be associated with significant changes in hemodynamics, especially hypotension. Hypotension following aortic unclamping may be a result of any combination of events including: (1) hypovolemia, (2) reactive hyperemia, (3) washout of acid from the ischemic areas below the clamp, (4) acid metabolites, (5) release of vasoactive substances, and/or as reported by Roizen et al. (6) an allergic reaction to the graft material.[103] The use of TEE, CVP, PCWP, or a combination of these monitors is useful in assessing adequacy of volume status prior to removing the aortic cross-clamp. The PCWP is generally raised above normal values just prior to clamp release to counteract the effects of acid washout, reactive hyperemia, etc. Administration of sodium bicarbonate is usually not necessary prior to removal of the cross-clamp. Casthely et al. have reported that in dogs, the administration of superoxide dismutase (a free radical scavenger) significantly decreased the cardiovascular changes associated with release of an aortic cross-clamp, whereas the administration of sodium bicarbonate produced no beneficial effects.[77] Raising filling pressure too long before release of the cross-clamp may place an undue and potentially deleterious work load on the heart. Communication with the surgeon for proper timing of the fluid load is warranted as is slow release of the aortic cross-clamp.

Slogoff and Keats have reported that the occurrence of intraoperative ischemia (CABG patients) as evidenced by ST segment changes is associated with postoperative myocardial infarctions.[104, 105] However, Mangano et al. reported that the occurrence of intraoperative ischemia was not an independent predictor of postoperative myocardial infarction in noncardiac surgical patients.[106] In this same study, Mangano et al. reported that postoperative ischemia is often precipitated by tachycardia and that the presence of postoperative ischemia during the first 48 hours after surgery was associated with a ninefold increase in the incidence of a major ischemia-related event such as myocardial infarction, unstable angina, or a cardiac-related death in patients who had undergone noncardiac surgery.[106] Of importance is that Mangano et al. reported that 47% of the ischemic events, 48% of the cases of congestive heart failure, and 13% of the episodes of ventricular tachycardia occurred after the third postoperative day.[106]

Reviews such as that of Mangano demonstrating the prevalence of cardiac-related events in the postoperative period have tended to shift the focus of preventing untoward cardiovascular-related events to the postoperative period.[107] Tuman et al. reported that patients who had received a combined general/epidural anesthetic for major vascular surgery had an attenuated hypercoagulable state postoperatively when compared to patients who had received a general anesthetic and that this diminution of their hypercoagulable state resulted in a lower incidence of thrombotic events of peripheral arterial grafts, coronary arteries, or deep vein thrombosis.[108] The authors speculate that the use of epidural anesthesia/analgesia in the postoperative period may be associated with a decrease in stress-mediated release of angiotension and catecholamines. In turn, platelet aggregation may be affected and the catabolism of proteins may be attenuated in conjunction with the possibility of increased antithrombin III levels and lower fibrinogen levels.[108]

Reeder et al. reported an association between postoperative myocardial ischemia and nocturnal hypoxia.[109] Reeder et al. also reported in this limited study of these patients that arterial oxygen saturation was lowest on the third postoperative day and that periods of hypoxemia were not detected clinically.[109] Hung et al. reported a significant association between sleep apnea and myocardial infarction.[110]

It would appear that a greater degree of emphasis will be focused on the postoperative period in an effort to devise treatment options to decrease the adverse effects of the stress response postoperatively, to decrease the hypercoagulable state postoperatively, to provide better and more consistent analgesia, to define the need for observation units, to define the duration of observation and risk, etc.

Anesthetic Considerations

The role that a specific anesthetic plays in overall outcome is a subject of continual controversy. In a recent article, Forrest et al. reported the role of various general anesthetic techniques on severe outcomes in a total of 17,201 patients undergoing a variety of surgical procedures.[111] The authors reported that halothane, isoflurane, and fentanyl were all associated with a significantly greater incidence of severe complications when compared to the control anesthetic (enflurane). The probabilities of any severe cardiovascular outcomes were 5.2%, 5.9%, 6.0%, and 3.8% for isoflurane, fentanyl, halothane, and enflurane, respectively.[111] The authors point out, however, that the individual anesthesiologist administering the anesthetic may possibly affect outcome more than the specific anesthetic technique per se. It should also be noted that the definition of severe outcome included tachycardia, hypertension, and dysrhythmias. If these factors for isoflurane, fentanyl, and halothane, respectively were deleted, then it appears that there would have been no significant difference between these agents and enflurane. The role of the individual anesthesiologist and his significance is familiar to us from the study of Slogoff et al.[112]

What is important is that the stress responses associated with surgery are attenuated. The stress response is associated with increases in serum levels of prolactin, growth hormone, adrenocorticotropic hormone, antidiuretic hormone, cortisol, aldosterone, renin, epinephrine, and norepinephrine. Alleviation of stress is a continuum that begins with the preoperative visit and ends with the discharge of the patient from the hospital. All phases of that continuum are important to the patient's well-being and eventual outcome. A number of investigators have reported the importance of preoperative visits and preparation in decreasing patient anxiety and level of stress and the potential for a decrease in perioperative complications as a result.[113–116] It is therefore difficult to conclude that a given anesthetic technique per se is the major determinant of outcome without controlling

TABLE 8.
Anesthetic Technique and Outcome

Series	Technique	Comment
Yeager et al.[121]	Epidural + Gen. vs. General	Fewer complications and lower cost in Epidural + General
Benefiel et al.	Isoflurane vs. Sufentanil	Fewer complications with Sufentanil
Haku et al.[123]	Epidural + Gen. vs. General	No difference
Crosby et al.[124]	Fentanyl vs. Sufentanil	No difference
Shah et al.[21]	Regional vs. General	No difference
Baron et al.[125]	Epidural + Gen. vs. General	No difference
Rivers et al.[126]	Epidural vs. General	No difference

interrelated variables such as preoperative preparation, depth of anesthesia, postoperative care, the individual anesthesiologist's response to predisposing changes in the patient's status, etc.

Halter and Pflug reported that plasma norepinephrine and epinephrine levels increased secondary to surgical stimulation and pain and that the increase in the rise of the levels of these catecholamines could be partially attenuated with spinal anesthesia, which produced a high thoracic somatosensory dermatome level. Conversely, a light general anesthetic may not attenuate the stress response to the same degree and may theoretically place the at risk patient in a more potentially compromising position.[117]

It should be remembered that the majority of adverse outcome events of either morbidity or mortality are cardiac-related and that the highest incidence of cardiac-related events occurs in the postoperative period.[6, 106, 118–120] When reviewing the body of literature available concerning anesthetic techniques for patients undergoing vascular surgery, there does not appear to be a best technique. Sample reports from the literature are presented in Table 8.

Yeager et al. reported that in 53 high-risk patients undergoing surgical procedures, the use of epidural plus general anesthesia resulted in a significantly lower overall postoperative complication rate, incidence of cardiovascular failure was significantly reduced, and hospital costs were significantly lower when compared to a group of patients who had received general anesthesia alone.[121] Cortisol excretion was lower in the epidural plus general group than in the general anesthesia alone group, indicating a more effective blunting of the stress response in the epidural plus general group. It is key to note that the method of providing analgesia in the postoperative period was markedly different between the groups. The combined group received epidural local anesthetics and/or narcotics while the general anesthesia group received parenteral narcotics on an as-needed basis. Management of stress in the postoperative period may have been dramatically different and could possibly impact outcome. In the Yeager et al. study, fentanyl with or without nitrous served as the base of the general anesthetic technique.

Benefiel et al. reported their findings comparing sufentanil vs. isoflurane for 96 patients undergoing aortic reconstruction (Benefiel et al., personal communication, 1986). The authors reported that the sufentanil group experienced a significantly lower incidence of both congestive heart failure and renal insufficiency postoperatively and postulated that sufentanil is protective (Benefiel et al., personal communication, 1986). Unfortunately the authors offered no explanation for these findings.

Aortic cross-clamp times, incidence of post-clamp hypotension, renal function during surgery, plasma catecholamine levels etc., were not reported. As in the Yeager et al. study, there is no assurance that the depth of anesthesia in the two groups were indeed equal. Additionally, postoperative analgesia was managed differently in the two groups in the Benefiel et al. study. The more recent studies by Haku et al., Crosby et al., Shah et al., Baron et al., and Rivers et al., which have compared epidural plus general vs. general, fentanyl vs. sufentanil, regional vs. general, epidural plus general vs. general, and epidural vs. general, respectively, have all failed to demonstrate that the anesthetic technique was associated with a significant effect on outcome.[21, 123–126] In a recent study in dogs, Spahn et al. were unable to demonstrate an influence of anesthesia on the threshold of pacing-induced ischemia when comparing halothane, isoflurane, and fentanyl/midazolam anesthesia techniques.[127]

From a theoretical standpoint, regional anesthesia may be associated with potential benefits. Davis et al. and Klassen et al. have reported that epidural anesthesia is associated with an improved endocardial/epicardial blood flow ratio in the setting of experimentally produced coronary stenosis in animal models.[128, 129] In a study involving patients with coronary artery disease, Blomberg et al. reported that high thoracic epidural anesthesia (T1 to T6) was associated with an increase in the diameter of stenotic areas of coronary arteries, although coronary perfusion pressure, coronary blood flow distribution, myocardial oxygen consumption, and lactate extraction were not altered significantly.[130] Baron et al. and Saada et al. have reported conflicting data concerning the effects of lumbar epidural anesthesia on myocardial performance.[131, 132]

The difference in early reports demonstrating a significant difference in pulmonary parameters postoperatively may have been related more to the postoperative management of pain rather than to the intraoperative anesthetic technique. Adequate pain control postoperatively with the use of intrathecal narcotics, epidural analgesics, local anesthetics, regional field blocks, intrapleural thoracic local anesthetics, and patient-controlled anesthesia systems have all been reported with varying degrees of success.

A major potential risk of regional anesthesia is the development of an

TABLE 9.
Risk of Peridural Hematoma

Series	Complications/ Patients	Comments
Cunningham et al.[23]	0/100	None
Rao and El-Etr[133]	0/4011	Heparin dose: 2,600 ± 400 units every 6 hr. remove catheter when coagulation studies normal
Ruff and Dougherty[134]	5/342	Traumatic, on aspirin
Odoom and Sih[122]	0/1000	ACT* < 200 sec, no hemophilia, leukemia, or thrombocytopenia
Baron et al.[112]	0/912	Heparin dose to activated partial thromboplastin time 2.5 × normal
Dickman et al.[135]	2 cases	Thrombolysis therapy or on long-term heparin

*ACT = activated coagulation time.

epidural hematoma. A number of series are presented in Table 9. In Rao and El Etra's series, a total of 847 spinals and 3,164 epidurals were performed without any evidence of an epidural hematoma.[133] However, the authors cancelled surgery for 24 hours if blood was encountered during needle or catheter insertion, moderate doses of heparin were administered (2,600 ± 400 units every 6 hours), and the catheters were removed when coagulation studies approached baseline values. The risk of a peridural hematoma is a genuine concern and a number of authors have reported either a series or case reports of patients who have had peridural hematomas.[134, 135] In many of the cases presented, the patients have been on aspirin therapy, have had a traumatic needle or catheter insertion, were receiving heparin before the procedure, or had received thrombolytic therapy. It is imperative to observe the patient for signs and symptoms of a peridural hematoma, to evaluate the patient in an expeditious fashion, and decompress the spinal cord surgically if necessary.

Predicting Risk

Over the years, a number of authors have examined a variety of factors in an effort to be able to predict perioperative morbidity and mortality. The

TABLE 10.
Goldman Cardiac Risk Index*

Variable	Point Score
History	
Age > 70 yr	5
Preoperative myocardial infarction in previous 6 mo	10
Physical examination	
S3 gallop or jugular venous distention	11
Important valvular aortic stenosis	3
Electrocardiogram	
Rhythm other than sinus or PACs on last preoperative electrocardiogram	7
>5 premature ventricular contractions/min documented at any time before surgery	7
General status (any of the following)	3
$Po_2 < 60$ or $Pco_2 > 50$ mm Hg	
$K < 3.0$ or $HCO_3 < 20$ mEq/L	
Blood urea nitrogen > 50 or creatinine > 3.0 mg/dL	
Abnormal aspartate aminotransferase, signs of chronic liver disease or patient bedridden from noncardiac causes	
Operation	
Intraperitoneal, intrathoracic, or aortic operation	3
Emergency operation	4
Total possible points	53

*From Goldman L et al: *N Engl J Med* 29:845–850, 1977. Used by permission.

TABLE 11.
CRI vs. Dripps ASA*

Classification	No. of Patients	No or Minor Complications	Life-Threatening Complications
CRI			
Class I	537	532	4 (0.7%)
Class II	316	295	16 (5%)
Class III	130	112	15 (11%)
Class IV	18	4	4 (22%)
Dripps			
ASA I, II	537	527	7 (2%)
ASA III	323	302	13 (4%)
ASA IV	112	87	19 (17%)

*From Goldman et al: *N Engl J Med* 294:845–850, 1977. Used by permission.

Dripps ASA classification published in 1963 is one such system that is familiar to all anesthesiologists. Another familiar classification system is the cardiac risk index (CRI) published by Goldman et al. in 1977 (Table 10).[1] Of interest is the comparison in that paper between the CRI and the Dripps ASA classification with the same patients. A comparison of the data is presented in Table 11. From the data it would appear that the outcome in Dripps ASA I and ASA II patients combined is similar to that of the CRI class I patients, that ASA III patients resemble the CRI class II patients, and that ASA IV patients resemble the outcome of a combining of CRI class III and IV patients.

In 1980, Del Guercio and Cohn presented an evaluation of the Automated Physiologic Profile previously described by Cohn in 1975 (Fig 2).[136, 137] Patients are placed in one of four stages based on hemodynamic measurements and blood gas analysis performed prior to surgery. Of the 148 patients studied, 23% (34 patients) were classified as belonging to stage 4. Of these 34 patients, 7 underwent a lesser surgical procedure than

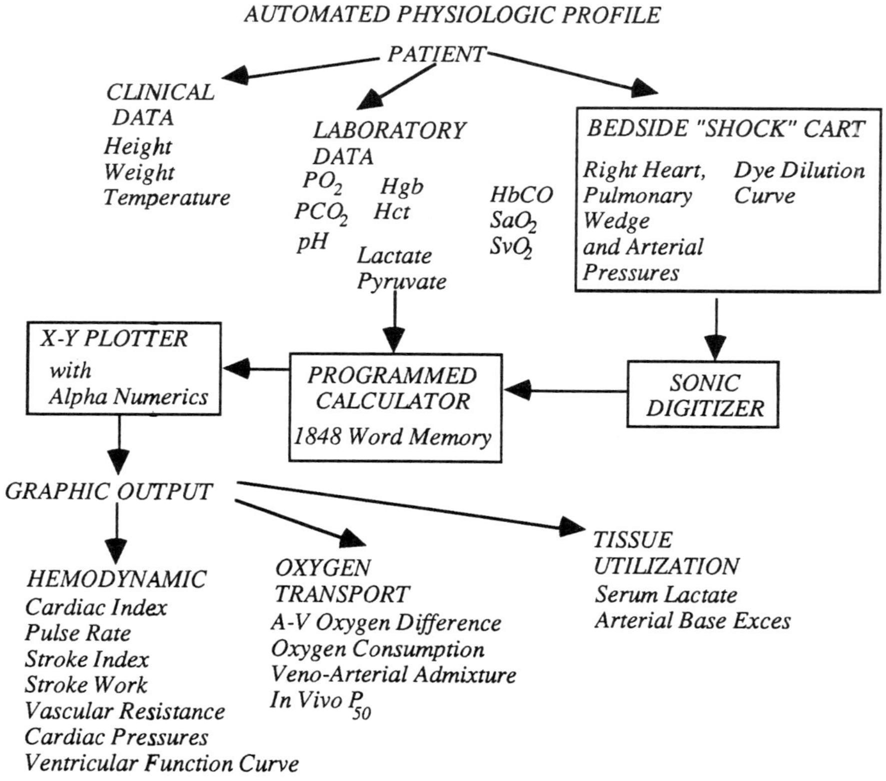

FIG 2.
Data obtained from automated physiologic profile. (From Cohn JD, Engler PE, Del Guercis LRM: *Crit Care Med* 3:52, 1975. Used by permission.)

TABLE 12.
Montreal Heart Institute Risk Factors*

Poor LV function (ejection fraction < 0.30 or LVEDP > 18 mm Hg)
CHF
Unstable angina or recent MI (<6 wk)
Age over 65
Severe obesity (body-mass index > 20)†
Repeat surgery
Emergency surgery
Other significant or uncontrolled systemic disturbances

*From Paiement B et al: *Can Anaesth Soc J* 30:61–68, 1983. Used by permission.
†Body mass index defined as weight (Kg)/height^2 (m).

TABLE 13.
Detsky Modified Cardiac Risk Index*

Variable	Point Score
Coronary artery disease	
Myocardial infarction ≤6 months	10
Myocardial infarction >6 months	5
Angina (Canadian cardiovascular society class)	
III	10
IV	20
Unstable angina <6 months	10
Alveolar pulmonary edema	
Within 1 wk	10
Ever	5
Valvular disease	
Suspected critical aortic stenosis	20
Dysrhythmia	
Rhythm other than sinus, with or without atrial ectopy	5
Presence of >5 PVCs/min at any time	5
Poor general medical status	5
Age >70 yr	5
Emergency surgical procedure	10

*From Detsky AS et al: *J Gen Intern Med* 1:211–219, 1986. Used by permission.

planned and all of these patients survived; in 19 patients, surgery was cancelled; but 8 patients in stage 4 underwent the proposed surgical procedure and all of these patients died. Multivariant discriminant analysis of data from the CASS was also published in 1980.[138] This was a cooperative study of 15 institutions, which examined 6,176 patients undergoing coronary artery bypass graft (CABG) between 1975 and 1978. Predictive variables for operative mortality were age, female sex, increased heart size, and congestive heart failure in addition to a left main artery stenosis ≥ 90%, marked wall motion abnormalities, rales, and an elevated LVEDP. With CASS data, the CASS principal investigators and their associates reported that CABG appeared not to prolong life nor to prevent a myocardial infarction in patients who were either asymptomatic or who had mild angina when compared to medical therapy during the 5-year period following angiography.[139]

The Montreal Heart Institute risk classification was published in 1983.[140] In this study of 500 open heart surgery patients, eight risk factors were identified (Table 12). Based on these factors patients were assigned to one of three groups: normal risk (no risk factors), increased risk (one risk factor), or high risk (more than one risk factor). The respective early mortality risk in these 500 patients was 0.4% in the normal risk group, 3.1% in the increased risk group, and 12.2% in the high risk group. Detsky et al. published a modified version of the cardiac risk index (Table 13).[27] Abnormal laboratory data such as renal function studies, electrolyte levels, and blood gas analyses are not accounted for in the Detsky et al. modified CRI. Greater emphasis is placed on the cardiac status, age, general health, and emergency nature of the surgery.

A potential shortcoming of any general risk factor index is the application of that index to a specific patient population or a specific set of surgical procedures. Jeffrey et al. reported that when the Goldman cardiac risk index was applied to 99 patients undergoing abdominal aortic procedures, the CRI underestimated the observed complication rate in this patient population (Table 14).[7]

In 1987, Eagle et al. published the results of their evaluation of 61 patients undergoing vascular surgery.[34] In this study, the authors evaluated various indices for validity of predicting complications in their patients (Table 15). The Goldman cardiac risk index, a prior myocardial infarction, and diabetes mellitus were not found to be predictable risk factors. Conversely, a history of CHF, the Dripps index, Q waves or nonspecific S-T wave changes on the ECG, and redistribution on a thallium scan were all found to be predictive. In a study of 30 patients requiring urgent or emergent vascular surgery within 6 weeks of a myocardial infarction, Rivers et al. reported a procedural mortality rate of 10% and a cardiac complication rate of 17%.[141] When comparing their observed complication rate of 33% in Goldman class IV patients to the predicted rate of 78%, the difference was attributed to monitoring and postoperative care. It would appear that no individual risk index will necessarily be able to accurately identify the po-

TABLE 14.
Jeffrey Data vs. Goldman CRI*

	Abdominal Aortic Patients		Goldman Group		
Class	**No. of Patients**	**Cardiac Complications**	**No. of Patients**	**Cardiac Complications**	***P***
1	56	4 (7%)	537	5 (1%)	.01
2	35	4 (11%)	316	21 (7%)	NS
3	8	3 (38%)	130	18 (14%)	NS
Total	99	11 (12%)	983	44 (4%)	.01

*From Jeffrey CC et al: *Anesthesiology* 58:462–464, 1983. Used by permission.

TABLE 15.
Eagle: Risk Predictors*

Clinical Descriptors	Cardiac Ischemic Event	No Cardiac Ischemic Event	*P*
Male	68 ± 8	64 ± 9	.2
Age yr (means + SD)	*n* = 8	*n* = 53	
History of angina	8 (100)	43 (81)	.2
Prior congestive heart failure	3 (38)	12 (27)	.3
Prior myocardial infarction	2 (25)	2 (4)	.02
Diabetes mellitus	4 (50)	13 (24)	.09
Q wave on ECG	2 (25)	4 (8)	.2
Nonspecific ST-T changes on ECG	5 F(63)	9 (17)	.01
Dripps-American Surgical Association index score	3.0	2.46	.04
Goldman index score	4.8 ± 2.8	4.5 ± 2.6	.3
Ischemic ECG changes during dipyridamole administration	2 (25)	5 (9)	.2
Chest pain during dipyridamole administration	3 (38)	5 (9)	.03
Fixed defect on thallium scan	6 (75)	27 (51)	.2
Reversible defect on thallium scan	8 (100)	10 (19)	<.001

*From Eagle KA et al: *JAMA* 257:2185–2189, 1987. Used by permission.

tential for perioperative cardiac or other complications in individualized patient or operation subsets.

Many patients now present for endovascular procedures such as balloon angioplasty, laser surgery, atherectomy, etc. Although many of these procedures are performed outside of the operating room and often are performed under sedation and local anesthesia, it is important that we have an understanding of the goals and potential risks in these various procedures.

Endovascular Surgery

Endovascular surgery began in the 1960s with the introduction of balloon angioplasty. This device has been both modified and redesigned and is now an integral part of the treatment of the patient with peripheral vascular disease. The concept of treating patients with vascular disease without the significant morbidity and mortality of surgery has resulted in the development of many devices that aid in treatment. Over the past several years, there has been an explosion of intravascular devices designed to manage peripheral vascular and coronary disease. The ability to treat vascular disease without significant operative intervention and achieve similar long-term results as with conventional surgical treatment has been the goal of all these devices. The initial wave of enthusiasm greeting these devices, however, has not been replaced with skepticism and cautious reappraisal as the long-term results of all these devices can only be termed disappointing. There is still some limited applicability for these devices and, more importantly, there is still a definite need for further investigation and refinement of these techniques since there is clearly a place for them in the future treatment of the patient with peripheral vascular disease.

The current armamentarium of the endovascular surgeon consists of several devices, including balloon angioplasty, angioscopy, atherectomy, and laser. In addition there are some new modalities currently being developed that will also be presented, including intravascular stents, intravascular ultrasound, and intravascular graft placement. The indications for use and the long-term results will be discussed as well as several new applications. Special intraoperative problems encountered with each of these will also be presented. These techniques have some applications in the current treatment of vascular disease and may have potential benefits in the future; however, it must be recognized that careful evaluation and investigation of all techniques are necessary to determine not only short-term results but long-term patency.

Angioplasty

Angioplasty was first introduced as a technique by Dotter in 1964 when he treated an elderly woman with gangrene who refused surgical intervention.[142] In 1965, Dotter modified this technique by employing a Fogarty embolectomy catheter to dilate an iliac artery lesion. Since those early interventions, many advances and modifications have occurred, resulting in the current technique of guide wire-directed balloon angioplasty with polyethylene balloons. These balloons allow the radial direction of forces, thus not permitting the force to be directed away from the primary lesions. Angioplasty was initially thought to function by compressing the atherosclerotic plaque, resulting in an increase in the diameter of the lumen. However, now it has been demonstrated that angioplasty functions by disrupting the plaque at its thinnest portion and dilating the underlying adventitia. After dilatation, the vessel will remodel with time. This results in a larger channel for flow.[143] The two most common complications of balloon angioplasty are intimal flaps, which can result in acute occlusion, and myointimal hyperplasia.

Angioplasty was originally a technique used in those situations in which the patient was deemed an unsuitable surgical candidate. However, with increasing experience, it has become a separate modality in the treatment of vascular disease. Indeed, it is now thought by some to be overutilized, especially in the patient who presents with minimal symptoms of claudication. The aggressive nature of the angiographers in the use of balloon dilatation is reflected in their patient selections. Spence et al. reported their indications for balloon dilatation as 81% for patients with claudication and 19% for those with rest pain.[144] This is the exact opposite numbers that are reported by most vascular surgeons, since nearly 80% of revascularizations are for limb-threatening ischemia. The indications for angioplasty should include: (1) intermittent claudication of sufficient severity that it adversely affects the patient's lifestyle; (2) pain at rest; (3) ischemic tissue changes including ulceration and gangrene; (4) impaired distal wound healing; and (5) simplification of surgical revascularization. Contraindications for balloon angioplasty include: (1) availability of a safer, simpler, less time-consuming or more effective surgical alternative; (2) distal embolization syndrome (blue toe syndrome) or deep ulcerations; (3) embolic occlusions; (4) long segments of diffuse disease; (5) long occlusions; and (6) acute thrombotic occlusions.[145] Misuse or inappropriate use of this modality can have catastrophic consequences. It should be especially noted that the presence of a lesion is not an indication for angioplasty.

Angioplasty can be performed as either a separate procedure in the radiology suite or it can be performed in the operating room either alone or in combination with a reconstructive procedure. If both angioplasty and surgical reconstruction are required to treat multilevel disease, it is usually best to perform the angioplasty several days prior to the operative procedure to determine the outcome of the balloon intervention. On occasion, however, it may be necessary to treat both lesions simultaneously since a lesion may not be recognized as hemodynamically significant until revascularization has been performed. In these situations, operative angioplasty may have to be performed. If a lesion is found at arteriography, the significance can be investigated with the measurement of a pressure gradient across the stenosis. If there is no gradient or the findings are equivocal, then further evaluation of the stenosis can be performed with the intraarterial administration of a vasodilator.[146] Occasionally, the patient will have significant outflow disease, which will cause the angiographic studies to be falsely negative, and only after revascularization will the gradient will be recognized. Evaluation of inflow lesions at surgery is equivalent to angiographic studies. Determination of the blood pressure across the stenosis can demonstrate whether or not the stenosis is significant. Again, if the initial pressure findings are somewhat equivocal, then a vasodilator can be administered to further determine its significance. If the stenosis is significant, then this lesion can be considered for balloon angioplasty.[147]

The long-term results from angioplasty indicate that in certain situations it has a significant benefit. However the variability of reporting initial technical success and long-term patency have clouded the data. Some reports do not include initial technical failures in their analysis of long-term patency. The initial failure rate of angioplasty has been reported to range from 5% for short segment iliac stenosis to 30% for significant femoral and popliteal disease.[148–150] Other studies only present the patients' symptoms and do not have any objective criteria on which to evaluate long-term patency. Tegtmeyer et al. had objective follow-up (i.e., ankle/brachial indices [ABIs] or measurement of pressure gradients) in only 39% of their patients.[148] This is especially interesting since the majority of angioplasty procedures are performed for claudication, which often improves only with an exercise program. The results of any balloon procedure should be confirmed with vascular laboratory evaluation. Diminishing ABIs or lessening of the flow within the vessel should be considered as an indication of a failing angioplasty and should be aggressively evaluated.

Even with these limitations in the reporting of data, there is a definite benefit of angioplasty in certain situations. The best results with angioplasty occur in the larger arteries. Angioplasty of limited iliac lesions has the best initial success and long-term patency reports. Several studies indicate that the initial technical success rate is 90% to 95% with 1-, 3-, and 5-year patency rates of 90%, 80%, and 60%, respectively.[148, 149, 151] Angioplasty also has been shown to have a benefit in superficial femoral artery disease, although the results are not as good as those in iliac arteries. The initial success rate is usually 80% to 85% and the 1-, 3-, and 5-year patency rates are 75%, 65%, and 45%, respectively.[152, 153] Balloon dilatation has been attempted in the tibial vessels with some success. Veith et al. reported on a series of 53 patients who had a technical success rate of 72%; however, long-term patency was not reported.[154] This modality is technically feasible but should only be utilized in very isolated cases until more information is available.

The morbidity rate of balloon angioplasty generally has been stated to range from 5% to 15%, with a mortality rate of approximately 1% to 2%. It is generally accepted that this rate decreases with the increasing experience of the interventionalist. The most common complication is that of groin hematoma or a pseudoaneurysm of the entry vessel. The more significant complications include embolization, thrombosis, and vessel rupture. Fortunately, these complications occur less frequently. However a recent report suggests that the complication rate may be as high as 26% with a 13% incidence of significant complications.[155] These complications can necessitate either urgent or emergent surgery, often in an unstable patient or a patient that was deemed as unsuitable for surgical intervention. It must always be recognized that a patient who is being evaluated for angioplasty must also be evaluated as a potential surgical candidate since the failed interventional procedure may lead to surgery. Obviously, angioplasty can be a double-edged sword.

Angioscopy

Direct visualization of the arterial tree has the potential to offer significant advantages in the treatment of arterial disease. The development of a small diameter angioscope, which has good resolution, has increased the attrac-

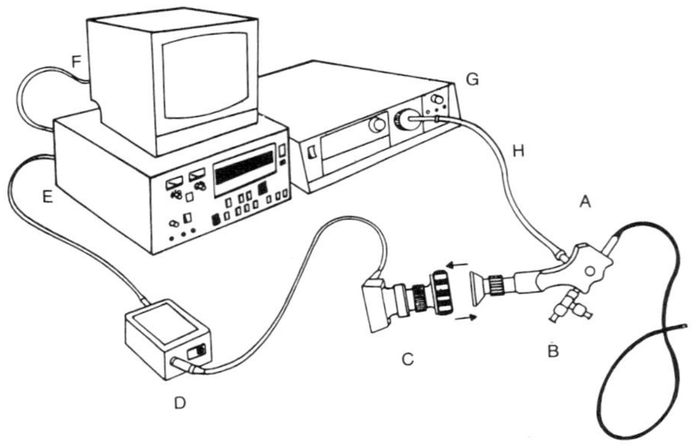

FIG 3.
Components of an angioscopic system: *A,* angioscope; *B,* irrigation port; *C,* miniature camera; *D,* camera control unit; *E,* videocassette recorder; *F,* monitor; *G,* light source, *H,* light source cable. (From Hernandez JJ, Quinones-Baldrich WJ: Angioscopy: Essential, desirable, and optional components. In Moore WS, Ahn SS, editors: *Endovascular surgery.* Philadelphia, 1989, Saunders. Used by permission.)

tiveness of intraoperative angioscopy. The performance of angioscopy requires three essential components: (1) the angioscope; (2) the light source; and (3) an irrigation system (Fig 3). Angioscopy has been found to be useful in thrombectomies, inspection of anastomoses, and in the performance of the in-situ bypass.[156–158] In addition, many other possible uses for angioscopy currently are being investigated.

Angioscopes are currently available either as disposable or reusable instruments. The disposable angioscopes offer the potential for less expensive equipment. However, the reusable angioscopes have better optics and have some steering capabilities. The only major limitations to the reusable angioscopes are the significant loss of time associated with damage to the instruments and the cost of the system, which can be as much as $50,000. Angioscopes have been reduced in size to such an extent that now almost all vascular procedures are accessible for evaluation. The currently available angioscopes can usually be coupled to video display screens, which are in use in most operating theaters. Each system, however, requires a light source that is usually recommended by the manufacturer and can be a significant expense. The lack of an irrigation system, which will be discussed in somewhat more detail in the complication section, was initially a major problem with angioscopy since a significant volume of fluid was administered to the patient during the procedure. Currently, there are several systems available that regulate the administration of fluid during angioscopy.

Angioscopy is most often performed at surgery. The technique involves the isolation of the vessel that has been selected for the introduction of the angioscope. Control of the normal blood flow can be accomplished in one of two ways. In evaluating a more proximal lesion, a balloon occlusion catheter can be introduced that will obstruct the inflow.[17] The irrigation system will then control collateral flow. Distal evaluation can be accomplished with occlusion of the inflow with standard vascular clamps and then distal visualization with the irrigation system to control the collateral flow provided by side branches. The patient requires continual close monitoring with special attention to the length of ischemia time and the amount of fluid administered.

The use of angioscopy in the performance of a femoral distal in-situ bypass has been described well. Miller et al. described their experience with angioscopy and found a significant difference between blind valvulectomy and angioscopically directed valve lysis.[159] A study by Gilbertson et al. states that angioscopy was superior to intraoperative angiography in determining technical problems with the graft.[160] Recently, a cooperative study reported its results with angioscopy to both lyse the valves and occlude the side branches during the performance of the in-situ bypass, thus obviating the long flap incision.[161] The major limitation was the length of time required for the procedure and the inability to occlude the smaller branches. While this is currently investigational, if perfected it could offer significant advantages over the current technique. In addition to the lysis of the valves and the inspection of the vein, the angioscope allows the surgeon to visualize the distal anastomosis evaluating it for technical problems.

Angioscopy also has significant advantages during thrombectomies and embolectomies. Intraoperative arteriograms may miss vessel injuries, such as intimal tears or dissections. Often arteriography cannot depict the presence of residual thrombus. Angioscopy can demonstrate if the procedure has been adequate and also allows evaluation for distal embolization. It can give additional information about significant atherosclerotic disease or myointimal hyperplasia, which will result in early failure of any thrombectomy. Techniques are currently being developed that will allow the endovascular treatment of lesions found at angioscopy.[162]

Angioscopy can depict any anastomosis, which can determine the technical adequacy of the repair. Its use in in-situ grafting has already been described. It also has been used in aortoiliac and aortofemoral grafting. Other less frequent locations for its use include the renal arteries after transaortic renal artery endarterectomy and carotid evaluation following carotid endarterectomy.[163, 164] These experiences have been limited, and at this time should be considered investigational. However, as the experience increases, there will be more and more utilization of the angioscope.

Complications from angioscopy have been relatively minor. To maintain a bloodless field, fluids were originally administered under pressure through the angioscope. This was accomplished by delivering intravenous fluids into the vascular tree with a pressure bag. Early complications with angioscopy were mostly related to the significant volume administered to the patient during the procedure, resulting in a number of patients developing pulmonary edema. Currently, the development of irrigation systems allows delivery of minimal fluids while maintaining a clear vascular field. Van Steigman et al. reported an average of 277 mL for an angioscopic procedure with a range of 100 to 750 mL.[165] A second potential complication results from the passage of the angioscope, which can cause significant vessel injury. There is a direct relationship between the size of the vessel and the potential for injury with the smaller vessels being more susceptible to injury. Damage to the endothelium can also occur and results in a reduction of prostacyclin production. This was demonstrated by Hashizume et al.[166] Repeated traumatic passages of the angioscope resulted in a significant reduction in the production of prostacyclin, which required 3 to 4 weeks for recovery. There have also been reports of remote organ injury resulting from ischemia time to perform the procedure and distal embolization. However, with careful technique, the overall incidence of injury continues to be remarkably low.[167]

Angioscopy has potential to be of great benefit in the evaluation and treatment of peripheral vascular disease. The ability to directly visualize the vascular system allows for the recognition of technical problems before they have the opportunity to induce thrombosis. It determines the significance of both proximal and distal disease to better assist in the determination of the best operative therapy. However, repeated passage of the angioscope may induce endothelial damage, which could possibly initiate either aggressive atherosclerosis or neointimal hyperplasia. Angioscopy has significant potential but the true value of this technique will require long-term evaluation.

Atherectomy

The ability to mechanically remove atherosclerotic plaque without operative intervention is the ultimate goal of all atherectomy devices. Currently this procedure is performed in either the radiology suite or the operating room by either the interventional radiologist, the cardiologist, or the vascular surgeon. There are four catheters available for clinical use: (1) the Simpson Atherocath (Devices for Vascular Intervention, Inc.); (2) the Kensey catheter; (3) the Auth Rotablator (Heart Technology, Inc.); and (4) the transluminal endarterectomy catheter (TEC [Interventional Technologies, Inc.]). All four catheters remove the atherosclerotic plaque from the vessel wall, the difference being the technique of removal and the handling of the plaque after it is removed.

The only system currently in widespread use is the Simpson atherocath, which has both a peripheral and coronary capability. It has been used in both the treatment of stenotic lesions and occlusions. As with all of the endovascular devices, larger vessels achieve a better long-term result. The Simpson therocath has a side-biting channel. The atherectomy catheter can be introduced either percutaneously or with direct vessel vision in the operating room; however, the procedure requires fluoroscopy. Catheter size ranges from 4 F to 11 F. The Simpson atherocath either has a guide wire attached to the distal end or can be passed over a guide wire. The plaque is traversed and the open port of the Simpson atherocath approximated to the most significant lesion. The catheter position is maintained by

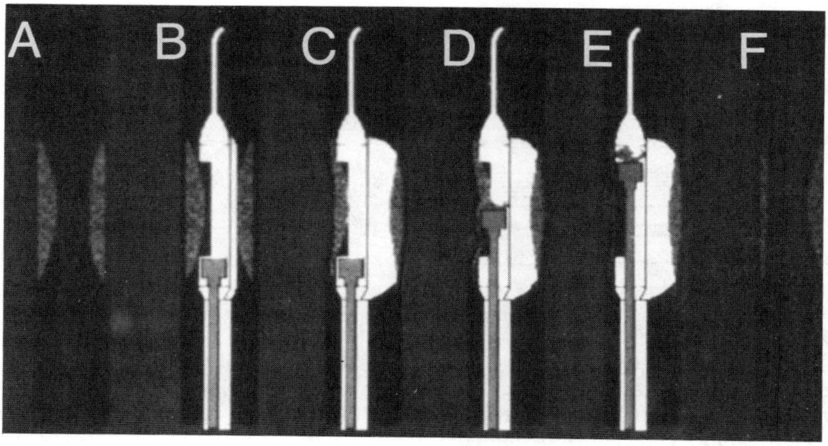

FIG 4.
The Simpson Atherocath and the atherectomy procedure. *A,* The lesion prior to passage of the catheter. *B,* The catheter passed across the lesion. *C,* The balloon inflated to maintain the catheter's position. *D,* The cutter is advanced. *E,* The specimen is trapped in the housing. *F,* The post-atherectomy vessel demonstrating improvement in the diameter of the vascular channel. (From Hinohara T et al: Transluminal atherectomy: The Simpson atherectomy catheter. In Moore WS, Ahn SS, editors: *Endovascular surgery.* Philadelphia, 1989, Saunders. Used by permission.)

inflation of the balloon and the atherocath is engaged serially, removing small sections of plaque (Fig 4). This results in the removal of significant plaque and balloon dilatation of the vessel. Early results have demonstrated the technical ability of this catheter with initial success rates of 90%.[168] Short-term results have also been promising with minimal 6 month restenosis. A recent study also presented a 1-year patency rate of more than 85%; however, these results are in contrast with another study that states that at 1 year the outcome is somewhat less promising since 25% of patients require either surgery or repeat atherectomy.[169, 170] Again, the major problem with all these studies is the selection of patients since the majority are undergoing these procedures for claudication.[171]

The second atherectomy device is the Kensey catheter (Fig 5). Due to several technical problems, the system currently has had only limited clinical use. This is a rotational catheter, which does not require a guide wire system. This offers the advantage of functioning in an obstructed blood vessel. The atherectomy device is currently used in an operative theater only and comes in 5-F and 8-F catheters. The catheter system requires fluoroscopy to evaluate the progress of the procedure and to evaluate outcome. The Kensey catheter functions as a high-speed rotational catheter, reaching speeds of 100,000 rpm. This obliterates the plaque as it opens the channel, hopefully reducing the risk of distal embolization. A recent study indicated that embolization did not occur early in clinical trials.[172] The high rotational speed also produces significant heat and pressure

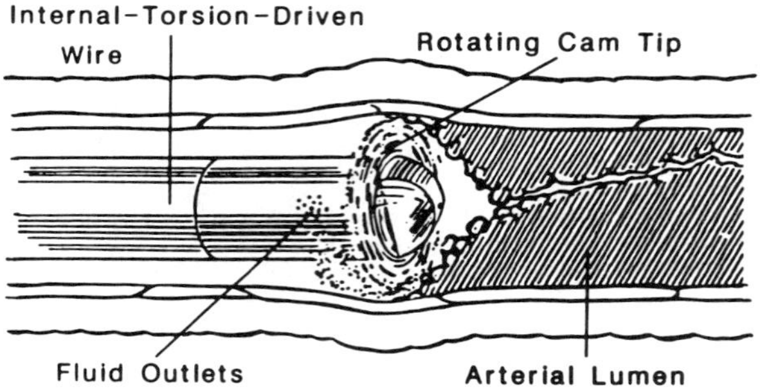

FIG 5.
The Kensey atherectomy catheter. This is a rotational catheter that will seek out the path of least resistance, tracking from the normal lumen to the more diseased lumen. Without the benefit of the guide wire, it can be seen why the major complication of this catheter is perforation. (From Snyder SO Jr et al: *J Vasc Surg* 8:541–543, 1988. Used by permission.)

within the lumen of the vessel, which can also result in vessel dilatation. The major complication of the procedure has been a significant rate of perforation, which has required either termination of the procedure or operative intervention. A limited series of patients reported on by Snyder et al. demonstrated only a 61% (14/23) initial success rate with the majority of failures caused by perforation.[173] A recent report on the Kensey catheter states that there was only a 37% patency rate at 19 months and the necessity of surgical intervention was not altered.[174]

The Auth Rotoblator is also a high-speed rotational atherectomy device. The major difference is a guide wire capability, which appears to reduce the perforation rate. The design is a high-speed rotational burr imbedded with multiple diamond chips (Fig 6). This drill achieves a rotational speed of 100,000 to 200,000 rpm. The basic tenant is that the plaque will be reduced to such small particles that there will be no distal embolization. Unfortunately, this has not been the case since the major complicating factor with the rotoblator has been the occurrence of distal emboli.[175] A recent report on an animal model, however, suggests that the pattern of distal embolization may not differ much than what occurs following angioplasty.[176] The potential therapeutic use of the Auth Rotoblator still awaits the results of significant clinical trials. Although this device has been recently approved for use, it must still be regarded as investigational.

The TEC is also a rotational system but functions at a much lower speed (750 rpm). Larger segments of debris are formed; however, this system is designed to remove the plaque. The catheter is connected to a vacuum chamber, which removes the debris as it is being formed. This system is designed in 5F through 9F sizes, allowing access to all vessels from the iliac arteries to the infrapopliteal arteries. The TEC can be used alone or in conjunction with balloon angioplasty. There are minimal clinical data available, but early clinical trials in a small sample population indicate that the system

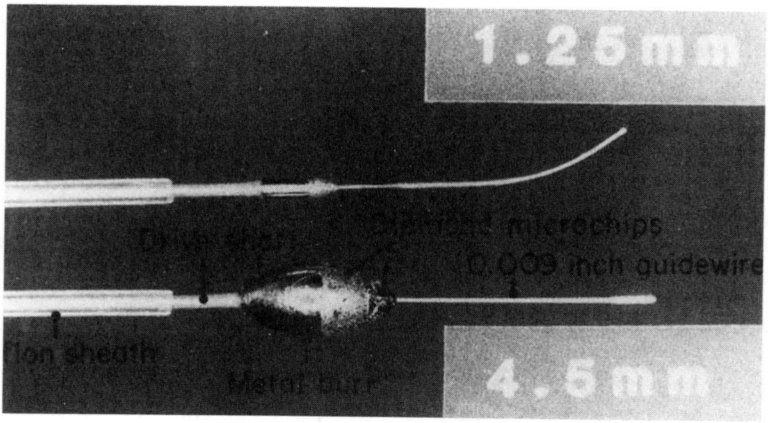

FIG 6.
The Rotablator. Shown are the 1.25-mm and the 4.5-mm atherectomy catheters. Notice the diamond microchips embedded into the distal portion of the 4.5 burr. (From Ahn SS: The rotablator—high-speed rotary atherectomy: Indications, technique, results, and complications. In Moore WS, Ahn SS, editors: *Endovascular surgery*. Philadelphia, 1989, Saunders. Used by permission.)

is technically able to open both stenosis and short occlusions; however, 6-month patency rates demonstrate 20% restenosis (Sketch et al., personal communication, 1990). As with the Auth Rotablator, final determination of the clinical value of the TEC will depend on long-term clinical trials in a much larger patient population.

The ability to mechanically remove atherosclerotic plaque with a minimally invasive technique could potentially offer significant benefit to the patient with vascular disease. These patients tend to have a multitude of medical problems and are at increased risk for surgical intervention. However, the currently available atherectomy devices have not been the salvation that was initially promised. The long-term results are not much better than those with balloon angioplasty. In addition, with the risk of distal embolization, perforation, and subsequent neointimal hyperplasia, they may actually worsen the lesion or convert a stable situation into one that requires surgical intervention. The true use of these instruments in the treatment of vascular surgery demands extended clinical trials with excellent objective long-term patency evaluation.

Laser

The word laser is actually an acronym for *l*ight *a*mplification by the *s*timulated *e*mission of *r*adiation. Laser surgery was initially presented as a technique to open completely obstructed blood vessels without surgery; that is, surgery without scalpels. This concept was presented to the public, prior to any significant long-term clinical trials, as a treatment for significant peripheral vascular disease without conventional surgical intervention. The initial studies suggested that the technique was technically feasible and based on those data, and the significant marketing potential, every facility in the United States rushed to become laser-capable. Unfortunately, studies with long-term patency reports suggest that laser does not add anything to the current treatment of atherosclerosis and that in some instances, it may actually accelerate the process. Indeed, after the initial wave of enthusiasm for laser with its intense marketing campaign, endovascular laser surgery is undergoing careful critical reappraisal.

The majority of lasers now available utilizes thermal energy, the primary types being the argon laser, the CO_2 laser, and the yttrium-aluminum-garnet crystal laser. These instruments utilize laser energy either directly on the lesion or to heat a metal probe that is directed at the lesion. This energy causes either disintegration of the structure of the plaque or ablation of the plaque. The heat generated by the laser can range from 60°C to several hundred degrees centigrade. Initially these catheters were associated with a rather significant perforation rate and the channel that was created was limited.[177, 178] These systems now have been coupled with balloon angioplasty (laser-assisted balloon angioplasty [LABA] to reduce the energy required to open the vessel and to increase the lumen of the vessel. This should decrease the perforation rate and increase the long-term patency results. As the technique improves, the perforation rate should decrease, but a recent report indicated that perforation still occurred in 33% of their procedures.[179] The long-term patency results with these techniques have also been disappointing.[174, 180, 181] Most studies fail to show any benefit over balloon angioplasty. Recent reports document less than a 50% patency rate at 12 months.[182] Even those studies that support the use of laser have significant problems. A recent multicenter trial reported that the major indication for the procedure is claudication and the long-term results are no better than those with balloon angioplasty.[183] An overall review of the literature reveals that the major complication rate of LABA continues to be 10%, and only 50% to 60% or less of the arteries that were successfully opened remained open past 1 year.[174, 177–184] The majority of the failures require surgery; thus, on one aspect the use of laser therapy may have actually increased the need for surgical intervention.

Recent developments in laser technology include the clinical trials of the excited dimer (Excimer) laser and the MCM Smart laser. The Excimer laser employs short duration, high energy pulses of ultraviolet light, which results in tissue ablation with minimal thermal energy. The hope of this laser is that the significant problems encountered with the high energy, and thus heat, generated from thermal probes would be eliminated. Two recent clinical studies have not demonstrated a significant advantage.[185, 186] In the study by McCarthy et al., there was only a 58% initial technical success rate and only a 47% 9-month patency rate of those arteries that were able to be canalized. The MCM smart laser, in simplistic form, is designed to recognize atherosclerotic disease through spectroscopy and then utilize an argon probe to destroy the atherosclerotic plaque. This technique has much promise but early results continue to have significant technical complications.[187]

The use of laser to remove atherosclerotic plaque has some very attractive potential. Unfortunately, the initial reports have been somewhat disappointing. The initial marketing campaign with laser surgery has now given way to some very sobering prospective studies, which suggest that the long-term patency rates of laser cases may not be comparable to those of simple balloon angioplasty. It has been suggested that laser may cause an aggressive atherosclerotic process in the vessel after treatment. Clearly, more significant work with laser must be performed before laser therapy becomes a significant part of the treatment of atherosclerotic peripheral vascular disease.

Intravascular Stents

Significant recurrent atherosclerotic disease can occur either immediately after or very shortly after an interventional procedure. To prevent an acute or short-term occlusion, intravascular stents were developed to maintain immediate patency after treatment. Currently, there are several stents beginning clinical investigation. The Palmaz stent is placed via an angioplasty balloon. The stent/catheter apparatus is positioned with fluoroscopic control, and the stent is fixed into position by expansion of the balloon. The original study described improvement in a small patient population with a follow-up period of only 6 to 12 months. Fourteen of the patients in this series were treated for claudication and only one for threatened limb loss.[188] This paper did not address the question of neointimal hyperplasia. Another early report indicates that the placement of the stents in the iliac artery position is technically feasible and that early patency results are adequate.[189] However, again, the major problem with stent placement continues to be the severe neointimal hyperplasia they incite; thus, long-term patency still remains a critical issue.

Another type of stent is the self-expanding stent.[190] The Wallstent represents this type of self-expandable stent. The Wallstent has been used extensively in Europe and a recent study from Germany reported on the use of the stent in both iliac arteries and the superficial femoral arteries. Again early reports show good results but severe neointimal hyperplasia occurred in 14%, resulting in further treatment.[191] In another study, Bertrand et al., using the Medivent stent, reported a 67% incidence of restenosis over 2 years.[192] Also available are thermal expansions stents, which are extremely pliable at room temperature but revert to their original configuration. The nitinol stent, composed of an alloy of nickel and tantalum, functions in this manner. The major problem continues to be significant neointimal hyperplasia.[193]

Stents have also been used in venous obstruction. Recent developments also include the biodegradable stent and stents that have been endothelial-seeded.[193] Both of these techniques are an attempt to manage the significant problem of neointimal hyperplasia; however, minimal data on their use are currently available. Intravascular stents may have significant use in the future management of peripheral vascular disease; however, the overall benefit will not be achieved until the significant problem of neointimal hyperplasia is resolved.

Intravascular Ultrasound

The ability to visualize the internal aspect of both arteries and veins and to determine the presence and absence of lesions has been the driving force behind the development of intravascular ultrasound (IVS).[194–196] IVS incorporates small ultrasonic transducers on the tips of catheters. This permits a cylindrical phased array in the vessel. IVS has been demonstrated to be superior to single plane angiography in the evaluation of the vascular system.[197] Its ability to depict defects and vessel diameter is equivalent to that of angioscopy. Several recent studies have presented potential uses for this device. Neville et al. reported on an experimental model in which IVS was successful in the treatment of arterial intimal defects.[198] Cayvelle et al. utilized IVS in monitoring intravascular stent placement.[199] Several authors have reported on the use of IVS in venous disease, specifically in determining the level of vena cava occlusion.[200, 201] The major difficulty with IVS at present is that the small size of the catheter, and thus the transducer, requires a fairly high frequency probe. This has resulted in some problems with image distortion.[202] Intravascular ultrasound may have some definite therapeutic advantages over some currently available techniques in the endovascular surgery management of peripheral vascular disease; however, significant investigation is still required.

Percutaneous Intravascular Graft Placement

Early experimental studies currently are being performed to determine if abdominal aortic aneurysms can be treated with percutaneous intravascular graft placement. This technique involves placing a graft through a femoral catheter and expanding it via a balloon.[203] The graft is then stabilized with the placement of stents into the aortic wall. This technique has been demonstrated successfully in the animal model and recently a series was reported from Brazil.[204] Five patients were treated, four of whom had successful placement of a graft, the fifth requiring standard repair since the graft was placed in the incorrect position. No other significant problems developed, demonstrating the technical feasibility of the technique. The ability to treat aneurysmal disease in this fashion would eliminate the need for surgery, reducing the morbidity and mortality associated with the disease and the surgical treatment, it is hoped. This technique still requires further investigation, including long-term follow-up.

Summary

The concept of managing peripheral vascular disease without surgery is very attractive. Unfortunately, many of the new modalities never achieved their initial promise. Angioplasty has demonstrated significant benefit in the management of isolated iliac artery stenosis and isolated superficial femoral artery stenosis. However, atherectomy and laser have not had the initial overwhelming benefit that was hoped for. In fact in several studies, these instruments have actually worsened the disease process, sometimes resulting in urgent surgical intervention. Many of these devices were rushed into the market due to commercial pressure rather than for scientific value. The results from the use of these instruments are now demonstrating that there are some significant problems that must be addressed. There is a role for endovascular surgery, but it will take additional prospective clinical trials to determine what that role will be. The outcome must not only consider who was helped; that is, the percentage of patients with claudication who improved and the limb salvage rate, but the number of patients who experienced a significant worsening of their disease state due to the noninvasive intervention. A procedure cannot be deemed successful if it converts a significant number of patients with stable claudication into patients who require operative intervention. The long-term results, including morbidity and mortality of the procedure, must be compared to the results obtained surgically to determine if there is a clear benefit of use of these procedures over surgery. It is imperative that the development of new techniques and the utilization of these techniques be removed from the realm of marketing and studied in well-designed clinical trials.

References

1. Goldman L et al: Multifactorial index of cardiac risk in non-cardiac surgical procedures. *N Engl J Med* 297:845–850, 1977.
2. Goldman L: Multifactorial index of cardiac risk in non-cardiac surgery: Ten-year status report. *J Cardiothorac Anesth* 1:237–244, 1987.
3. Eagle KA et al: Combining clinical and thallium data optimizes preoperative assessment of cardiac risk before major vascular surgery. *Ann Intern Med* 110:859–866, 1989.
4. Logue RB, Kaplan JA: The cardiac patient and noncardiac surgery. *Curr Probl Cardiol* 7:1–49, 1982.
5. Roizen MF, Sohn YJ, Stoney RJ: Intraoperative management of the patient requiring supraceliac aortic occlusion. In Wilson SE et al, editors: *Vascular surgery. Principals and practice.* New York, 1987, McGraw-Hill, pp 312–321.
6. Diehl JT et al: Complications of abdominal aortic reconstruction: Analysis of perioperative risk factors in 557 patients. *Ann Surg* 197:49–56, 1983.
7. Jeffrey CC et al: A prospective evaluation of cardiac risk. *Anesthesiology* 58:462–464, 1983.
8. Hertzer NR et al: Coronary artery disease in peripheral vascular patients: A classification of 100 coronary angiograms and results of surgical management. *Ann Surg* 199:223–233, 1984.
9. Raby KE et al: Correlation between preoperative ischemia and major cardiac events after peripheral vascular surgery. *N Engl J Med* 321:1296–1300, 1989.

10. Rao TLK, Jacobs KG, El-Etr AA: Reinfarction following anesthesia in patients with myocardial infarction. *Anesthesiology* 59:499–505, 1983.
11. Gotto AM, Farmer JA: Risk factors for coronary artery disease. In Braunwald E, editor: *Heart disease*. Philadelphia, 1988, Saunders, p 1153.
12. Bedford RF, Feinstein B: Hospital admission blood pressure, a predictor for hypertension following endotracheal intubation. *Anesth Analg* 59:357–370, 1980.
13. Hartford M et al: Cardiovascular and renal effects of long-term antihypertensive treatment. *JAMA* 259:2553–2557, 1988.
14. Stone JG et al: Myocardial ischemia in untreated hypertensive patients: Effect of a single small dose of a beta-adrenergic blocking agent. *Anesthesiology* 68:495–500, 1988.
15. Mangano DT: Assessment of risk for cardiac and noncardiac surgical procedures. In Duke PC, editor: myocardial ischemia and performance. *Anesthesiology Clin North Am* 9:521–552, 1991.
16. Goldman L et al: Cardiac risk and complications in noncardiac surgery. *Medicine* 57:357–370, 1978.
17. Steen PA, Tinker JH, Tarhan S: Myocardial reinfarction after anesthesia and surgery. *JAMA* 239:2566–2570, 1978.
18. Tarhan S et al: Myocardial infarction after general anesthesia. *JAMA* 220:1451–1454, 1972.
19. Von Knorring JV: Postoperative myocardial infarction: A prospective study in high-risk group of surgical patients. *Surgery* 90:55–60, 1981.
20. Rivers SP et al: Safety of peripheral vascular surgery after recent acute myocardial infarction. *J Vasc Surg* 11:70–76, 1990.
21. Shah KB et al: Reevaluation of perioperative myocardial infarction in patients with prior myocardial infarction undergoing noncardiac operations. *Anesth Analg* 71:231–235, 1990.
22. Domaingue CM, Davies MJ, Cronin DK: Cardiovascular risk factors in patients for vascular surgery. *Anesth Intensive Care* 10:324–327, 1982.
23. Cunningham FO, Egan JM, Ianahara T: Continuous epidural analgesia in abdominal vascular surgery—A review of 100 consecutive cases. *Am J Surg* 139:624–627, 1980.
24. Schulze RA Jr et al: Ventricular arrhythmias in the late hospital phase of acute myocardial infarction: Relation to left ventricular function detected by gated cardiac blood pool scanning. *Circulation* 52:1006–1011, 1975.
25. Schulze RA Jr, Strauss HW, Pitt B: Sudden death in the year following myocardial infarction: Relation to ventricular premature contractions in the late hospital phase and left ventricular ejection fraction. *Am J Med* 62:192–199, 1977.
26. Pasternack PF et al: The value of silent myocardial ischemia monitoring in the prediction of perioperative myocardial infarction in patients undergoing peripheral vascular surgery. *J Vasc Surg* 10:617–625, 1989.
27. Detsky AS et al: Predicting cardiac complications in patients undergoing noncardiac surgery. *J Gen Intern Med* 1:211–219, 1986.
28. Boucher CA et al: Determination of cardiac risk by dipyridamole-thallium imaging before peripheral vascular surgery. *N Engl J Med* 312:389–394, 1985.
29. Mangano DT et al: Dipyridamole-thallium—201 scintigraphy as a preoperative screening test, a reexamination of its predictive value. *Circulation* 84:493–502, 1991.
30. Cutler BS et al: Applicability and interpretation of electrocardiographic stress

testing in patients with peripheral vascular disease. *Am J Surg* 141:501–506, 1981.
31. McPhail N et al: The use of preoperative exercise testing to predict cardiac complications after arterial reconstruction. *J Vasc Surg* 7:60–68, 1988.
32. Gerson MC et al: Cardiac prognosis in noncardiac geriatric surgery. *Ann Intern Med* 103:832–837, 1985.
33. Leppo J et al: Noninvasive evaluation of cardiac risk before elective vascular surgery. *J Am Coll Cardiol* 9:269–276, 1987.
34. Eagle KA et al: Dipyridamole-thallium scanning in patients undergoing vascular surgery. *JAMA* 257:2185–2189, 1987.
35. Lane SE et al: Predictive value of quantitative dipyridamole-thallium scintigraphy in assessing cardiovascular risk after vascular surgery in diabetes mellitus. *Am J Cardiol* 64:1275–1279, 1989.
36. Marwick TH, Underwood DA: Dipyridamole-thallium imaging may not be a reliable screening test for coronary artery disease in patients undergoing vascular surgery. *Clin Cardiol* 13:14–18, 1990.
37. Cambria RP et al: The impact of selective use of dipyridomole-thallium scans and surgical factors on the current morbidity of aortic surgery. *J Vasc Surg* 15:43–51, 1992.
38. Younis LT et al: Prognostic importance of silent myocardial ischemia detected by intravenous dipyridamole-thallium myocardial imaging in asymptomatic patients with coronary artery disease. *J Am Coll Cardiol* 14:1635–1641, 1989.
39. Hertzer NR et al: Routine coronary angiography prior to elective aortic reconstruction: Results of a selective myocardial revascularization in patients with peripheral vascular disease. *Arch Surg* 114:1336–1344, 1979.
40. Beven EG: Routine coronary angiography in patients undergoing surgery for abdominal aortic aneurysm and lower extremity occlusive disease. *J Vasc Surg* 3:682–684, 1986.
41. Leppo J et al: Thallium-201 myocardial scintigraphy in patients with triple-vessel disease and ischemic exercise stress tests. *Circulation* 59:714–721, 1979.
42. Crawford E et al: Graft replacement of aneurysm in descending thoracic aorta: Results without bypass or shunting. *Surgery* 89:73–85, 1981.
43. Carlson DE, Karp RB, Kouchoukos NT: Surgical treatment of aneurysms of the descending thoracic aorta: An analysis of 85 patients. *Ann Thorac Surg* 35:58–69, 1983.
44. Najafi H et al: Descending aortic aneurysmectomy without adjuncts to avoid ischemia. *Ann Thorac Surg* 30:326–335, 1980.
45. Alpert RA et al: Intraoperative urinary output does not predict postoperative renal function in patients undergoing abdominal aortic revascularization. *Surgery* 95:707–711, 1984.
46. Gornick CC Jr, Kjellstrand CM: Acute renal failure complicating aortic aneurysm surgery. *Nephron* 35:145–157, 1983.
47. Gelman S et al: Regional blood flow during cross-clamping of the thoracic aorta and infusion of sodium nitroprusside. *J Thorac Cardiovasc Surg* 85:287–291, 1983.
48. Gamulin Z et al: Effects of infrarenal aortic cross-clamping on renal hemodynamics in humans. *Anesthesiology* 61:394–399, 1984.
49. Hollier L et al: Thoracoabdominal aortic aneurysm repair—analysis of postoperative morbidity. *Arch Surg* 123:871–875, 1988.

50. Marquez JM et al: Renal function and cardiovascular responses during positive airway pressure. *Anesthesiology* 50:393–398, 1979.
51. Cousins MJ et al: Metabolism and renal effects of enflurane in man. *Anesthesiology* 44:44–53, 1976.
52. Gellman S, Fowler KC, Smith LR: Regional blood flow during isoflurane and halothane anesthesia. *Anesth Analg* 63:557–565, 1984.
53. Hunter JM, Jones RS, Utting JE: Effect of anaesthesia with nitrous oxide in oxygen and fentanyl on renal function in the artificially ventilated dog. *Br J Anaesth* 52:343–348, 1980.
54. Priano LL: Effects of high-dose fentanyl on renal hemodynamics in conscious dogs. *Can Anaesth Soc J* 30:10–18, 1983.
55. Merin RG et al: Comparison of the effects of isoflurane and desflurane on cardiovascular dynamics and regional blood flow in the chronically instrumented dog. *Anesthesiology* 74:568–574, 1991.
56. Seguro AC et al: Effect of potassium depletion on ischemic renal failure. *Nephron* 51:350–354, 1989.
57. Hughes JM et al: Diuresis and natriuresis during continuous dopamine-1 receptor stimulation. *Hypertension* 11:1–69, 1988.
58. Elliott WJ et al: Renal and hemodynamic effects of intravenous fenoldopam versus nitroprusside in severe hypertension. *Circulation* 81:970–977, 1990.
59. Russell JD, Churchill DN: Calcium antagonists and acute renal failure. *Am J Med* 87:306–315, 1989.
60. Loutzenhiser RD, Epstein M: Renal hemodynamic effects of calcium antagonists. *Am J Med* 82:23–28, 1987.
61. Ratych RE, Bulkley GB: Free radical medicated post ischemic reperfusion injury in the kidney. *J Free Radicals Biol Med* 2:311–319, 1986.
62. Kaufman RP et al: Inhibition of thromboxane (Tx) synthesis by free radical scavengers. *J Trauma* 28:458–564, 1988.
63. Griffiths IR et al: Spinal cord compression and blood flow. *Neurology* 28:1145–1151, 1978.
64. Elliot J et al: Spinal cord ischemia: Secondary to surgery of the abdominal aorta. In Bernhard V, Towne J, editors: *Complication in vascular surgery*. Orlando, Fl, 1985, Grune & Stratton.
65. Katz N et al: Incremental risk factors for spinal cord injury following operation for acute traumatic aortic transection. *J Thorac Cardiovasc Surg* 81:669–674, 1981.
66. Casthely PA et al: Anaesthesia for aortic arch aneurysm repair: Experience with 17 patients. *Can Anaesth Soc J* 132:23–28, 1985.
67. McCullough JL, Hollier LH, Nugent M: Paraplegia after thoracic aortic occlusion: Influence of cerebrospinal fluid drainage. *J Vasc Surg* 7:153–160, 1988.
68. Svennson LG et al: Influence of aortic shunts, laminectomy, papaverine, calcium channel blocker, allopurinol, and superoxide dismutase on spinal cord blood flow and paraplegia in baboons. *Ann Surg* 204:38–47, 1986.
69. Svensson LG, Grum DF, Bednarski M: Appraisal of CSF alterations during aortic surgery with intrathecal papaverine administration and CSF drainage. *J Vasc Surg* 11:423–429, 1990.
70. Grum DF, Svensson LG: Changes in cerebrospinal fluid pressure and spinal cord perfusion pressure prior to cross-clamping of the thoracic aorta in humans. *J Cardiothorac Vasc Anesth* 5:331–336, 1991.
71. Svensson LG et al: Intrathecal papaverine for the prevention of paraplegia

after operation on the thoracic or thoracoabdominal aorta. *J Thorac Cardiovasc Surg* 96:823–829, 1988.
72. Hill AC et al: The effect of verapamil on cerebral cortical and spinal cord blood flow during proximal descending thoracic aortic occlusion. *J Trauma* 28:1214–1219, 1988.
73. Laschinger JC et al: Prevention of ischemic spinal cord injury following aortic cross-clamping: Use of cortiosteroids. *Ann Thorac Surg* 38:500–507, 1984.
74. Vacanti FX, Ames A III: Mild hypothermia and Mg^{++} protect against irreversible damage during CNS ischemia. *Stroke* 15:695–698, 1984.
75. Kass IS, Cottrell JE, Chambers G: Magnesium and cobalt, not nimodipine protect neurons against anoxic damage in the rat hippocampal slice. *Anesthesiology* 69:710–715, 1988.
76. Gambling DR, Birmingham CL, Jenkins LC: Magnesium and the anaesthetist. *Can J Anaesth* 35:644–654, 1988.
77. Casthely PA et al: Superoxide dismutase and hemodynamic changes following aortic cross clamp release. *J Cardiothorac Anesth* 2:450–454, 1988.
78. Casthely PA et al: Comparison of superoxide dismutase, thopental, and nimodipine for maintenance of somatosensory evoked responses during aortic cross clamping and declamping in dogs. *J Cardiothorac Anesth* 2:792–797, 1988.
79. Breckwoldt WL et al: Spinal cord protection during aortic occlusion: Efficacy of intrathecal tetracaine. *Ann Thorac Surg* 51:959–963, 1991.
80. Laschinger JC, Izumoto H, Kouchoukos NT: Evolving concepts in prevention of spinal cord injury during operations on the descending thoracic and thoracoabdominal aorta. *Ann Thorac Surg* 44:667–674, 1987.
81. Shine T, Nugent M: Sodium nitroprusside decreases spinal cord perfusion pressure during descending thoracic aortic cross-clamping in the dog. *J Cardiothorac Anesth* 4:185–193, 1990.
82. Laschinger JC et al: Direct noninvasive monitoring of spinal cord motor function during thoracic aortic occlusion: Use of motor evoked potentials. *J Vasc Surg* 7:161–171, 1988.
83. Sheng F et al: Determinants of gastrointestinal complications in aortic surgery. *Vasc Surg* 6:257–267, 1987.
84. Johnson WC, Nabseth DC: Visceral infarction following aortic surgery. *Ann Surg* 180:312–318, 1974.
85. Hudson JC et al: Ibuprofen pretreatment inhibits prostocyclin release during abdominal exploration in aortic surgery. *Anesthesiology* 72:443–449, 1990.
86. Seltzer JL et al: The hemodynamic response to traction on the abdominal mesentery. *Anesthesiology* 63:96–99, 1985.
87. London M et al: Intraoperative myocardial ischemia: Localization by continuous 12 lead electrocardiography. *Anesthesiology* 69:232–241, 1988.
88. Tuman KJ et al: Effect of pulmonary artery catheterization on outcome in patients undergoing coronary artery surgery. *Anesthesiology* 70:199–206, 1989.
89. Ansley DM et al: The relationship between central venous pressure and pulmonary capillary wedge pressure during aortic surgery. *Can J Anaesth* 34:594–600, 1987.
90. Berlauk JF et al: Preoperative optimization of cardiovascular hemodynamics improves outcome in peripheral vascular surgery: A prospective randomized clinical trial. *Ann Surg* 214:289–299, 1991.
91. Frank SM et al: Right and left arm blood pressure discrepancies in vascular surgery patients. *Anesthesiology* 75:457–463, 1991.

92. Roizen MF et al: Monitoring with two-dimensional transesophageal echocardiography. Comparison of myocardial function in patients undergoing suprarenal-infraceliac, or infrarenal aortic occlusion. *J Vasc Surg* 1:300–305, 1984.
93. Attia RR et al: Myocardial ischemia due to infrarenal aortic cross-clamping during aortic surgery in patients with severe coronary disease. *Circulation* 53:961–965, 1976.
94. Kouchoukos NT et al: Hemodynamic effects of aortic clamping and decompression with a temporary shunt for resection of the descending thoracic aorta. *Surgery* 85:25–30, 1979.
95. Buffington CW et al: The prevalence of steal-prone coronary anatomy in patients with coronary artery disease: An analysis of the coronary artery surgery study registry. *Anesthesiology* 69:721–727, 1988.
96. Reiz S et al: Isoflurane—a powerful coronary vasodilator in patients with coronary artery disease. *Anesthesiology* 59:91–97, 1983.
97. Moffitt EA et al: Myocardial metabolism and hemodynamic responses with isoflurane anesthesia for coronary arterial surgery. *Anesth Analg* 65:53–61, 1986.
98. Buffington CW et al: Isoflurane induces coronary steal in a canine model of chronic coronary occlusion. *Anesthesiology* 66:280–292, 1987.
99. Pagel PS et al: Comparison of the systemic and coronary hemodynamic actions of desflurane, isoflurane, halothane and enflurane in the chronically instrumented dog. *Anesthesiology* 74:539–551, 1991.
100. Hartman JC et al: Influence of desflurane on regional distribution of coronary blood flow in a chronically instrumented canine model of multivessel coronary artery obstruction. *Anesth Analg* 72:289–299, 1991.
101. Goldstein RE: Coronary vascular responses to vasodilator drugs. *Prog Cardiovasc Dis* 24:419–436, 1982.
102. Bache J, Dymek OJ: Local and regional regulation of coronary vascular tone. *Prog Cardiovasc Dis* 24:191–212, 1981.
103. Roizen MF et al: Anaphylactoid reactions to vascular graft material presenting with vasodilation and subsequent disseminated intravascular coagulation. *Anesthesiology* 71:331–338, 1989.
104. Slogoff S, Keats AS: Does perioperative myocardial ischemia lead to postoperative myocardial infarction? *Anesthesiology* 62:107–114, 1985.
105. Slogoff S, Keats AS: Further observations on perioperative myocardial ischemia. *Anesthesiology* 65:539–542, 1986.
106. Mangano DT et al: Association of perioperative myocardial ischemia with cardiac morbidity and mortality in men undergoing noncardiac surgery. *N Engl J Med* 323:1781–1787, 1990.
107. Mangano DT: Perioperative cardiac morbidity (review). *Anesthesiology* 72:153–184, 1990.
108. Tuman KJ et al: Effects of epidural anesthesia and analgesia on coagulation and outcome after major vascular surgery. *Anesth Analg* 73:696–704, 1991.
109. Reeder MK et al: Postoperative myocardial ischemia: Temporal association with nocturnal hypoxaemia. *Br J Anesth* 67:626–631, 1991.
110. Hung J et al: Association of sleep apnoea with myocardial infarction in men. *Lancet* 336:261–264, 1990.
111. Forest JB et al: Multicenter study of general anesthesia III. Predictors of severe perioperative adverse outcomes. *Anesthesiology* 76:3–15, 1992.
112. Baron HC et al: Continuous epidural analgesia in the herarinized vascular

surgical patient; A retrospective review of 912 patients. *J Vasc Surg* 6:144–146, 1987.

113. Egbert LD et al: The value of the preoperative visit by an anesthetist: A study of doctor-patient rapport. *JAMA* 185:553–555, 1963.
114. Egbert LD et al: Reduction of postoperative pain by encouragement and instruction of patients: A study of doctor-patient rapport. *N Engl J Med* 270:825–827, 1964.
115. Wolfer JA, Davis CA: Assessment of surgical patients' preoperative emotional condition and postoperative welfare. *Nurs Res* 19:402–411, 1970.
116. Anderson EA: Preoperative preparation for cardiac surgery facilitates recovery, reduces psychological distress, and reduces the incidence of acute postoperative hypertension. *J Consult Clin Psychol* 55:513–520, 1987.
117. Pflug AE, Halter JB: Effect of spinal anesthesia on adrenergic tone and the neuroendocrine responses to surgical stress in humans. *Anesthesiology* 55:120–126, 1981.
118. Breslow MJ et al: Epidural morphine decreases postoperative hypertension by attenuating sympathetic nervous system hyperactivity. *JAMA* 261:3577–3581, 1989.
119. Reigel MM et al: Late survival in abdominal aortic aneurysm patients: The role of selective myocardial revascularization on the basis of clinical symptoms. *J Vasc Surg* 5:222–227, 1987.
120. Rettke Sr et al: Significance of mildly elevated creatinine kinase (myocardial band) activity after elective abdominal aortic aneurysmectomy. *J Cardiothorac Vasc Anesth* 5:425–430, 1991.
121. Yeager MP et al: Epidural anesthesia and analgesia in high-risk surgical patients. *Anesthesiology* 66:729–736, 1987.
122. Odoom JA, Sih IL: Epidural analgesia and anticoagulant therapy: Experience with one thousand cases of continuous epidurals. *Anaesthesia* 38:254–259, 1983.
123. Haku E, Hayashi M, Kato H: Anesthetic management of abdominal aortic surgery: A retrospective review of perioperative complications. *J Cardiothorac Anesth* 3:587–591, 1989.
124. Crosby ET et al: A randomized double blind comparison of fentanyl and sufentanil oxygen anesthesia for abdominal aortic surgery. *J Cardiothorac Anesth* 4:168–176, 1990.
125. Baron JF et al: Combined epidural and general anesthesia versus general anesthesia for abdominal aortic surgery. *Anesthesiology* 75:611–618, 1991.
126. Rivers SP et al: Epidural versus general anesthesia for infrainguinal arterial reconstruction. *J Vasc Surg* 14:764–770, 1991.
127. Spahn DR et al: Influence of anesthesia on the threshold of pacing-induced ischemia. *Anesth Analg* 74:14–25, 1992.
128. Klassen GA et al: Effect of acute sympathectomy by epidural anesthesia on the canine coronary circulation. *Anesthesiology* 52:8–14, 1980.
129. Davis RF, DeBoer LWV, Maroko PR: Thoracic epidural anesthesia reduces myocardial infarct size after coronary artery occlusion in dogs. *Anesth Analg* 65:711–717, 1986.
130. Blomberg S et al: Effects of thoracic epidural anesthesia on coronary artery disease. *Anesthesiology* 73:840–847, 1990.
131. Baron JF et al: Left ventricular global and regional function during lumbar epidural anesthesia in patients with and without angina pectoris. Influence of volume loading. *Anesthesiology* 66:621–627, 1987.

132. Saada M et al: Abnormalities in myocardial segmental wall motion during lumbar epidural anesthesia. *Anesthesiology* 71:26–32, 1989.
133. Rao TLK, El-Etr AA: Anticoagulation following placement of epidural and subarachnoid catheters: An evaluation of neurological sequelae. *Anesthesiology* 55:618–620, 1981.
134. Ruff RL, Dougherty JH Jr: Complication of lumbar puncture followed by anticoagulation. *Stroke* 12:879–881, 1981.
135. Dickman CA et al: Spinal epidural hematoma associated with epidural anesthesia: Complications of systemic heparinization in patients preceiving peripheral vascular thrombolytic therapy. *Anesthesiology* 72:942–950, 1990.
136. Cohn JD, Engler PE, Del Guercio LRM: The automated physiologic profile. *Crit Care Med* 3:51–58, 1975.
137. De Guercio LRM, Cohn JD: Monitoring operative risk in the elderly. *JAMA* 243:1350–1355, 1980.
138. Kennedy JW et al: Multivariate discriminant analysis of the clinical and angiographic predictors of operative mortality from the collaborative study in coronary artery surgery (CASS). *J Thorac Cardiovasc Surg* 80:876–887, 1980.
139. CASS Principal investigators and their associates: Myocardial infarction and mortality in the coronary artery surgery study (CASS) randomized trial. *N Engl J Med* 310:750–758, 1984.
140. Paiement B et al: A simple classification of the risk in cardiac surgery. *Can Anaesth Soc J* 30:61–68, 1983.
141. Rivers SP et al: Safety of peripheral vascular surgery after recent acute myocardial infarction. *J Vasc Surg* 11:70–76, 1990.
142. Dotter CT, Judkins MP. Transluminal treatment of arteriosclerotic obstruction: Description of a new technic and a preliminary report of its application. *Circulation* 30:654–670, 1974.
143. Zarins CK et al: Arterial disruption and remodeling following balloon dilatation. *Surgery* 92:1086–1095, 1982.
144. Spence R et al: Long-term results of transluminal angioplasty of the iliac and femoral arteries. *Arch Surg* 116:1377–1385, 1981.
145. Deutsch LS: Techniques of percutaneous balloon angioplasty including aortoiliac and femoropopliteal systems: Indications, results, and complications. In Moore WS, Ahn SS, editors: *Endovascular surgery.* Philadelphia, 1989, Saunders, pp 163–208.
146. Flanigan DP et al: Aortofemoral or femoropopliteal revascularization? A prospective evaluation of the papaverine test. *J Vasc Surg* 1:215–219, 1984.
147. Pfeiffer RB Jr, String ST: Adjunctive use of the balloon dilatation catheter during vascular reconstructive procedures. *J Vasc Surg* 3:841–845, 1986.
148. Tegtmeyer CJ et al: Results and complications of angioplasty in aortoiliac disease. *Circulation* 83(suppl 1):53–60, 1991.
149. Wilson SE, Wolf GL, Cross AP and the principal investigators of Veterans Administration Cooperative Study No 199: Percutaneous transluminal angioplasty vs. operation for peripheral arteriosclerosis: Report of a prospective randomized trial in a selected group of patients. *J Vasc Surg* 9:1–9, 1989.
150. Becker G, Katzen B, Dake M: Noncoronary angioplasty. *Radiology* 170:921–940, 1989.
151. Johnston KW et al: 5-year results of a prospective study of percutaneous transluminal angioplasty. *Ann Surg* 206:403–413, 1987.
152. Hewes R et al: Long-term results of superficial femoral artery angioplasty. *AJR* 146:1025–1029, 1986.

153. Milford MA et al: Femoropopliteal percutaneous transluminal angioplasty for limb salvage. *J Vasc Surg* 8:292–299, 1988.
154. Bakal CW et al: Percutaneous transluminal angioplasty of the infrapopliteal arteries: Results in 53 patients. *AJR* 154:171–174, 1990.
155. Weibull H et al: Complications after percutaneous transluminal angioplasty in the iliac, femoral, and popliteal arteries. *J Vasc Surg* 5:681–686, 1987.
156. White GH et al: Intraoperative video angioscopy compared with arteriography during peripheral vascular operations. *J Vasc Surg* 6:488–495, 1987.
157. Fleisher HL III et al: Angioscopically monitored saphenous vein valvulotomy. *J Vasc Surg* 4:360–364, 1986.
158. Vollmar JF, Hutschenreiter S: Vascular endoscopy for thromboendarterectomy. In Moore WS, Ahn SS, editors: *Endovascular surgery.* Philadelphia, 1989, Saunders, pp 87–94.
159. Miller A et al: Angioscopically directed valvulotomy: A new valvulotome and technique. *J Vasc Surg* 13:813–821, 1991.
160. Gilbertson JJ et al: A blinded comparison of angiography, angioscopy, and duplex scanning in the intraoperative evaluation of in situ saphenous vein bypass grafts. *J Vasc Surg* 15:121–129, 1992.
161. Rosenthal D et al: Endovascular in situ femoropopliteal bypass: A multicenter preliminary report. *J Vasc Surg* (submitted).
162. White GH et al: Endoscopic intravascular surgery removes intraluminal flaps, dissections, and thrombus. *J Vasc Surg* 11:280–288, 1990.
163. Mehigan JT, Decampli WM: Angioscopic control of carotid endarterectomy. In Moore WS, Ahn SS, editors: *Endovascular surgery.* Philadelphia, 1989, Saunders, pp 95–99.
164. Vollmar JF, Loeprecht H, Hutschenreiter S: Advances in vascular endoscopy. *Thorac Cardiovasc Surg* 35:334–341, 1987.
165. Van Stiegmann G et al: Flexible angioscopy seems faster and more specific than arteriography. *Arch Surg* 122:279–282, 1987.
166. Hashizume M et al: Intimal response of saphenous vein to intraluminal trauma by simulated angioscopic insertion. *J Vasc Surg* 5:862–868, 1987.
167. Towne JB: Complications of vascular endoscopy. In Moore WS, Ahn SS, editors: *Endovascular surgery.* Philadelphia, 1989, Saunders, pp 114–117.
168. Hinohara T et al: Directional atherectomy: New approaches for treatment of obstructive coronary and peripheral vascular disease. *Circulation* 81:79–91, 1990.
169. von Pölnitz A et al: Percutaneous peripheral atherectomy: Angiographic and clinical follow-up of 60 patients. *J Am Coll Cardiol* 15:682–688, 1990.
170. Graor RA, Whitlow PL: Transluminal atherectomy for occlusive peripheral vascular disease. *J Am Coll Cardiol* 15:1552–2558, 1990.
171. Dalman RL, Taylor LM, Porter JM: Current status of endovascular procedures for treatment of lower extremity atherosclerotic occlusive. *Curr Probl Surg* 28:103–124, 1991.
172. Kensey KR et al: Recanalization of obstructed arteries with a flexible, rotating tip catheter. *Radiology* 165:387–389, 1987.
173. Snyder SO Jr et al: The Kensey catheter: Preliminary results with a transluminal atherectomy tool. *J Vasc Surg* 8:541–543, 1988.
174. Cull DL et al: Experience with laser-assisted balloon angioplasty and a rotary angioplasty instrument: Lessons learned. *J Vasc Surg* 14:332–339, 1991.
175. Prevosti LG et al: Particulate debris from rotational atherectomy: Size, distribution, and physiological effect. *Circulation* 78:83, 1988.

176. Titus BG, Auth DC, Ritchie JL: Distal embolization during mechanical thrombolysis: Rotational thrombectomy vs balloon angioplasty. *Cathet Cardiovasc Diag* 19:279–285, 1990.
177. Ginsburg R: Laser angioplasty as an adjunct to balloon dilatation. In Moore WS, Ahn SS, editors: *Endovascular surgery,* Philadelphia, 1989, Saunders, pp 389–401.
178. Matsumoto T, Okamura T, Rajyaguru V: Laser arterial disobstructive procedures in 148 lower extremities. *J Vasc Surg* 10:169–177, 1989.
179. Wright JG et al: Laser angioplasty for limb salvage: Observations on early results. *J Vasc Surg* 10:29–38, 1989.
180. Perler BA et al: Percutaneous laser probe femoropopliteal angioplasty: A preliminary experience. *J Vasc Surg* 10:351–357, 1989.
181. Pilger E et al: Nd:YAG laser with sapphire tip combined with balloon angioplasty in peripheral arterial occlusions long term results. *Circulation* 83:141–147, 1991.
182. Sanborn TA et al: Peripheral laser-assisted balloon angioplasty: Initial multicenter experience in 219 peripheral arteries. *Arch Surg* 124:1099–1103, 1989.
183. Rosenthal D et al: Thermal laser-assisted balloon angioplasty of the superficial femoral artery: A multicenter review of 602 cases. *J Vasc Surg* 14:152–159, 1991.
184. Miller BF et al: Surveillance for recurrent stenosis after endovascular procedures. *Arch Surg* 126:867–872, 1991.
185. McCarthy WJ et al: Excimer laser-assisted femoral angioplasty: Early results. *J Vasc Surg* 13:607–614, 1991.
186. Litvack F et al: Percutaneous excimer-laser and excimer-laser assisted angioplasty of the lower extremities: Results of initial clinical trial. *Radiology* 172:331–335, 1989.
187. Geschwind HJ et al: Results and follow-up after percutaneous pulsed laser-assisted balloon angioplasty guided by spectroscopy. *Circulation* 83:787–796, 1991.
188. Palmaz JC et al: Intraluminal stents in atherosclerotic iliac artery stenosis: Preliminary report of a multicenter study. *Radiology* 168:727–731, 1988.
189. Cikrit DF et al: Early experience with the Palmaz expandable intraluminal stent in iliac artery stenosis. *Ann Vasc Surg* 5:150–155, 1991.
190. Joffre F, Rousseau H, Puel J: Arterial stenting. *J Intervent Radiol* 4:155–159, 1989.
191. Günther RW et al: Iliac and femoral artery stenoses and occlusions: Treatment with intravascular stents. *Radiology* 172:725–730, 1989.
192. Bertrand ME, Rickards AF, Serruys PW: Coronary stent implantation for primary and secondary prevention of restenosis after PTCA. Results of a pilot multicenter trial. *Eur Heart J* 9:55, 1988.
193. Penn IM, Levine SL, Schatz RA: Intravascular stents as an adjunct to endovascular intervention. In Moore WS, Ahn SS, editors: *Endovascular surgery.* Philadelphia, 1989, Saunders, pp 258–277.
194. Nissen SE et al: Application of a new phased-array ultrasound imaging catheter in the assessment of vascular dimensions: In vivo comparison to cineangiography. *Circulation* 81:660–666, 1990.
195. Isner JM et al: Percutaneous intravascular US as adjunct to catheter-based interventions: Preliminary experience in patients with peripheral vascular disease. *Radiology* 175:61–70, 1990.

196. Pandian NG et al: Intravascular high frequency two-dimensional ultrasound detection of arterial dissection and intimal flaps. *Am J Cardiol* 65:1278–1280, 1990.
197. Tabbara M et al: In vivo human comparison of intravascular ultrasonography and angiography. *J Vasc Surg* 14:496–504, 1991.
198. Neville RF Jr et al: Endovascular management of arterial intimal defects: An experimental comparison by arteriography, angioscopy, and intravascular ultrasonography. *J Vasc Surg* 13:496–502, 1991.
199. Cavaye DM et al: Intraluminal ultrasound assessment of vascular stent deployment. *Ann Vasc Surg* 5:241–246, 1991.
200. Sarfati PO et al: Intraoperative ultrasonography for location of proximal limit of inferior vena caval thrombosis. *Ann Vasc Surg* 5:459–461, 1991.
201. Cavaye DM et al: Intravascular ultrasound imaging of an acute dissecting aortic aneurysm: A case report. *J Vasc Surg* 13:510–512, 1991.
202. West AI: Endovascular ultrasound. In Moore WS, Ahn SS, editors: *Endovascular surgery*. Philadelphia, 1989, Saunders, pp 518–525.
203. Mirich D et al: Percutaneously placed endovascular grafts for aortic aneurysms: Feasibility study. *Radiology* 170:1033–1037, 1989.
204. Parodi JC, Palmaz JC, Barone HD: Transfemoral intraluminal graft implantation for abdominal aortic aneurysms. *Ann Vasc Surg* 5:491–499, 1991.

Oxygen Delivery and Utilization in the Critically Ill

Aurel C. Cernaianu, M.D., F.I.C.S.

Assistant Professor of Surgery, University of Medicine and Dentistry of New Jersey, Robert Wood Johnson Medical School at Camden, Director, Research Programs, Division of Cardiothoracic Surgery and Department of Anesthesiology, Cooper Hospital/University Medical Center, Camden, New Jersey

Anthony J. DelRossi, M.D., F.A.C.S.

Associate Professor of Surgery, University of Medicine and Dentistry of New Jersey, Robert Wood Johnson Medical School at Camden, Chairman, Department of Surgery, Head, Division of Cardiothoracic Surgery, Cooper Hospital/University Medical Center, Camden, New Jersey

Critically ill patients are characterized by dramatic physiologic changes that ultimately may affect tissue perfusion and oxygenation. Generally, all hemodynamic and respiratory monitoring in patients in the intensive care unit (ICU) should focus on evaluation of perfusion. As Shoemaker defines in a recent editorial,[1] "Oxygen transport measurements constitute an important approach to evaluate perfusion in acute circulatory problems." Since the amount of oxygen consumed by the subcellular organelles directly correlates with tissue integrity,[2–5] the assessment of oxygen transport parameters has become particularly interesting to those caring for critically ill patients. The oxygen transport system, oxygen utilization, and its components are increasingly part of the monitoring arsenal used in the ICU.

The Oxygen Transport System

The transport of oxygen to the tissue comprises the amount of oxygen delivered (Do_2) and the volume of oxygen consumed intracellularly ($\dot{V}o_2$). Measurable factors that influence the adequacy of oxygen transport are hemoglobin concentration (Hb), the percentage of Hb saturation with oxygen (Sao_2), cardiac output ($\dot{Q}$), $\dot{V}o_2$, and the affinity of Hb for oxygen (P_{50}). In addition, oxygen transport is influenced by the distribution of perfusion.[6]

In healthy individuals, oxygen supply may be increased to meet excessive demands during increased activity or stress. The components of the oxygen transport system and their normal values are shown in Table 1.

TABLE 1.
Components of the Oxygen Transport System

Component*	Calculation Formula	Normal Value†
$C(a-\bar{v})O_2$	$CaO_2 - C\bar{v}O_2$	3.5–5 mL/dL
$C\bar{v}O_2$	$(Hb \times 1.35 \times S\bar{v}O_2) + (P\bar{v}O_2 \times 0.003)$	15 mL/dL
SaO_2	Measured	100%
CaO_2	$(Hb \times 1.36 \times SaO_2) + (PaO_2 \times 0.003)$	20 mL/dL
DO_2	$CaO_2 \times Q \times 10$	1,000 mL/min
$\dot{V}O_2$	$Q \times C(a-\bar{v})O_2 \times 10$	110–150 mL/min/m^2
$S\bar{v}O_2$	$1 - \dot{V}O_2/DO_2$	75%
PaO_2	Measured	90–105 mm Hg
$PaCO_2$	Measured	35–45 mm Hg
$\dot{V}O_2/DO_2$	—	22%–30%
P_{50}	Calculated	27 mm Hg
Qs/Qt	$(CcO_2 - CaO_2)/(CcO_2 - C\bar{v}O_2)$	6%
PaO_2	Measured	40–45 mm Hg

*SaO_2 = arterial oxygen saturation; CaO_2 = arterial oxygen content; DO_2 = oxygen delivery; $\dot{V}O_2$ = oxygen consumption; $S\bar{v}O_2$ = mixed venous oxygen saturation; $P\bar{v}O_2$ = mixed venous PO_2; PaO_2 = arterial PO_2; Q = cardiac output; Hb = hemoglobin concentration; Qs/Qt = intrapulmonary shunt, VO_2/DO_2 = oxygen extraction.
†Normal implies: Hb = 15 g/dL; SaO_2 = 1; Q = 5 L/min.

The normal oxygen transport system and its components are presented in Figure 1.[7] It should be stressed that these assumptions are made to describe the oxygen transport system in a global way and do not give any information about tissue oxygenation of specific vital organs. Since the assessment of oxygen transport variables is a newly emerging concept, there is much debate as to the optimal value of the individual components of the system, particularly the appropriate Hb concentration (Fig 2);[8] the position of the oxyhemoglobin dissociation curve, which influences oxygen on- and off-loading with an impact on oxygen availability (Fig 3)[6]; and the requirements for oxygen tension, cardiac output, and variability of blood volume.

Hb uptake and the release of oxygen has been analyzed in the past. Figure 4 represents the relationship between oxygen saturation and its partial pressure. Anemia and related changes in blood viscosity and vessel tone have all been described as influencing factors in oxygen transport.[9, 10] A decrease in hematocrit (Hct) may trigger compensatory mechanisms that will either increase cardiac output or the oxygen extraction. Metabolic factors have been also implicated as regulating factors of oxygen transport in severe anemia.[11] The Hct level has been associated with survival[12] and

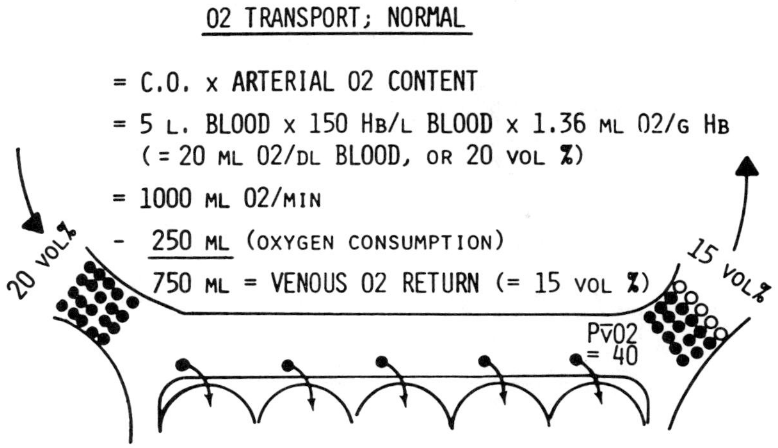

FIG 1.
Normal oxygen transport, giving normal values for oxygen consumption and venous oxygen content. *Solid dots* represent oxygen in mL/dL. (From Snyder JV, Carroll GC: *Curr Probl Surg* 19:650–719, 1982. Used by permission.)

hyperviscosity due to polycythemia has been correlated with impairment of cerebral blood flow[13] and occlusive vascular accidents.[14] Hemodilution to an Hct level of 25% to 30% has been shown to improve flow in the microcirculation and improve hemodynamics and oxygen transport in patients undergoing cardiac[15, 16] or vascular surgery.[17] Hemodilution can generally be tolerated because Do_2 is normally in excess of that actually required by

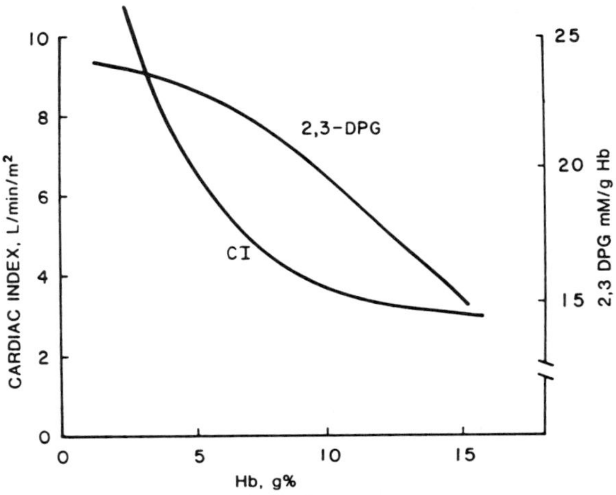

FIG 2.
Effect of anemia on cardiac index and 2,3-DPG. (From Finch CA, Lenfant C: *N Engl J Med* 286:407–415, 1972. Used by permission.)

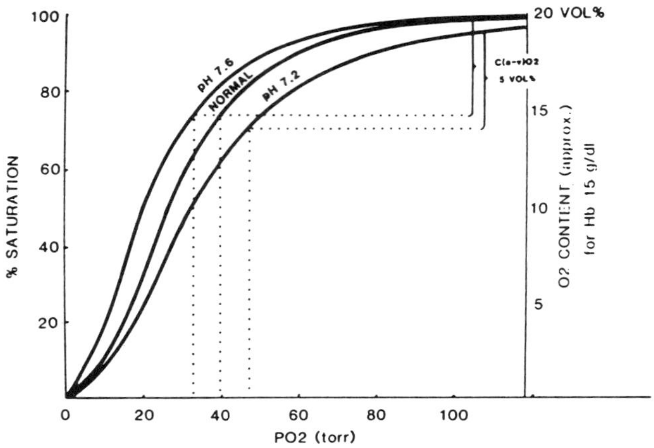

FIG 3.
Shifts in the oxyhemoglobin curve. When Hb is normal, Pa_{O_2} is 100 mm Hg (torr) and other factors are constant, $C\bar{v}_{O_2}$ remains 5 mL/dL less than Ca_{O_2} and $P\bar{v}_{O_2}$ is about 32, 40, and 48 mm Hg when the oxyhemoglobin dissociation curve is in the positions illustrated. (From Snyder JV: Oxygen transport: The model and reality. In Snyder JV, Pinsky MR, editors: *Oxygen transport in the critically ill patient.* St Louis, 1992, Mosby–Year Book, pp 3–15. Used by permission.)

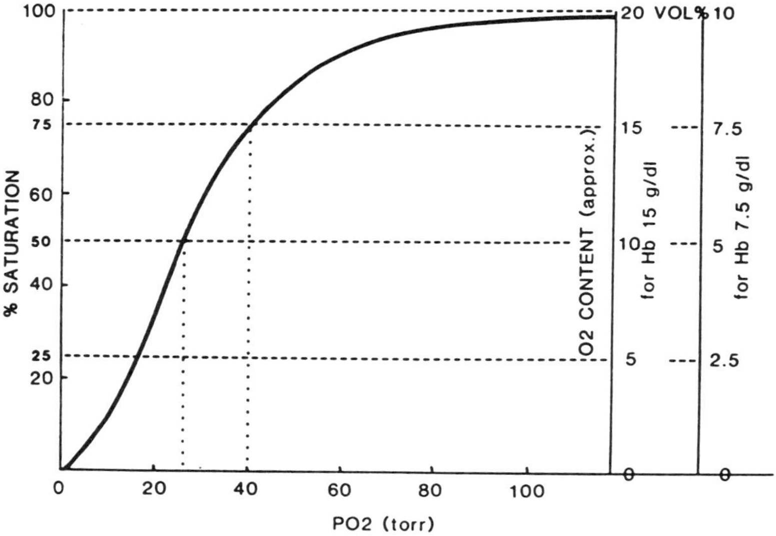

FIG 4.
The normal relationship between oxygen saturation and partial pressure. A new axis has been added for specific levels of hemoglobin to estimate the effect of a change in $C(a-\bar{v}_{O_2})$ on $P\bar{v}_{O_2}$. (From Snyder JV: Oxygen transport: The model and reality. In Snyder JV, Pinsky MR, editors: *Oxygen transport in the critically ill patient.* St Louis, 1992, Mosby–Year Book, pp 3–15. Used by permission.)

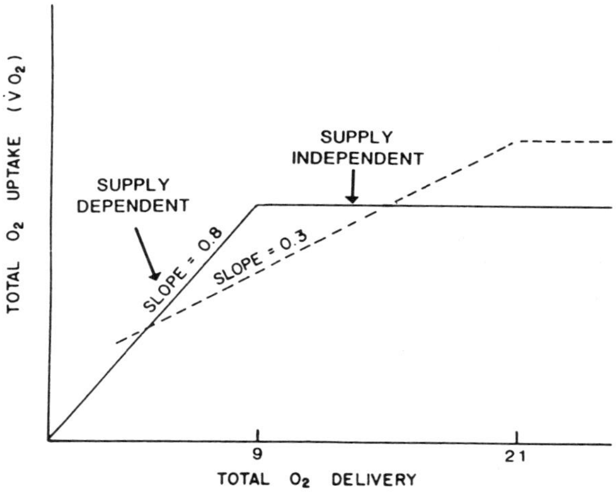

FIG 5.
Oxygen uptake ($\dot{V}O_2$) as a function of total oxygen delivery for healthy patients *(solid line)* and those with adult respiratory distress syndrome *(dotted line)*. Oxygen delivery must increase 2½-fold above normal values to supply independent $\dot{V}O_2$ in patients with adult respiratory distress syndrome. (From Cain SM: *Am J Med Sci* 288:199–124, 1984. Used by permission.)

tissue. On the other hand, exercise capacity may be enhanced when a slightly increased Hct is present.[18] Fluid loading may increase $\dot{V}O_2$ and demonstrate an oxygen uptake deficit, particularly in the hyperactive patient.[19] Pace et al.[20] have shown that critical DO_2 remains practically the same for either an anemic or hypoxic type of anemia.

The shape of the oxyhemoglobin dissociation curve (see Fig 3) is regulated by 2,3-diphosphoglyceric acid and pH. P_{50} represents the point of 50% Hb saturation with oxygen and corresponds to a PaO_2 of 27 ± 3 mm Hg.[21] Since the stored red blood cells (RBCs) and many of the Hb-based RBC substitutes have a low P_{50}, the improvement of P_{50} of these products has become a major research interest.[21] A change of only 2 mm Hg in $P\bar{v}O_2$ from the normal value may result in a change in cardiac output up to 1.12 L.[22] A rightward shift of the curve is produced by hypercarbia with resultant decreases in CaO_2, SaO_2, and $S\bar{v}O_2$ if $\dot{V}O_2$ and PaO_2 remain unchanged. In this situation, the partial pressure of oxygen in capillaries is a factor in maintaining tissue oxygenation.[6] The theoretical advantage of a right-shifted oxyhemoglobin dissociation curve is that a greater DO_2 is possible at a PO_2 lower than 50 mm Hg than in a left-shifted curve.[23] At low PaO_2 (30 to 40 mm Hg), there is a tendency of the curve to shift to the left. Some shift is caused by alkalosis with a resultant slight increase in arterial and venous content. However, large drops in $P\bar{v}O_2$ with potential tissue hypoxia may also be seen if $C(a - \bar{v})O_2$ remains constant. The left shift is generally better tolerated because compensatory mechanisms such as increase in blood flow to regional organs, have taken effect. Oxygen dysfunction asso-

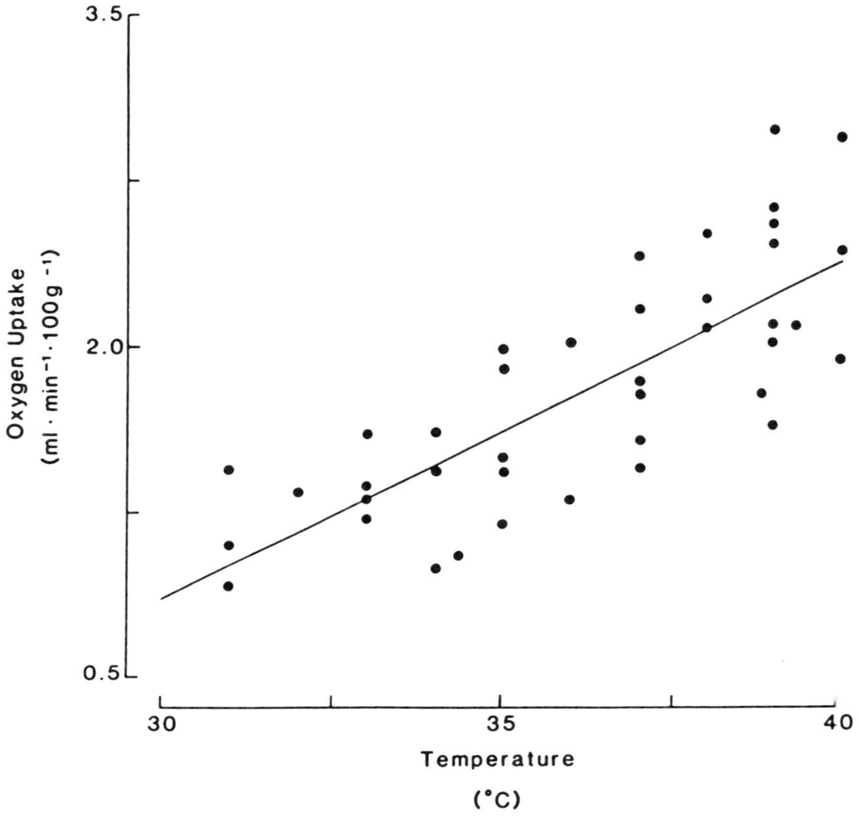

FIG 6.
Relationship between temperature and oxygen uptake in ileal tissue. (From Kvietys PR et al: *Am J Physiol* 249:246, 1985. Used by permission.)

ciated with a left-shifted oxyhemoglobin curve has been discussed by Woodson and colleagues.[24–26]

The induction of a shift from left to right has been used to improve Do_2 with resultant reduction of myocardial necrosis in animal models of coronary ischemia.[27] The affinity of Hb for oxygen may also be influenced by electrolyte imbalance, particularly hypophosphatemia, low or high pH, multiple transfusion with acid-citrate-dextrose (ACD)-preserved blood products, or the administration of particular drugs, especially methylprednisolone,[28] inotropes, and vasodilators.[29]

Under normal conditions, the Do_2 is a phenomenon that provides sufficient tissue oxygenation.[30] Critical Do_2 has been defined as the level below which uptake is related to delivery and above which no matter how great the increase in Do_2, $\dot{V}o_2$ remains constant.[31, 32] Figure 5[33] shows the theoretical relationship between $\dot{V}o_2$ and Do_2 in healthy subjects (solid lines) and patients with adult respiratory distress syndrome (dotted lines). Cain[33] has found that $\dot{V}O_2$ becomes supply-dependent below a DO_2 of approximately 9 mL/min/kg. At higher levels, $\dot{V}O_2$ is independent of DO_2. Studies by the same investigator[34] have shown that arachidonic acid metabolites, neutrophils, complement cascade activation, and oxygen radicals may impede cellular oxygen uptake. Also, the presence of intracellular or extracellular edema, microemboli, or accumulation of tissue metabolites may interfere with $\dot{V}O_2$.[35] Other factors that have been shown to cause alterations in tissue $\dot{V}O_2$ are an increase in body temperature (Fig 6),[36] intraorgan or interorgan blood flow maldistribution, and increased activity of the endocrine system. These factors all create an additional metabolic tissue demand.

Adequate arterial oxygen saturation (SaO_2) is maintained at a PaO_2 over 60 mmHg (see Fig 3). Although this artificial level of oxygenation is acceptable for healthy individuals, anemia or low pH may change this relationship. Only 2% or less of the total amount of oxygen transported is dissolved. Negligible under normal conditions, the dissolved oxygen becomes an important oxygenation factor in severe anemia (Hb less than 3 g/dL) or in shock. Roca and his associates have investigated maximal oxygen consumption ($\dot{V}O_{2max}$)[37] and its relationship to other components of tissue oxygenation in healthy subjects (Figs 7–10).[37] They postulated that $\dot{V}O_{2max}$ is limited by the rate of oxygen diffusion from the erythrocytes in the muscle capillaries to the muscle mitochondria. The authors found that in healthy subjects, $\dot{V}O_{2max}$ is limited by the interaction of convective DO_2, capillary blood flow (Fick's principle), and the diffusion of oxygen from the erythrocytes to the mitochondria (Fick's first law of diffusion). Convective DO_2 depends on blood flow, SaO_2, and Hb, and is an important factor in determining capillary PaO_2. On the other hand, the diffusive transport depends on capillary PaO_2 and tissue diffusion capacity for oxygen. Other components of the oxygen transport system such as microcirculation, resistance to flow, VO_2, and cardiac output and distribution of perfusion have been discussed in detail elsewhere.[6]

Types of Oxygen Supply Deficiency

The response of $\dot{V}O_2$ to changes in components of the oxygen transport system has been considered biphasic in experimental preparations of perfused organs.[38, 39] The definition of metabolic oxygen regulation has been considered by some investigators for the process of maintaining metabolic rate despite a decrease in oxygen supply. A metabolic conformity has also been described in lower vertebrates[40] (progressive decrease in $\dot{V}O_2$ as oxygen supply becomes less available).

Under controlled conditions, during anesthesia or mechanical ventilation, the $\dot{V}O_2$ rate remains initially independent of the components of the oxygen transport system. Then, as it decreases further, it becomes directly correlated to the oxygen transport. This biphasic response has been de-

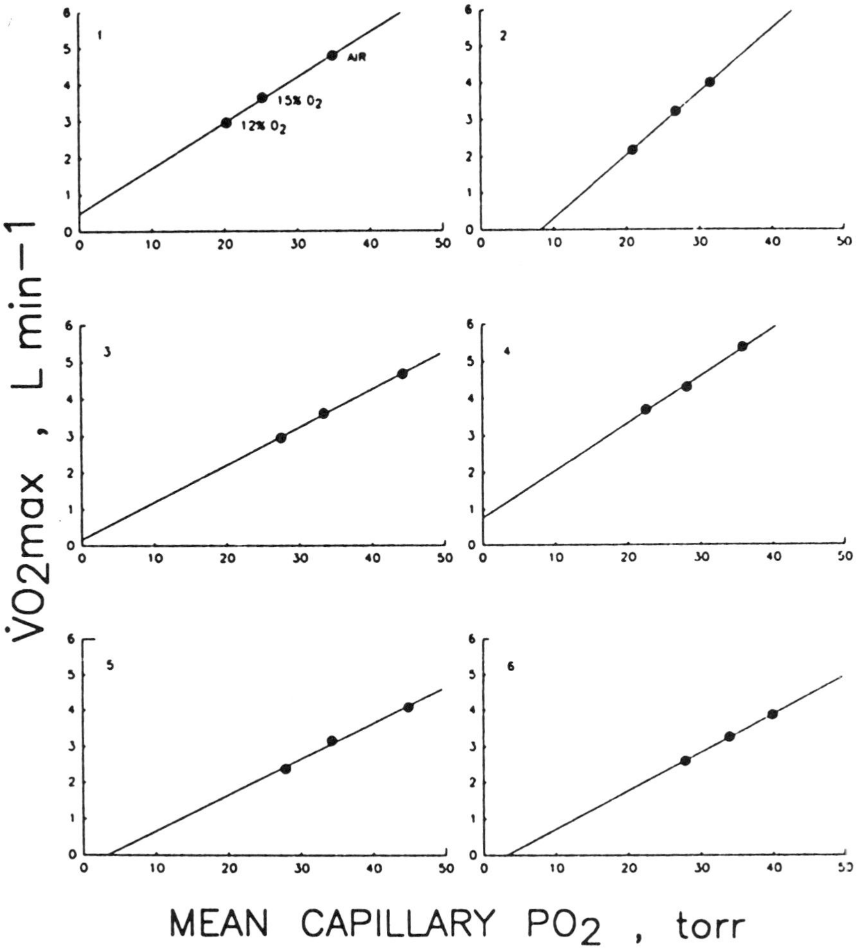

FIG 7.
Maximum O_2 uptake ($\dot{V}O_2max$, ordinate) and mean muscle capillary PO_2 (abscissa) fall together along a straight line through origin as FIO_2 fraction is reduced from air to 12% O_2. Measurements are at target work load producing $\dot{V}O_2max$. Each panel contains individual data for one subject. (Fran Roca J et al: *J Appl Physiol* 67:291–299, 1989. Used by permission.)

fined as physiologic oxygen supply dependency (see Fig 5). It is presumed that metabolic demands are met when VO_2 remains constant.[41]

Critical oxygen transport has been defined as the point at which $\dot{V}O_2$ begins to decrease (Fig 11).[41] Although no precise data related to this parameter are available in humans, it is estimated to be approximately 8 mL/min/kg in the anesthetized patient.[32] This term should be differentiated

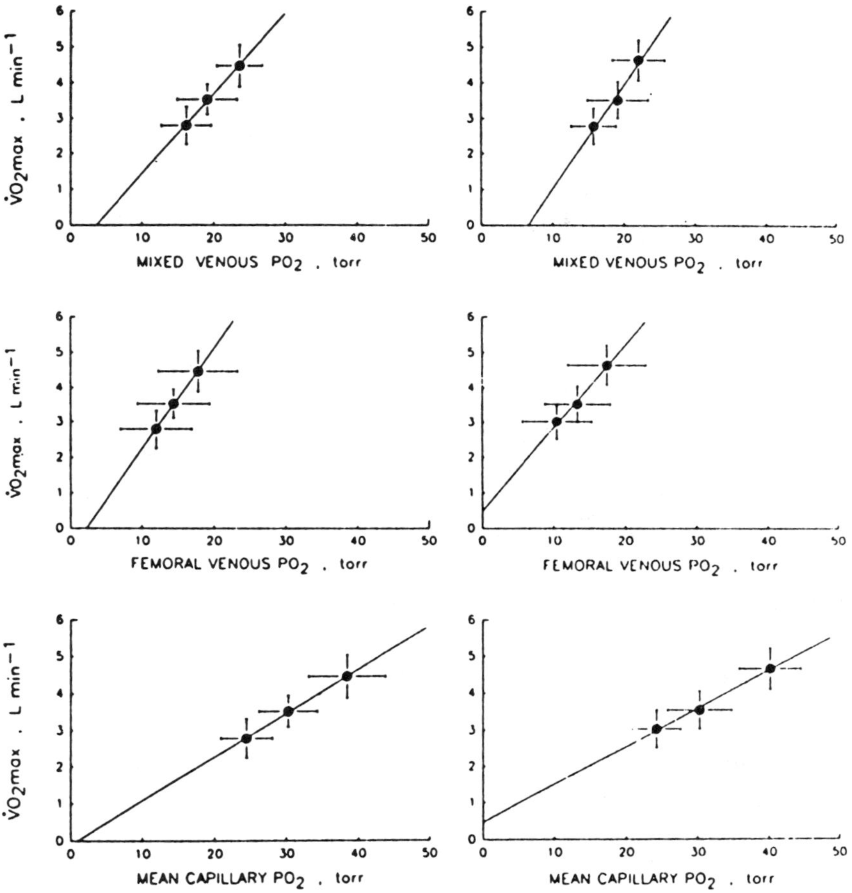

FIG 8.
Regression analyses between maximal O_2 uptake ($\dot{V}O_2max$, ordinate) and mixed venous, femoral venous, and mean capillary PO_2 (abscissa). Group mean results are given at target work load (left) and last minute work load (right). (From Roca J et al: *J Appl Physiol* 67:291–299, 1989. Used by permission.)

from that of critical PaO_2 (6.5 mmHg), which represents the minimum level of oxygenation that can maintain the process of mitochondrial oxidative phosphorylation.[42] The critical oxygen transport may be influenced by age, metabolic rate, and critical $\dot{V}O_2$.[39, 43]

Pathologic oxygen supply dependency has been described in a variety of critically ill patients[44–49] in whom $\dot{V}O_2$ seems to be dependent on many of the components of the oxygen transport system. As shown in Figure 11, the $\dot{V}O_2/DO_2$ ratio is low, with a direct correlation between the $\dot{V}O_2$ and systemic oxygen transport.

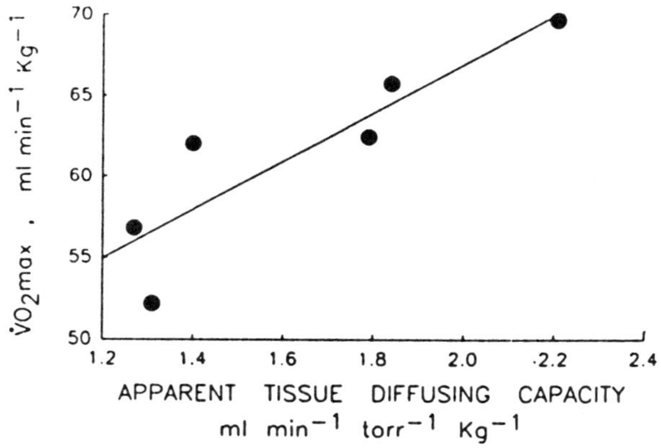

FIG 9.
Relationship between maximum O_2 uptake ($\dot{V}O_2max$, ordinate) and calculated apparent O_2 tissue diffusing capacity (abscissa). Correlation between these variables was found, suggesting that subjects with higher VO_2max have higher apparent O_2 tissue diffusing capacity. (From Roca J et al: *J Appl Physiol* 67:291–299, 1989. Used by permission.)

Clinical Assessment of Oxygen Transport

The measurement of oxygen transport variables in conjunction with cardiorespiratory indicators may help in clinical management. Usually, the adequacy of the oxygen transport system is assessed by measuring the $\dot{V}O_2$ or by testing for metabolic markers. Direct measurement of $\dot{V}O_2$ can be ob-

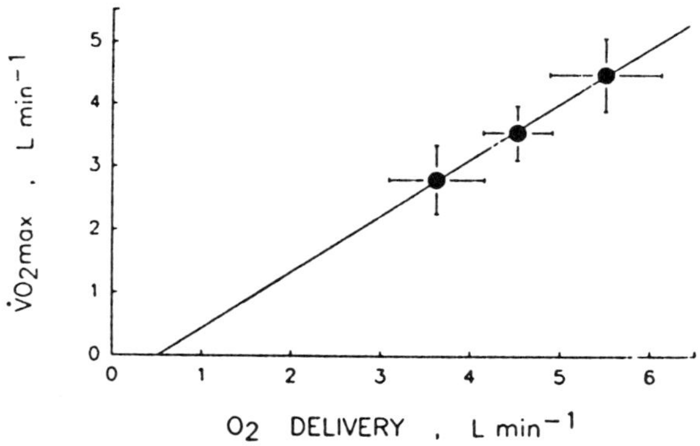

FIG 10.
Maximum O_2 uptake ($\dot{V}O_2max$, ordinate) and O_2 delivery (abscissa) are linearly related through origin as inspiratory O_2 fraction is reduced. Group mean results are given at target work load. (From Roca J et al: *J Appl Physiol* 67:291–299, 1989. Used by permission.)

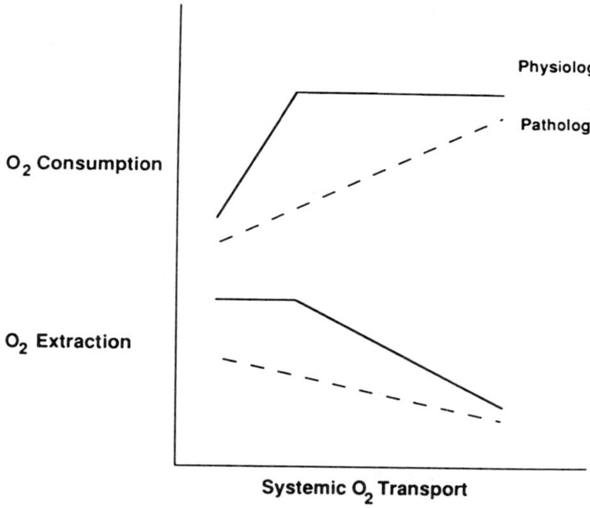

FIG 11.
Schema showing the relationship of systemic oxygen transport of oxygen extraction and $\dot{V}O_2$ physiologic relationship is characterized by an independent and dependent portion of the $\dot{V}O_2$ response when oxygen transport is altered. When systemic oxygen transport is high, oxygen extraction is low, and oxygen extraction rapidly increases as oxygen transport is reduced. This is in contrast to the pathologic response observed in patients with a variety of conditions. In these patients, oxygen extraction remains low when oxygen transport is decreased so that $\dot{V}O_2$ has an apparent dependence on oxygen transport through a very wide range. (From Lister G: Oxygen supply/demand in the critically ill. In Taylor RW, Shoemaker WC, editors: *Critical care state of the art.* Anaheim, Calif, 1991, Society of Critical Care Medicine, pp 311–350. Used by permission.)

tained by analyzing the volume and composition of inspired and expired gases over a known time:

$$\dot{V}O_2 = \frac{(V_{ins} \times FiO_2) - (V_{exp} \times FeO_2)}{t}$$

where V_{insp} is the inspired volume, V_{exp} is the expired volume, FiO_2 and FeO_2 are the fraction of inspired and expired oxygen, and t represents the time.

Errors in this measurement may be introduced by deficiencies in gas content analysis, or in patients on mechanical ventilation (FiO_2 may vary during the respiratory cycle), or by inaccurate measurement of gas volumes during spirometry. When anesthetics are added to treatment, the Haldane equation:

$$V_{insp} = \frac{V_{exp} \times FeN_2}{FiN_2},$$

(where $FiN_2 = 1 - FiO_2$, and $FeN_2 = 1 - FeO_2 - FeCO_2$; FiN_2 and FeN_2 are the fractions of nitrogen in inspired and expired gases), which assumes the absence of other gases than oxygen, carbon dioxide, and nitrogen, may not be accurate. Other situations like metabolic disturbances, intoxication, or multiorgan system failure, are all sources for error in the measurement of $\dot{V}O_2$.

Direct measurement of $\dot{V}O_2$ with a closed system can also be obtained by the patient breathing 100% oxygen through a circuit in which the rate exchange of CO_2 may be quantified:

$$\dot{V}O_2 = \frac{\Delta V}{t \times FiO_2} \text{ at STP}$$

where ΔV represents change in volume, and STP is standard temperature and pressure. Pitfalls in interpretation and errors with this method have been described by Quan et al.[50] and Chapler et al.[51] Problems have been also reported in patients with abnormal airway anatomy and in those with decreased lung compliance.[52]

Direct measurement of $\dot{V}O_2$ in patients with sepsis who are on mechanical ventilation has been used and described by Houtchens and Westenskow[53] using a volume oxygen measuring device. Because of inherited problems with direct measurement, the calculation of $\dot{V}O_2$ from

$$\dot{V}O_2 = Q \times C(a - \bar{v})O_2$$

has become more practical, particularly in patients in whom pulmonary artery catheters are already in place for other hemodynamic measurements. Pitfalls and errors with this method are documented elsewhere.[54]

Metabolic markers are used in conjunction with other oxygen transport variables to assess the adequacy of tissue oxygenation. The changes in $\dot{V}O_2$, $\dot{V}O_2/DO_2$, arterial pH, and lactate concentration are shown in Figure 12.[41] Earlier investigations[55, 56] have found that blood lactate concentration is the premier marker of anaerobic metabolism. Some investigators have shown that elevation of $\dot{V}O_2$ following increases in DO_2 occurs predominantly in patients with lactic acidosis.[57–59] However, Silverman[60] argues that considerable intersubject variation occurs in the level of $\dot{V}O_2$ required to relieve an existing tissue oxygen debt. In his study on 17 critically ill patients, changes in lactate levels did not correlate with either changes in $\dot{V}O_2$ or the absolute postintervention (fluid administration, RBCs, or dobutamine infusion) $\dot{V}O_2$ level, and the attainment of any specific $\dot{V}O_2$ value does not ensure the reversal of an ongoing oxygen debt. The author suggested that therapeutic interventions should be tailored to the patient's tissue needs and guided by an assessment of an oxygen debt (e.g., lactate level) rather than absolute $\dot{V}O_2$ measurements. Since lactate metabolism takes place in the liver, states that are accompanied by hepatic impairment may present with an increased blood lactate concentration. The lactate to pyruvate ratio has been advocated by some investigators[53] to be a better marker of hypoxia, since an increase in lactate only may result from other reasons than tissue ischemia, such as hyperglycemia,[61] hyperventilation,[62] and administration of catecholamines.[63]

Arterial acidemia could be considered a marker of tissue hypoxia[55]; however, many compensatory buffering mechanisms exist. A detailed re-

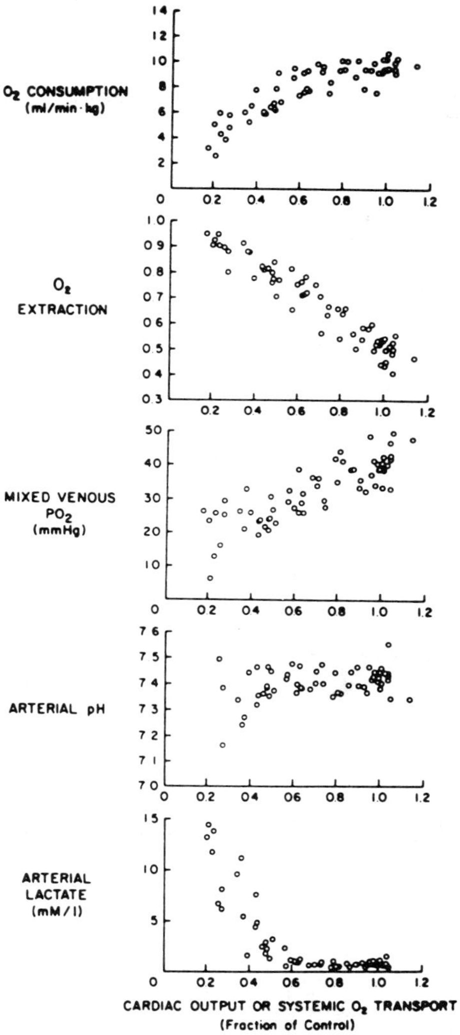

FIG 12.
Changes in $\dot{V}O_2$, oxygen extraction, $P\bar{v}O_2$ arterial pH, and arterial lactate concentration as cardiac output is progressively reduced in five conscious lambs. Cardiac output and systemic oxygen transport are shown as a fraction of control or baseline values on the X axis. (From Lister G: Oxygen supply/demand in the critically ill. In Taylor RW, Shoemaker WC, editors: *Critical care state of the art.* Anaheim, Calif, 1991, Society of Critical Care Medicine, pp 311–350. Used by permission.)

view related to lactic acidemia and critical illness has been published recently.[56] Weil et al.[64] demonstrated the superiority of venous pH as a marker of tissue hypoxia, particularly in mild hypoxic states.[65]

Systemic $\dot{V}O_2$ may be altered in the presence of changes in body temperature, general anesthesia, as a response to injury, and during shock. Every 1°C elevation in body temperature corresponds to a 10% to 13% increase in $\dot{V}O_2$.[66] During hypothermic cardiopulmonary bypass, $\dot{V}O_2$ decreases below normal values with a concomitant 7% decrease in $\dot{V}O_2$ for 1°C.[67, 68] During fever, there is a transient increase in $\dot{V}O_2$. Postoperative shivering has been associated with a 100% increase in $\dot{V}O_2$, and this should be considered in the case of debilitated patients or in those with scarce reserves. Treatment with sedatives and/or neuromuscular blockers may ameliorate this problem.[69] General anesthesia decreases $\dot{V}O_2$ due to loss of hypothalamic temperature regulation, reduced muscle tone and heat generation.[70, 71]

Injury is characterized by changes in metabolic activity. Early after injury, $\dot{V}O_2$ decreases (shock phase) to be followed by an increase in metabolic activity and a correspondent increase in $\dot{V}O_2$ (flow phase). Skeletal trauma may present with a 30% increase in $\dot{V}O_2$, whereas patients with burns or those with sepsis may exceed a 100% increase in $\dot{V}O_2$.[72] All metabolic changes induced by agitation, fever, or the application of therapeutic interventions in the ICU should be considered during the evaluation of $\dot{V}O_2$ in critically ill patients.

During shock, the oxygen transport system is either not able to deliver enough oxygen to the tissues or is impaired. Successful resuscitation has been characterized by a greater than normal increase in $\dot{V}O_2$ and has been associated with increased survival.[73] Monitoring $\dot{V}O_2$ during low output shock may detect early signs of irreversible hemodynamic decompensation.[74] The inability of a high output state to deliver oxygen to the tissues has been connected to maldistribution and imperfect cellular oxygen utilization rather than to derangement of total systemic oxygen transport.[53, 75] Shoemaker et al.[73] have demonstrated that resuscitation efforts that do not improve $\dot{V}O_2$ provide a very poor prognosis. This outcome has been associated with loss of cell integrity, particularly at the respiratory cellular level.

Oxygen Debt-Induced Cellular Alterations

Hypoxic tissue is characterized by a series of alterations of cellular and subcellular tissue perfusion and tissue metabolism, as well as cellular structure and function. Intense neurohormonal activity coupled with hemodynamic disturbances and changes in the microcirculation and release of various vasoactive agents have been implicated in the pathophysiologic mechanism of trauma and shock-induced hypoxic states. All these conditions will eventually decrease the circulating volume, resulting in transient or irreversible changes at the subcellular level.

The mitochondria is the place where electron transport-linked reactions provide approximately 95% of the total body's energy needs under normal conditions. To accomplish this function, the available cellular oxygen should surpass 90%. The lack of oxygen may produce cellular damage, manifested by either a deficit in electron transport-linked carriers,[76] or by a lack of metabolic substrates with resultant deleterious effects on the cellular energy supply.[77]

During severe hypoxia, as well as after death and cessation of cell function, the mitochondria continue with different rates of substrate metabolism. The ability to utilize alpha-ketoglutarate for example, which enters indirectly into the electron transport system from the tricarboxylic acid cycle, is highly depressed. By contrast, the use of succinate substrate, which passes directly from the tricarboxylic acid cycle into the electron transport system, continues with a lesser degree of suppression. The succinate system is located in the inner mitochondrial membrane and may contribute to functional stability.[78] The alpha-ketoglutarate system is located inside the matrix and needs a complex organization of enzymes which then make it more sensitive to alterations produced by reduced oxygen.[79]

The hypoxia-induced depression in mitochondrial metabolism has been related to an alteration in the relationship between nicotinamide-adenine dinucleotide (NAD) and the electron transport phosphorylation system, and a derangement in the coupling process between phosphorylation and oxidation through electron transport. The result is a decrease in the respiratory control ratio (RCR). Factors that might interfere with the maintenance and production of energy during cellular ischemia include mitochondrial swelling, vulnerability of the alpha-ketoglutarate system, failure to recycle due to decreased available energy, increased mitochondrial calcium levels, extramitochondrial inhibition of other factors such as free fatty acids (FFA) or altered adenine triphosphatase activity.[77] There is a significant reduction in mitochondrial redoxidation potential in hemorrhagic shock[80] with a reduction in the mitochondrial NAD^+/NADH ratio. This represents a decrease in the rate of oxidative phosphorylation. The tricarboxylic acid cycle is inhibited because of a reduction of the ratio of oxaloacetate to malate.[81]

It is estimated that only 10% of normal mitochondrial NAD is sufficient to maintain respiration and phosphorylation capacity.[82] However, the addition of exogenous NAD did not restore the respiratory control activities in experimental studies.[83]

During shock and ischemia, intramitochondrial Mg^{2+} decreases (plasma Mg^{2+} increases), suggesting that this element is no longer bound and that alterations exist at the level of the mitochondrial membrane. Mg^{2+} takes part in the process of coenzyme A and thiamine pyrophosphate synthesis.

In contrast, the mitochondrial levels of Ca^{2+} are increased during cellular hypoxia.[84] The influx of Ca^{2+} is considered a sign of cell swelling and inhibition of mitochondrial production of ATP. An inhibiting mitochondrial mechanism has been associated with the presence of elevated amount of FFAs. Hepatic ischemia and reperfusion presents with increased levels of FFAs.[85] The addition of albumin may, however, restore the RCR in mitochondria isolated from ischemic hearts.[86]

The energy-linked shuttle mechanisms that help the translocation of ATP from the inner mitochondrial site of the oxidative phosphorylation to the cytoplasm, and the return of adenosine diphosphate and inorganic phosphate to the mitochondria for resynthesis of ATP, have been found to be altered during shock and hypoxia.[81, 87] Other intracellular alterations seen during shock and hypoxia have been detailed elsewhere.[77]

The reversibility of mitochondrial dysfunction depends on the extent of the damage of the mitochondrial membranes, as well as the duration of the hypoxic impact. If the mitochondrial membranes are intact, it is possible that improvement of $Sa{O_2}$ may re-establish the electron transfer system and the production of energy. There are, however, instances when ischemia creates permanent damage to the mitochondrial membranes, particularly if hypoxia extended beyond a critical time. There is much debate whether organs such as the brain and heart may tolerate more extensive hypoxic insults or if the ischemic tolerance seen in these organs result from circulatory priorities and redistribution of cardiac output. In these circumstances, circulation in the vital organs is maintained at the expense of other vascular beds.

Monitoring Tissue Oxygenation

It seems that the reversal of ischemic cellular sequelae is a function of prompt assessment of tissue oxygenation and the application of interventions that allow the enhancement of $D{O_2}$ and tissue oxygen utilization. ICU monitoring has been developed to detect significant new changes in the patient's status and to measure the effect of therapeutic interventions. It is now considered that therapy for critically ill patients needs to be based not only on pathophysiology, but also on monitoring and outcome predictions.[88]

Shoemaker et al.[88] have presented comparative elements of traditional monitoring based on vital signs, Hct, central venous pressure, and urine output, and the pathophysiologic approach based on the significance of hemodynamic and oxygen transport patterns for critically ill patients. They conclude that "an appropriate decision tree helps achieve therapeutic goals expeditiously by providing a coherent, organized patient management plan. This plan should maintain the patient in an optimal hemodynamic state without allowing hypoxia from blood volume, hemodynamic, and oxygen transport deficits to develop."

Recent advances in technology allow the assessment of the oxygen transport system in at least three ways: perfusion, oxygen utilization, and oxygen content. Mixed venous oxygen pressure ($P\bar{v}{O_2}$) may adequately reflect tissue perfusion and oxygenation[89]; however, it becomes an unreliable indicator in those with hepatic disease or occlusive vascular disease.[90] Probably the most popular tool for assessing tissue oxygenation is the oxygen electrode, a part of many technologies such as the blood gas analyzer, the pulse oximeter, or measurement of the transcutaneous oxygen tension.[91] The multi-wire surface electrode has been developed by Kessler and Lübbers[92] to provide more sites (multiple measurements) for sampling of oxygen levels. Its use in the ICU is presently limited.

Mass spectroscopy has been used for differentiating gases based on molecular weight. The instrument can simultaneously measure a variety of gases and its application is expanding for assessment of oxygenation of particular organs at risk,[93] or for the measurement of various metabolic markers.[94]

Nuclear magnetic resonance (NMR) spectroscopy allows the noninvasive measurement of phosphorus-containing metabolites, such as ATP, phosphocreatine (PCr), and inorganic phosphorus (Pi) as well as intracellular pH.[95–99] Another noninvasive method for assessment of cellular metabolism is positron emission tomography (PET). This technology is based on quantification of labeled tracers.[100, 101]

With the use of more liberal invasive monitoring for critically ill patients, the assessment of global tissue oxygenation through the measurement of mixed venous oxygen saturation ($S\bar{v}O_2$) is now available.[89] An expanded discussion on the principles of $S\bar{v}O_2$ measurement and its clinical value and patient treatment applications has been recently published elsewhere.[102, 103]

Summary

Monitoring of critically ill patients must provide hemodynamic and oxygen transport information, which should give the health care provider an understanding of the underlying pathophysiology, and should be useful in the application of intensive care therapy. The biological significance of these assessments is of utmost importance for the ultimate goal—the improved outcome. In the ICU, the assessment of tissue oxygenation may become a crucial method to identifying problems during the evaluation of applied therapy. It is important to stress that a new concept may emerge, i.e., that therapy should be directed towards augmentation of hemodynamic and oxygen transport variables rather than return of these parameters to the normal ranges.

References

1. Shoemaker WC: Tissue perfusion and oxygenation: A primary problem in acute circulatory failure and shock status. *Crit Care Med* 19:595–596, 1991.
2. Erecinska M, Wilson DF: Regulation of cellular energy metabolism. *J Membr Biol* 70:1–14, 1982.
3. Chance B et al: Multiple controls of oxidative metabolism in living tissues as studied by phosphorus magnetic resonance. *Proc Natl Acad Sci USA* 83:9458–9462, 1986.
4. Katz LA et al: Relationship between phosphate metabolites and oxygen consumption of heart in vivo. *Am J Physiol* 256:265–274, 1989.

5. Van Beek JHGM, Westerhof N: Response time of mitochondrial oxygen consumption following stepwise changes in cardiac energy demand. In Piper J, Goldstick TK, Meyer M, editors: *Oxygen transport to tissue XII. Advances in experimental medicine and biology.* New York, 1990, Plenum, pp 415–422.
6. Snyder JV: Oxygen transport: The model and reality. In Snyder JV, Pinsky MR, editors: *Oxygen transport in the critically ill patient.* St Louis, 1992, Mosby–Year Book, pp 3–15.
7. Snyder JV, Carroll GC: Tissue oxygenation: A physiologic approach to a clinical problem. *Curr Probl Surg* 19:650–719, 1982.
8. Finch CA, Lenfant C: Oxygen transport in man. *N Engl J Med* 286:407–415, 1972.
9. Florenzano F et al: Left ventricular function in chronic anemia: evidence of noncatecholamine positive inotropic factor in the serum. *Am J Cardiol* 54:638–645, 1984.
10. Rand PW et al: Viscosity of normal human blood under normothermic and hypothermic conditions. *J Appl Physiol* 19:117–122, 1964.
11. Varat MA, Adolph RJ, Fowler NO: Fundamentals of clinical cardiology. *Am Heart J* 83:415, 1972.
12. Asmundsson T, Kilburn KH: Survival of acute respiratory failure: A study of 239 episodes. *Ann Intern Med* 70:471, 1969.
13. Humphrey PRD et al: Cerebral blood flow and viscosity in relative polycythemia. *Lancet* 2:873, 1979.
14. Pearson TC, Wetherly-Mein G: Vascular occlusive episodes and venous hematocrit in primary proliferative polycythemia. *Lancet* 2:1919, 1978.
15. Shah DM et al: Increased cardiac output and oxygen transport after intraoperative isovolumic hemodilution. *Arch Surg* 115:597–600, 1980.
16. Jobes DR, Gallagher J: Acute normovolemic hemodilution. *Int Anesthesiol Clin* 20:59–76, 1982.
17. Wolfe JHN et al: The effect of hemodilution upon patients with intermittent claudication. *Surg Gynecol Obstet* 160:347, 1985.
18. Woodson RD: Hemoglobin concentration and exercise capacity. *Am Rev Respir Dis* 129:72, 1984.
19. Haupt MT, Gilbert EM, Carlson RW: Fluid loading increases oxygen consumption in septic patients with lactic acidosis. *Am Rev Respir Dis* 131:912, 1985.
20. Pace NL, Stanley TH, Andriano KP: Transcutaneous PO_2 poorly estimates arterial PO_2 in adults during anesthesia. *Int J Clin Monit Comput* 1:227, 1985.
21. Harken AH, Woods M: The influence of oxyhemoglobin affinity on tissue oxygen consumption. *Ann Surg* 183:130–135, 1976.
22. Watkins GM et al: The left shifted oxyhemoglobin curve in sepsis: A preventable defect. *Ann Surg* 180:213, 1974.
23. Bryan-Brown CW: Oxygen transport and the oxyhemoglobin dissociation curve. In Berk JL, Sampliner JE, editors: *Handbook of critical care,* ed 2. Boston, 1982, Little, Brown, p 557.
24. Woodson RD: Physiological significance of oxygen dissociation curve shifts. *Crit Care Med* 7:368, 1979.
25. Woodson RD et al: Increased blood oxygen affinity decreases canine brain oxygen consumption. *J Lab Clin Med* 100:411, 1982.
26. Woodson RD, Aurebach S: Effect of increased oxygen affinity and anemia on cardiac output and its distribution. *J Appl Physiol* 53:1299, 1982.

27. Woodson RD: Importance of 2,3-DPG in banked blood: New data in animal models. In Collins JA, Murawski K, Shafer AW, editors: *Massive transfusion in surgery and trauma.* New York, 1982, Liss, pp 69–78.
28. Farber MO et al: Steroids, hypoxemia and oxygen transport. *Chest* 75:451–455, 1979.
29. Springer RR et al: Effects of changes in arterial carbon dioxide tension on oxygen consumption during cardiopulmonary bypass. *Chest* 75:549–554, 1979.
30. Wassaman K: Coupling of external and internal respiration. *Am Rev Respir Dis* 129:521, 1984.
31. Cain SM: Peripheral uptake and delivery in health and disease. *Clin Chest Med* 4:139, 1983.
32. Shibutani K et al: Critical level of oxygen delivery in anesthetized man. *Crit Care Med* 11:640, 1984.
33. Cain SM: Supply dependency of oxygen uptake in ARDS: Myth or reality? *Am J Med Sci* 288:119–124, 1984.
34. Cain SM: Effect of time and vasoconstriction tone on oxygen extraction during hypoxic-hypoxia. *J Appl Physiol* 45:219, 1978.
35. Granger DN et al: Effects of adenosine on intestinal hemodynamics, oxygen delivery and capillary fluid exchange. *Am J Physiol* 235:707, 1978.
36. Kvietys PR et al: Effects of temperature on ileal blood flow and oxygenation. *Am J Physiol* 249:246, 1985.
37. Roca J et al: Evidence for tissue diffusion limitation on VO_{2max} in normal humans. *J Appl Physiol* 67:291–299, 1989.
38. Adams RP, Dieleman LA, Cain SM: A critical value for oxygen transport in the rat. *J Appl Physiol* 53:660, 1982.
39. Fahey JT, Lister G: Postnatal changes in critical cardiac output and oxygen transport in conscious lambs. *Am J Physiol* 253:100, 1989.
40. Ultsch GR, Jackson DC, Moalli R: Metabolic oxygen conformity among lower vertebrates: The toadfish revisited. *J Comp Physiol* 142:439, 1981.
41. Lister G: Oxygen supply/demand in the critically ill. In Taylor RW, Shoemaker WC, editors: *Critical care state of the art.* Anaheim, Calif, 1991, Society of Critical Care Medicine, pp 311–350.
42. Jobsis FF, Lammana JC: Kinetic aspects of intracellular redox reactions. In Robin ED, editor: *Extrapulmonary manifestations of respiratory disease.* New York, 1978, Decker, pp 63–106.
43. Schumacker PT et al: Effects of hyperthermia and hypothermia on oxygen extraction by tissues during hypovolemia. *J Appl Physiol* 63:1246–1252, 1987.
44. Danek SJ et al: The dependence of oxygen uptake on oxygen delivery in the adult respiratory distress syndrome. *Am Rev Respir Dis* 122:387–395, 1980.
45. Mohsenifar Z et al: Relationship between O_2 delivery and O_2 consumption in the adult respiratory distress syndrome. *Chest* 84:267–271, 1983.
46. Annat G et al: Oxygen delivery and uptake in the adult respiratory distress syndrome. Lack of relationship when measured independently in patients with normal blood lactate concentrations. *Am Rev Respir Dis* 133:999–1001, 1986.
47. Bihari D et al: The effects of vasodilation with prostacyclin on oxygen delivery and uptake in critically ill patients. *N Engl J Med* 317:397–403, 1987.
48. Dorinsky PM et al: Relationships of oxygen uptake and oxygen delivery in respiratory failure not due to the adult respiratory distress syndrome. *Chest* 93:1013–1019, 1988.

49. Fenwick JC et al: Increased concentrations of plasma lactate predict pathological dependence of oxygen consumption on oxygen delivery in patients with adult respiratory distress syndrome. *J Crit Care* 5:81–86, 1990.
50. Quan SF et al: Changes in venous admixture with alterations of inspired oxygen concentration. *Anesthesiology* 52:477–482, 1980.
51. Chapler CK, Cain SM, Stainsby WN: The effect of hyperoxia on oxygen uptake during acute anemia. *Can J Physiol Pharmacol* 62:809–814, 1984.
52. Buran MJ: Oxygen consumption. In Snyder JV, Pinsky MR, editors: *Oxygen transport in the critically ill.* St Louis, 1987, Mosby–Year Book, pp 16–21.
53. Hontchens BA, Westenskow DR: Oxygen consumption in septic shock: Collective review. *Circ Shock* 13:361–384, 1984.
54. Nelson LD et al: Technical problems with data acquisition. In Snyder JV, Pinsky MR, editors: *Oxygen transport in the critically ill.* St Louis, 1987, Mosby Year Book, pp 205–234.
55. Cain SM: Oxygen deficit incurred during hypoxia and its relation to lactate and excess lactate. *Am J Physiol* 213:57–63, 1967.
56. Mizock LD, Falk JL: Lactic acidosis in critical illness. *Crit Care Med* 20:80–93, 1992.
57. Gilbert EM et al: The effect of fluid loading, blood transfusion and catecholamine infusion on oxygen consumption in patients with sepsis. *Am Rev Respir Dis* 134:873–878, 1986.
58. Kaufman BS, Rackow EC, Falk JL: The relationship between oxygen delivery and consumption during fluid loading in patients with trauma and septic shock. *Chest* 85:336–340, 1984.
59. Vincent JL et al: Oxygen uptake/supply dependency: Effects of a short-term infusion. *Am Rev Respir Dis* 142:2–7, 1990.
60. Silverman HJ: Lack of relationship between induced changes in oxygen consumption and changes in lactate levels. *Chest* 100:1012–1015, 1991.
61. Huckabee WE: Relationship of pyruvate and lactate during anaerobic metabolism. I. Effects of infusion of pyruvate or glucose and of hyperventilation. *J Clin Invest* 37:244, 1958.
62. Takano N: Blood lactate accumulation and its causative factors during passive hyperventilation in dogs. *Jpn J Physiol* 16:481–496, 1966.
63. Eldridge F et al: Effect of respiratory alkalosis on blood lactate and pyruvate in humans. *J Appl Physiol* 22:461–468, 1967.
64. Weil MH et al: Difference in acid-base state between venous and arterial blood during cardiopulmonary resuscitation. *N Engl J Med* 315:153–156, 1986.
65. Fahey JT, Lister G: Response to low cardiac output: Developmental differences in metabolism during oxygen deficit and recovery in lambs. *Pediatr Res* 26:180–187, 1989.
66. Beisel W, Wannemacher RW, Neufeld HA: Relation of fever to energy expenditure. In Ross Laboratories (ed): *Assessment of energy metabolism in health and disease.* Columbus, Ohio, 1980, Ross Conference on Medical Research, p 144.
67. Harris EA, Seelye ER, Squire AW: Oxygen consumption during cardiopulmonary bypass with moderate hypothermia in man. *Br J Anaesth* 43:1113–1120, 1971.
68. Fox LS et al: Relationship of whole body oxygen consumption to perfusion flow rate during hypothermic cardiopulmonary bypass. *J Thorac Cardiovasc Surg* 83:239–248, 1982.

69. Rodiguez JL et al: Physiologic requirements during rewarming: Suppression of the shivering response. *Crit Care Med* 11:490–497, 1983.
70. Roc CF et al: The influence of body temperature in early postoperation oxygen consumption. *Surgery* 60:85, 1966.
71. Waxman K, Shoemaker WC: Physiologic responses to massive intraoperative hemorrhage. *Arch Surg* 117:470–475, 1982.
72. Kinney JM et al: Tissue fuel and weight loss after injury. *J Clin Path* 23:65–72, 1970.
73. Shoemaker WC, Appel C, Bland RD: Use of physiologic monitoring to predict outcome and assist in clinical decisions in critically ill postoperative patients. *Am J Surg* 146:43–50, 1983.
74. Abraham E et al: Sequential cardiorespiratory pattern in septic shock. *Crit Care Med* 11:799–803, 1983.
75. Shah DM, Newell JC, Saba TM: Defects in peripheral oxygen utilization following trauma and shock. *Arch Surg* 116:1277–1281, 1981.
76. Williamson JR: Mitochondrial metabolism and cell regulation. In Parker L, Gomez-Poyon, editors: *Mitochondria: bioenergetics and membrane structure.* New York, 1976, Academic, pp 79–107.
77. Chandry IH: Cellular mechanism in shock and ischemia and their correction. *Am J Physiol* 245:117–134, 1968.
78. Lardy H, Ferguson SM: Oxidative phosphorylation in mitochondria. *Annu Rev Biochem* 38:911–1034, 1969.
79. Moss GS, Erve PP, Schumer W: Effect of endotoxin on mitochondrial respiration. *Surg Forum* 20:24–26, 1969.
80. Kraven T et al: Improved survival and metabolic changes in a rat shock model produced by ATP-$MgCl_2$. *Curr Surg* 36:435–437, 1979.
81. Ozawa K: Energy metabolism. In Cowley RA, Trump BF, editors: *Pathophysiology of shock and ischemia.* Baltimore, 1982, Williams & Wilkins, pp 74–83.
82. MacLennon DH, Tzagoloff A: Effect of diphosphopyridine nucleotide deficiency on respiration, respiratory control and phosphorylation in mitochondria. *J Biol Chem* 214:1933–1937, 1966.
83. Bleu AE et al: Cellular alterations with shock and ischemia. *Angiology* 25:31–41, 1974.
84. Mela L: Mitochondrial function in shock, ischemia and hypoxia. In Cowley RA, Trump BF, editors: *Pathophysiology of shock, anoxia and ischemia.* Baltimore, 1982, Williams & Wilkins, pp 84–95.
85. Okawa M, Clemens MG, Chansky H: Studies on the mechanism of beneficial effects of ATF-$MgCl_2$ following hepatic ischemia. *Am J Physiol* 244:695–702, 1983.
86. Higgins EF, Chan HP, Park FB: Deleterious effects of free fatty acids in mitochondria during acute myocardial ischemia. *Surg Forum* 31:10–12, 1980.
87. Schumer W: Localization of energy pathway block in shock. *Surgery* 64:55–59, 1968.
88. Shoemaker WC, Kram HB, Appel PL: Therapy of shock based on pathophysiology, monitoring and outcome prediction. *Crit Care Med* 18:519–525, 1990.
89. Birman H et al: Continuous monitoring of mixed venous oxygen saturation in hemodynamically unstable patients. *Chest* 86:753–756, 1984.
90. Cove JB: Monitoring of tissue oxygenation. In Snyder JR, Pinsky MR, editors: *Oxygen transport in the critically ill.* St Louis, 1987, Mosby–Year Book, pp 164–175.

91. Lübbers DW: Theoretical basis of the transcutaneous blood gas measurements. *Crit Care Med* 9:721, 1981.
92. Kessler M, Lübbers DW: Aufbau and Anwendungs möglichkeiten verschiedner PO_2-electroden. *Pflugers Arch Ges Physiol* 291:82, 1966.
93. Magovern GJ et al: Assessment of myocardial protection during global ischemia with myocardial gas tension monitoring. *Surgery* 92:373, 1982.
94. Weaver JC: Continuous monitoring of volatile metabolites by mass spectrometer. In Cohen JS, editor: *Noninvasive probes of tissue metabolism.* New York, 1982, Wiley, pp 25–47.
95. Meyer RA, Kushmerick MJ, Brown TR: Application of P-NMR spectroscopy to the study of striated muscle metabolism. *Am J Physiol* 242:C1–C11, 1982.
96. Koutcher JA, Burt CT: Principles of nuclear magnetic resonance. *J Nucl Med* 25:101–111, 1984.
97. Kushmerick MJ: Patterns in mammalian muscle energetics. *J Exp Biol* 115:165, 1985.
98. Adler S, Shoubridge E, Radda GK: Estimation of cellular pH gradients with P-NMR in intact rabbit renal tubular cells. *Am J Physiol* 247:188, 1984.
99. Civan MM et al: Intracellular pH of perfused single frog skin: Combined F- and P-NMR analysis. *Am J Physiol* 247:506, 1984.
100. Phelps ME, Schelbert HR, Mazziotta JC: Positron computed tomography for studies of myocardial and cerebral function. *Ann Intern Med* 98:339–359, 1983.
101. Ter-Pogossian MM, Raichle ME, Sobel BE: Positron emission tomography. *Sci Am* 243:170–181, 1980.
102. Cernaianu AC, Nelson LD: Continuous measurement of mixed venous saturation: Principles and clinical applications. In Shoemaker WC, Edwards DJ, Vincent JL, editors: *Oxygen transport—Principles and practice.* London, 1992, Saunders (in print).
103. Cernaianu AC et al: Continuous venous oximetry for hemodynamic and oxygen transport stability post cardiac surgery. *J Cardiovasc Surg* 33:14–20, 1992.

Clinical Dilemmas in Obstetrics

Christina Campbell, M.B., Ch.B.

Associate Professor of Anesthesia, Indiana University School of Medicine, Indianapolis, Indiana

The field of obstetrical anesthesia continues to challenge even those most resilient of anesthesiologists who remain committed to the provision of superior anesthesia for the parturient. On the surface, the subspecialty appears wonderfully dynamic. It certainly has embraced wholeheartedly the recent advances in our understanding of pain mechanisms and the application of neuraxial narcotics for acute pain management. Yet the field remains haunted by old and all-too-familiar problems that threaten not only advancement of specialized knowledge but worse, may jeopardize commitment by anesthesiologists to a field that, in fact, should expect only the highest level of anesthesia expertise. While it may appear anachronistic to be discussing old problems in a volume entitled *Advances in Anesthesia*, until some of these old problems are aired, discussed, and the appropriate corrective actions taken, there appears little opportunity for evolution of the so-called "Cinderella" specialty. This chapter will examine some of these clinical dilemmas currently faced by anesthesiologists in obstetrics.

How to Provide Obstetrical Anesthesia Coverage

Clinical Scenario 1

You are interviewing for a position as a staff anesthesiologist at a 200-bed private hospital in a small college town. The chief of staff of the hospital happens to be a member of a group with a very busy obstetrics practice. In confidence he expresses to you his dissatisfaction with the services presently provided by the anesthesia department. He asks for your opinions on the feasibility of providing 24-hour anesthesia coverage for the obstetrics floor.

The problem of how to provide appropriate anesthesia coverage for the obstetric suite is not new. The last national survey examining the availability of obstetric anesthesia personnel was conducted jointly by the American Society of Anesthesiologists Committee on Obstetrical Anesthesia and the Liaison Committee for Obstetrics and Gynecology of the American College of Obstetrics and Gynecology in 1986.[1] The results of this study indicated

TABLE 1.
Reasons for Noninvolvement of Anesthesiologists in Obstetrics*

Unpredictability of labor and delivery
Isolation of labor and delivery suites from the general operating rooms
Financial impracticality of small obstetric services
Increased risk of malpractice claims
Lower level of remuneration
Lack of mutual respect and appreciation for their respective problems between obstetricians and anesthesiologists
Stress created by consumerism

*Adapted from Gibbs CP et al: *Anesthesiology* 65:298–306, 1986.

persistent, serious deficiencies in the anesthesia care available to the majority of parturients in this country. At this time, Gibbs et al. reported anesthesiologists to be available full-time for the labor and delivery suite in only 21% of all hospitals surveyed, on nights and on weekends in only 15%. Furthermore, anesthesiologists administered anesthesia for 70% of cesarean deliveries but were involved with only 20% of vaginal deliveries. It is unlikely that the situation has improved appreciably. Indeed, the American Society of Anesthesiologists Consultation Program reports that currently one of the most frequent reasons for hospitals seeking their assistance (39% of all requested consultations) is because of the hospital's failure to secure adequate obstetrical anesthesia coverage.[2] If Indiana is representative of national trends, the situation may actually have deteriorated. In a recent study modeled along the lines of that of Gibbs et al., we found that anesthesiologists were available full-time for obstetric patients in only 14% of Indiana hospitals, and on nights and on weekends in only 11%.

At first glance, it is difficult to understand the reluctance of anesthesiologists to be involved in obstetrical coverage. A rational view might be that a mother and her infant would warrant and demand the best possible anesthesia care available. Showing more pragmatism, the various regulatory bodies have aspired to simple parity. Specifically, the Joint Commission on Accreditation of Healthcare Organizations (JCAHO),[3] the American Society of Anesthesiologists (ASA),[4] and the American College of Obstetricians and Gynecologists (ACOG)[5] have all indicated in independent statements that the quality of anesthesia care available to the obstetric patient should be the *same* as that for the surgical patient. Yet we seem to be failing even in providing for this goal. The Collaborative Survey of 1986,[1] in addition

TABLE 2.
Improving the Availability of Obstetrical Anesthesia

Improve hospital design: situate labor and delivery suites closer to the main operating room
Press for consolidation of obstetrical services (this is diametrically opposite to the current trend created by HMOs)
Offer financial subsidy, particularly in smaller, less busy units
Designate a director of obstetrical anesthesia
Arrange frequent continuing education programs for obstetricians and anesthesiologists to encourage mutual understanding

to gathering statistical data regarding availability of obstetrical anesthesia, also attempted to gain insight into possible reasons for anesthesiologists' reticence for involvement. Table 1 summarizes their findings. While it is doubtful that much can be done to improve on the unpredictability of labor and delivery, the other reasons cited could be viewed as potentially correctable. Some basic steps toward improving the availability of obstetrical anesthesia personnel are offered in Table 2.

The one glaringly obvious lesson apparent from the study of Gibbs et al. is that hospitals with fewer than 500 deliveries annually do not provide adequate anesthesia care or coverage. It is impractical to believe that these small obstetric units can sustain a reasonable work load, schedule, or income for even the most committed of anesthesiologists. In a hospital delivering 500 babies annually, it can be expected that there will be no deliveries in approximately 90 days, and only one in 125 days (Fig 1).[6] The single most effective measure, therefore, in luring anesthesiologists to the field would be to consolidate obstetric services into larger units. Unfortunately, the recent trend has been in exactly the opposite direction with many smaller hospitals attempting to attract the business of health maintenance organizations (HMOs) by offering obstetric services as part of those of a full service hospital. It is now estimated that 50% of the obstetric facilities in this country fall into the category of delivering less than 500 babies annually.

Key, however, to having anesthesia departments willing to provide obstetrical anesthesia coverage is having anesthesiologists who believe it is part of their practice responsibility. It is vital, therefore, for teachers of ob-

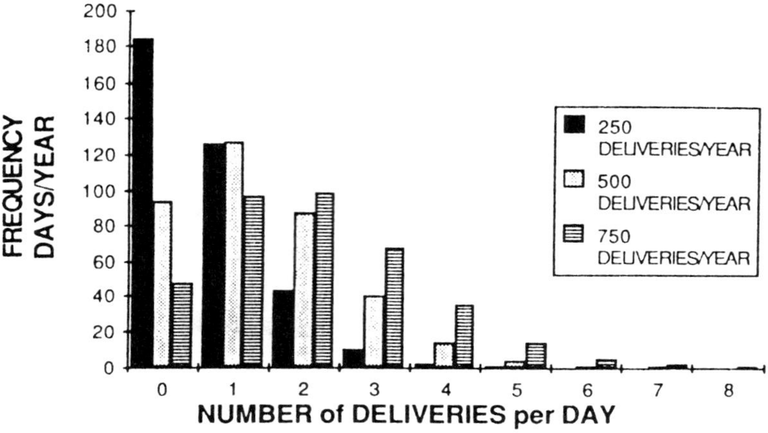

FIG 1.
Histogram showing the anticipated number of deliveries per day according to the number of deliveries per year. These data were derived using the Poisson equation for a random distribution of events in time. (From Levinson G, Shnider SM: *Anesthesiology* 65:245–246, 1986. Used by permission.)

stetric anesthesia to instill this sense of duty, and, it is hoped, some of their enthusiasm, into their trainees at an early stage. It is equally important to garner future support from fledgling obstetricians by impressing upon them early the desirability of having skilled anesthesia care available 24 hours a day, educating them about anesthetic techniques, and providing them with good role models of the consultant anesthesiologist.

Success in retaining superior anesthesia care for the labor and delivery suite is undoubtedly more likely, however, if one secures the services of anesthesiologists who not only enjoy, but are committed to responding to the unique needs of the obstetric patient. The other maladies linked to difficulty in attracting obstetrical anesthesia coverage—the increased risk of malpractice litigation, poor interpersonal relationships with obstetricians, and the added anxiety generated by patient consumerism—possibly could all be minimized by such an approach. It is well accepted that patients are much less likely to sue a physician they truly believe is interested in their well-being.[7] Anesthesia groups and hospital administrators would also be well served by designating a suitably qualified person to organize the obstetrical anesthesia service. In return for this added responsibility, this designate might receive a stipend so that he or she could fulfill the essential administrative, educator, and communicator roles without suffering income loss. The benefits that could accrue from having this single intermediary for all involved parties would almost certainly be outweighed by this comparatively small financial outlay.

There lurks on the horizon yet another threat to the future of equitable anesthesia availability for the parturient. Third-party insurance companies are, in some states, considering altering fee schedules for labor epidural analgesia. In instances in which initial placement of the epidural catheter is performed by an anesthesiologist, but subsequent "top-up" doses are performed by a member of the anesthesia care team, payment would cover only the time involved in catheter placement. Such misconceptions regarding subsequent responsibility for the patient must be challenged. The anesthesiologist's ability to care safely for more than one laboring patient simultaneously has, in the past, helped to compensate somewhat for the disparity between the time invested, that is the time spent covering the obstetrical suite, and that for which one could actually bill. Such an irresponsible action on the part of insurance companies would surely serve only to further jeopardize obstetrical anesthesia services. As things stand at the present, however, it is possible for anesthesia departments to find ways to cover the obstetrical suite with minimal financial hardship either by sharing the load or by supporting at least those who express a desire to do so.

Dilemmas Caused by Consumerism

Clinical Scenario 2

You have just joined a group of anesthesiologists practicing in a small community hospital. At your first staff meeting, in a gush of enthusiasm and naivete, you expressed an interest in obstetrics and were immediately elected director of obstetrical anesthesia. The first phone call that you receive on assuming your position is from an irate obstetrician wanting to know why you have written an NPO order for a patient who is anticipating an uncomplicated labor and vaginal delivery with epidural analgesia.

Should We Feed Patients in Labor?

The past decade or so has witnessed considerable change in the ways in which physicians, nursing personnel, and patients interact. There is now greater emphasis on interdependence for clinical decision-making, with many patients actually "shopping around" for those physicians whom they believe will be more accommodating to their input. Obstetrics has preceded most disciplines in its acceptance of this attitude. Sadly, as commonly occurs in similar circumstances, unquestioned acquiescence to patient demands may actually result in less optimal care of the patient, the price tag for possible improved patient satisfaction. A perfect example of this type of clinical situation is illustrated by the current debate being waged between obstetricians and obstetric anesthesiologists as to the prudence of allowing patients to eat during labor.[8–11] Proponents of a more liberal policy toward allowing oral intake during labor maintain that if the patient is allowed to take oral sustenance, she will be less stressed, less likely to require an intravenous line, and therefore less likely to need medical intervention. In a recent article, Elkington went further, stating that "there is neither evidence of benefit in withholding fluids nor evidence of risk in allowing them."[9] While it is now acknowledged that ice chips and small sips of water are unlikely to pose an additional hazard to the aspiration potential in the parturient and indeed may actually facilitate gastric emptying to some degree,[12] many anesthesiologists would take exception to Elkington's statement. Such a sweeping remark is seen, I believe, as a threat to opening the flood gates to total abandonment of NPO policies. Some natural easing of strict NPO policies has in fact occurred in recent times. Only 47% of 217 institutions surveyed in 1988 reported a strict NPO or "ice chips only" policy for their patients in labor[8] (Table 3). The deeper concern sparked by Elkington's statement is that it underscores our failure to educate both obstetricians and patients adequately about the risks of pulmonary aspiration of gastric contents. Abouleish and Merriman[11] have recently pointed out that even the clear fluids that are commonly offered to patients in labor may present an unnecessary additional risk due to their acidity (Table 4).

Advocates of oral feeding of patients in labor appear unwilling to accept

TABLE 3.
Survey Results of Institutional Eating and Drinking Policies*

Policy†	Percentage of Institutions
NPO	28.1
NPO except ice chips	18.9
Fluids (usually designated clear, may include soups and gelatin)	10.1
Ice chips and sips of water or clear fluids	8.8
Ice chips or popsicles, or lollipop or hard candy	8.3
Early labor, clear fluids; active labor, ice chips	5.5
Liquids and light eating as desired	5.5
Sips of clear fluids	4.1
Active labor, ice chips and clear fluids	1.8
Variable, depending on physician's or midwife's orders	1.8
Liquids and/or ice chips in early labor	1.4
Clear liquids and hard candy	0.9
Clear liquids with saltine crackers	0.9
Early labor, fluids ad lib; active labor, clear fluids	0.9
Ice chips and juices	0.5
Clear fluids, ice, popsicles	0.5
Liquids and nonparticulate nutrients	0.5
Early labor, eat lightly and drink	0.5
Primiparas, up to 300 mL; multiparas, clear liquids ad lib	0.5
Primiparas, intake seldom; multiparas, clear liquids	0.5

*Adapted from McKay S, Mahan C: *Birth* 15:222–229, 1988.
†Institutions with more liberal policies often specified NPO for women at risk or in whom a cesarean section was anticipated.

TABLE 4.
pH of Clear Fluids Used for Oral Intake During Labor*

Fluid	pH
Tap water	7.2
Fruit juices†	
Apple	3.65
Grape	3.20
Cranberry‡	2.70
Gatorade‡	
Orange	3.03
Lemonade	3.13

*From Abouleish E, Merriman T: *Anesth Analg* 73:674, 1991. Used by permission.
†Produced by Campbell Soup Co, Camden, NJ.
‡Produced by Quaker Oats, Chicago.

that significant morbidity and even mortalities still occur from the sequelae of pulmonary aspiration. Unlike other so-called developed countries, we do not have an organizsed, obligatory, national reporting system for maternal deaths. Instead, the statistics that are available to us on maternal aspiration are semi-reliable at best, but more likely grossly underrepresent the problem. Several recent, retrospective studies of maternal mortality have clearly shown that aspiration is an identifiable factor in as many as 25% of anesthesia-related deaths, with the latter accounting for approximately 5% to 10% of all reported maternal deaths[13–17] (Table 5). Additional cases of aspiration probably are missed by being categorized under "failed or difficult endotracheal intubation," since this is often the precipitating and more dramatic event. In an attempt to better define and quantitate maternal aspiration, Gibbs et al. in 1981 surveyed all members (approximately 600) of the Society of Obstetric Anesthesia and Perinatology.[18] Physicians from 123 institutions agreed to report on all cases of aspiration that occurred during a 1-year period. Twenty-one cases of aspiration were reported, all in association with general anesthesia, and all but 3 occurring during emergent or urgent procedures. Of the 19 cases in which it was used, endotracheal intubation was described as difficult in 14. In 2 instances, the outcome was death. If this sampling is representative of the problem, and the numbers extrapolated to include all obstetric facilities in this country (approximately 5,000), then the true incidence of pulmonary aspiration in the obstetric population may be quite daunting.

There remain two other areas in which generally held misconceptions persist. The first is that pulmonary aspiration of gastric contents occurs *only*

TABLE 5.
Sampling of Available Data on Anesthesia-Related Maternal Mortality as it Relates to Overall Maternal Mortality

Study	Period	Anesthesia-Related Deaths as a Percentage of Total Maternal Deaths
Report from the Maternal Mortality Collaborative, (a special interest group of the American College of Obstetricians and Gynecologists),[13] 19 reporting areas involved	1980–1985	5.9
Michigan maternal mortality study[14]	1972–1984	6.9
Report from North Carolina[15]	1981–1985	10
Report on national trends orchestrated by Centers for Disease Control[16]	1979–1986	4.8
Report on confidential inquiries into maternal deaths in England and Wales[17]	1979–1981	12.6

in the setting of an unprotected airway during the administration of general anesthesia. The potential risk is in fact present whenever upper airway reflexes are lost, with the parturient being especially vulnerable under these circumstances because of disruption of the normal anatomy of the gastroesophageal junction. Hence, aspiration has been known to complicate convulsions associated with local anesthetic toxicity and pregnancy-induced hypertension, and following high or total spinal anesthesia. Chadwick et al.[19] reported in his study of obstetric anesthesia malpractice claims that 2 of the 16 cases of pulmonary aspiration occurred in association with spinal anesthesia. The second misconception is that the routine use of antacids effectively nullifies potential aspiration morbidity. Antacids do nothing to decrease the incidence of aspiration, and even benign pulmonary aspirations (i.e., those involving nonparticulate liquids of relatively high pH) may result in significant hypoxemia for several hours.

Careful retrospective reviews of maternal morbidity and mortality, such as those provided by the England and Wales Triennial Reports on Confidential Inquiries into Maternal Deaths and the recent American Society of Anesthesiologists Closed Claims Project,[19] have supplied useful information regarding the epidemiology of aspiration. We now appreciate that while not exclusive to general anesthesia, it most commonly occurs in association with general anesthesia for emergency cesarean section where

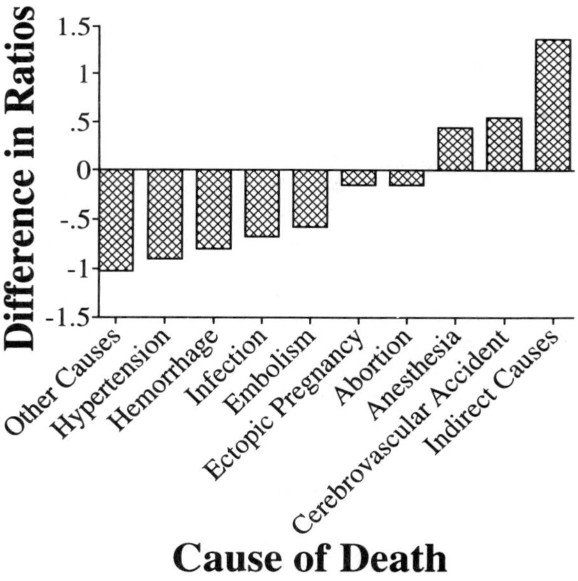

FIG 2.
Comparison between major causes of maternal deaths reported in Maternal Collaborative Study (1980–1985) and those reported nationally from 1974–1978. Note that the only causes to increase their contribution to overall maternal mortality are those related to anesthesia, cerebrovascular accidents, and indirect causes. (From Rochat RW et al: *Obstet Gynecol* 159:187–193, 1988. Used by permission.)

difficulty is encountered in securing the airway. Obesity and other maternal conditions such as diabetes mellitus and hypertension further increase the risks. Even the most experienced anesthesiologist will occasionally encounter difficulty with endotracheal intubation. It is essential therefore, that every member of the obstetric team be familiar with the difficult airway protocol, and that all the necessary equipment be readily at hand. With roughly one in four patients now undergoing delivery by cesarean section, and 50% of these women receiving general anesthesia, it is not surprising that anesthesia-related maternal mortality is only one of three categories that have actually *increased* their contribution to overall mortality in recent times (Fig 2).[13]

From the information that is available then, it seems that anesthesiologists are justified in maintaining a conservative stance on the potential for aspiration in patients in labor. Table 6 lists measures that should be incorporated into the treatment of the obstetric patient if morbidity and mortality from this complication are to be contained. Increased utilization of regional anesthetic techniques, together with routine prophylaxis of patients with nonparticulate antacid prior to any anesthetic or operative intervention, should improve maternal safety. However, as long as there remains

TABLE 6.
Steps to Minimize Pulmonary Aspiration in the Obstetric Patient

1. Allow patients in active labor only ice chips or small sips of water. Those patients at particular risk of an operative delivery should only receive sufficient quantities to keep them comfortable, and ideally should be NPO.
2. Carefully evaluate airway of all patients admitted to labor suite.
3. Avoid oversedation.
4. Use regional anesthesia and avoid general anesthesia whenever possible.
5. Preface any anesthetic or obstetric intervention (eg, immediately prior to initiation of epidural analgesia, or shortly before vaginal delivery) with 15 to 30 mL 0.3M sodium citrate solution or Bicitra.
6. Avoid hypotension, aortocaval compression, local anesthetic toxicity, and excessively high blocks.
7. In patients recognized as being at particular risk, e.g. the morbidly obese patient, consider use of ranitidine and metaclopramide.
8. Should general anesthesia become necessary, use a rapid-sequence intubation technique with cricoid pressure properly maintained until the endotracheal tube cuff has been inflated and end-tidal CO_2 sensed. Ideally an experienced anesthesiologist should be in attendance.
9. Educate all members of the obstetric team on a failed intubation drill.
10. On emergence from general anesthesia, extubate only when the patient is fully responsive with no evidence of residual neuromuscular blockade.
11. Provide appropriate continuous observation of all obstetric patients during labor, delivery, and the immediate postpartum period.

on record a single maternal death as a result of aspiration, this must be viewed as having been preventable and appropriate steps taken to minimize future occurrence. Such a simple step as restricting oral intake in patients in active labor to sips of water and ice chips would appear to be a reasonable approach. Stated more forcefully, it certainly makes little sense to add to gastric contents when anesthetic intervention is at all possible. Some might argue that the unpredictability of delivery makes this the case in every patient in labor. Education of patients and obstetrical staff as to the need for caution is obviously critical to our gaining their cooperation. The problem at present appears to be getting their ears to point in our direction!

Maintaining Good Standards of Anesthesia Care

Obstetricians, I fear, are not alone in succumbing to the influences of consumerism. Anesthesiologists too may feel pressure from a number of directions to minimize their presence in the labor and delivery suite. There is every temptation to gloss over the preanesthetic evaluation, or compromise safe regional anesthetic techniques, in order to "get the patient comfortable" and get out of the room quickly. Trends identified in a recent re-

TABLE 7.
Maternal Injuries in Obstetric Anesthesia Claims*

Injury	Non-Obstetric Claims, %	Maternal Injury Claims, %
Patient/maternal death	39	27†
Headache	1	15†
Pain during anesthesia	<0.5	11†
Patient/maternal nerve damage	16	11
Patient/maternal brain damage	13	9
Emotional distress	2	8‡
Back pain	1	6‡

*Adapted from Chadwick HS et al: *Anesthesiology* 74:242–249, 1991. Used by permission.
†$P \leq .01$.
‡$P \leq .05$.

view of obstetric malpractice claims could be explained by prevalence of this attitude. Results of a comparison of obstetric and nonobstetric anesthesia malpractice claims by Chadwick et al.[19] showed that the obstetric claims contained a disproportionately greater number of minor injuries (headache, backache, and emotional injury) and bad outcomes from local anesthetic toxicity during regional anesthesia (Table 7). It behooves the anesthesiologist then to get involved early, to participate in childbirth preparation classes and continuing education classes, so that accurate information is transmitted to expectant parents, and realistic attitudes about anesthesia are established beforehand. Likewise, in the labor room, the competent obstetric anesthesiologist will work at building a rapport with the patient while skillfully tailoring analgesia to her specific requirements. Patient attitudes appear often to be strongly influenced by nursing personnel, and gaining their support is essential to success.

Lastly, obstetric nurses may also fall prey to forces resulting in inferior care to the parturient. They, perhaps above others, feel the pressure to make the birth experience as unintrusive as possible. Unfortunately, when attempts to accommodate this are combined with a blasé view of the implications of anesthesia in an otherwise healthy woman, the stage is set for disaster. One area in which care has been known to be less than optimum in the past is in the postanesthesia care unit (PACU). Significant disparities frequently exist between the standard of care available in the obstetric PACU and that available in the general surgical PACU. This has prompted renewed efforts by regulatory bodies to improve compliance with established guidelines. The JCAHO,[3] the ASA,[20] and the ACOG have all reiterated their support of postobstetrical anesthesia care facilities, equipment, and personnel being held to the same standard as those available to the surgical patient.

What is the Appropriate Anesthetic Technique for Emergent Cesarean Section?

Clinical Scenario 3

As the anesthesiologist on call you are summoned to the obstetrics floor to provide anesthesia for an emergent cesarean section. An obese (105 kg) primigravid patient has been in labor for many hours. The obstetrician thinks that cesarean section is indicated because of a nonreassuring fetal heart rate pattern—late decelerations have been evident on the fetal monitor for 45 minutes. He wants to move quickly because the fetal scalp pH is 7.2. You are informed that apart from mild hypertension, she has no other medical problems.

The choice of anesthesia for emergent cesarean deliveries appears to be less clear-cut than in the past. In situations in which the fetus or the mother is in obvious dire distress, as for example umbilical cord prolapse with severe fetal bradycardia, maternal hemorrhage with hemodynamic instability, or catastrophic uterine rupture, the necessity and appropriateness of rapidly induced general anesthesia is unquestioned. More commonly, however, we are faced with being asked to administer anesthesia for emergency cesarean section with less distinct diagnostic implications because of fetal distress. Previously a bias toward using general anesthesia in such instances existed. This was based on the premise that timing was critical to optimizing neonatal outcome, and that even the short delay required to establish surgical anesthesia with a regional anesthetic technique was unacceptable. Decisions regarding anesthesia in cases of fetal distress have become less restrictive for a number of reasons. First, as has been discussed previously, significant maternal morbidity and mortality are known to be associated with general anesthesia for emergency cesarean section.[13–17] The major concerns are unexpected difficulty with endotracheal intubation and pulmonary aspiration of gastric contents. Airway difficulties are encountered with greater frequency in the obstetric population than in general surgical patients. Lyons[21] has reported that failed endotracheal intubation may be expected in 1 in 300 obstetric patients, compared to other studies indicating a frequency of 1 in 2,000 in surgical patients. There are a number of recognized factors which, in combination, may hinder visualization of the glottis in pregnancy.[22,23] Vascular engorgement and edema of upper airway structures often result in visual distortion and easy vulnerability of the tissue to bleeding and further edema. Laryngoscopy is often performed in less than ideal conditions with the patient already prepped and draped and tilted for uterine displacement. Obesity in the parturient can magnify these untoward conditions, as do the various hypertensive disorders of pregnancy. Inadequate attention to positioning in the obese patient may also result in loss of the atlantooccipital gap and, because of mammamegaly or excessive adiposity around the neck, shoulders, and face, impair both access to the airway and proper alignment of the pharyngeal and laryngeal axes. Added to these physical impediments are adverse physiolog-

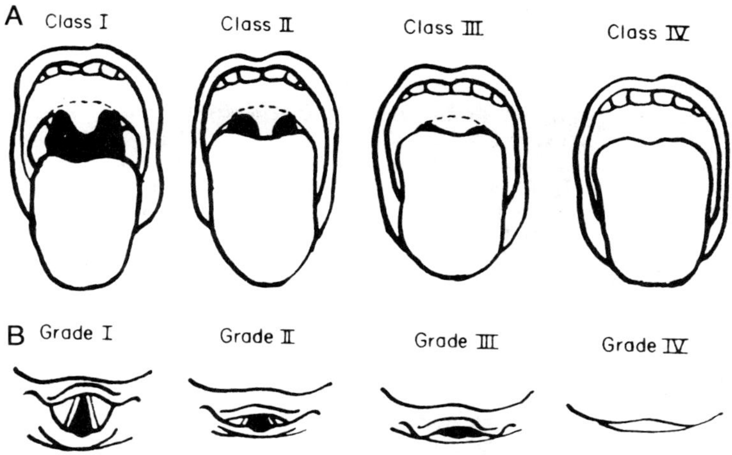

FIG 3.
A, pictorial classification of the pharyngeal structures. Note: class III patients, soft palate visible; class IV, soft palate not visible. **B,** the four grades of laryngoscopic view. (**A** Adapted from Mallampati SR et al: *Can Anaesth Soc J* 32:429–434, 1985; **B** from Cormack RS, Lehane J: *Anaesthesia* 39:1105–1111, 1984. Used by permission.)

ical effects. A decrease in functional residual capacity together with an increase in metabolic oxygen requirements increase the pressure on the anesthesiologist to accomplish intubation rapidly and in the face of precipitous declines in arterial oxygenation.

Anticipation of potential airway problems is obviously crucial to averting disastrous sequelae. Obstetricians should be encouraged to refer at risk patients for an anesthesia consultation during their pregnancy. In addition, careful antepartum assessment of all parturients by an anesthesiologist following admission to the labor suite would identify those individuals with obvious risk factors; for example, those with marked obesity, severe facial edema, a short neck, restricted neck mobility, a receding mandible, protruding incisors, or difficulty opening the mouth. In a retrospective review of cases of failed intubations in obstetric patients, Samsoon and Young[24] illustrated how useful simple preoperative examination of the oral cavity can be in predicting airway difficulty (Fig 3, Table 8). With a greater appreciation for the possibility of problems, a strategy could then be developed whereby the necessity for emergency induction of general anesthesia would be minimized. This might include the early placement of an epidural catheter and confirmation of its correct placement. Many obstetric anesthesiologists are also advocating a similar approach in any patient who is at a higher than usual risk of undergoing an operative delivery. Patients categorized thus might include those with preeclampsia, diabetes mellitus, breech presentations, multiple gestations, intrauterine growth retardation, and oligohydramnios.

TABLE 8.
Retrospective Analysis of the Airway Following Failed Intubation Attempts in Obstetric Patients*

Patient†	Intubation Risk Prior to C-Section	Clinical Assessment (Class)	Laryngoscopy (Grade)
Primipara, 25 years, emergency LSCS	Not expected	IV	IV
Primipara for ELSC, footling breech	Not expected	II	I
Primipara with compound presentation, emergency LSCS	Not expected	IV	III
Primipara with fetal distress	Not expected	IV	III
Primipara for LSCS, failure to progress	Not expected	IV	III
Primipara, 46 years, elective section	Not expected	IV	III–IV
Primipara, 28 years, elective section	Not expected	IV	III

*Adapted from Samsoon GLT, Young JRB: *Anaesthesia* 42:487–490, 1987. Used by permission.
†LSCS = lower segment cesarean section; ELSC = elective lower segment cesarean section.

Unfortunately, despite careful patient selection and preparation, occasional cases of unexpected airway difficulties will still occur. Following the recommendations of the 1978 to 1981 Report on Confidential Inquiries into Maternal Deaths in England and Wales,[17] greater provision was made for senior anesthetists to supervise anesthesia care in obstetric facilities. It was thought that a major contributory factor to airway difficulties in obstetric patients was inexperience on the part of the operator. Yet despite this increased supervision by seasoned individuals, instances of inability to secure the airway persisted. Lyons has reported that often such cases do not present any apparent anatomical reasons for the difficulty encountered ahead of time.[21] To best deal with airway emergencies, the entire obstetric team must be familiar with an established and acceptable contingency plan. Examples of suitable algorithms are available in recent publications.[21, 23, 25, 26] Previously, the recommendation had been, in instances of severe fetal distress, to proceed with cesarean delivery with mask inhalation anesthesia, provided that ventilation was judged to be adequate. A safer dictum might be to simply wake the patient and perform a regional anesthetic, or an awake intubation, unless the gravity of the situation man-

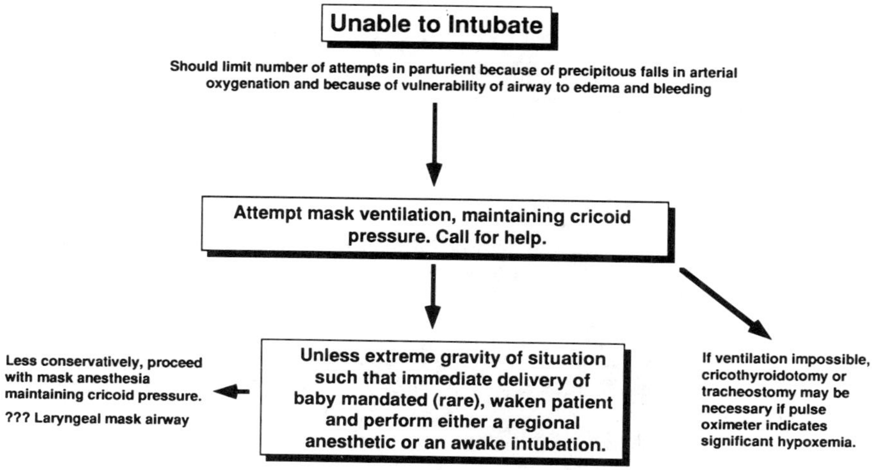

FIG 4.
Algorithm for management of failed intubation.

dates immediate delivery of the baby. As depicted in Figure 4, the latter situation is unusual and proceeding with a mask anesthetic may, in fact, be the less conservative approach as far as maternal safety is concerned. Obviously in cases of failed intubation, if efforts at mask ventilation are unsuccessful, then the patient should be wakened in any event. An emergency cricothyroidotomy or tracheotomy may be necessary to treat progressive hypoxemia.

Both anesthesiologists and obstetricians are beginning to question the wisdom of exposing a mother to the now recognized dangers of an emergent general anesthetic but especially if she is known to be at particular risk. Greater emphasis is being placed on increased utilization of regional anesthesia whenever possible. Marx et al.[27] reported on the successful use of spinal and epidural anesthesia for cesarean deliveries of fetuses demonstrating signs of fetal distress (either persistent heart rate abnormalities or a capillary pH of less than 7.20). The appropriateness of this shift in attitude and greater emphasis on maternal welfare has been solidified by recent studies of neonatal outcome, the second factor in the equation. Anesthesiologists should be familiar with the limitations of labor and delivery interventions to affect later development of the newborn. Only with an improved appreciation of relative risk vs. expected benefit can rational decisions regarding anesthesia be expected.

The diagnosis of fetal distress is often made by an individual obstetrician's interpretation of the continuous electronic fetal heart rate tracing. Anesthesiologists, in general, do not appreciate the lack of specificity of this method of assessment of fetal well-being. Continuous electronic monitoring of fetal heart rate (EFM) was introduced by Hon in the late 1960s. The purported benefit of such intense surveillance was earlier detection of fetal distress, thereby reducing the frequency and severity of perinatal asphyxia. Disenchantment with the technique by some came early however, when Havercamp et al.[28] reported that EFM showed no improvement over traditional auscultation techniques in its effect on immediate neonatal outcome but did increase the risk of cesarean delivery. This author noted a threefold increase in the cesarean section rate when obstetricians relied solely on continuous EFM to monitor the fetus and reacted to what they perceived to be "ominous fetal heart rate patterns" (defined as late decelerations, severe variable decelerations, tachycardia with total loss of short-term variability, or marked bradycardia that was not relieved by corrective measures in 15 to 30 minutes).

Next came the important realization that the contribution of intrapartum asphyxia to the incidence of mental retardation and cerebral palsy had been grossly overestimated.[29–35] Preexisting factors, including factors that antecede the pregnancy, appear to be of far greater significance.[31] The recent literature suggests that intrapartum events and obstetric management are contributory factors in less than 10% of cases of cerebral palsy.[29–31] Furthermore, previous studies linking neurological outcome with birth asphyxia have likely been misleading, with abnormal fetal heart rate patterns sometimes being produced by factors intrinsic to the fetus and not the result of preventable obstetric events.[33, 36]

Interpretation of studies on aspects of intrapartum fetal asphyxia have been made difficult by poor definition of the terms "fetal distress" and "asphyxia." Parer and Livingston[37] have placed emphasis on loss of fetal heart rate variability as evidence of the need for urgent delivery. He is of the opinion that diminished short-term variability, in combination with other ominous signs such as decelerations or bradycardia, is evidence that compensatory physiologic mechanisms (i.e., redistribution of cardiac output to vital organs, brain, heart, and adrenal glands) are being overwhelmed by severe or prolonged asphyxia. Others believe that a blood gas and acid-base assessment is necessary for the diagnosis, and only a significant metabolic acidemia produced by anaerobic metabolism can indicate asphyxia.[38, 39] What remains to be clarified is at what point in ongoing oxygen deprivation to the fetus permanent neurological injury can be expected. On the positive side, it does seem that mature, otherwise healthy human fetuses are able to withstand more severe and prolonged asphyxia than previously thought.[38–40] Whereas earlier studies suggested that infants were at risk when the umbilical artery pH fell below 7.2, recent data suggest that a pH value of 7.0 may be a more appropriate limit.[39] Furthermore, follow-up studies of even quite severely depressed infants show that the prognosis for long-term neurologic and cognitive function is good.[36] Only those infants demonstrating severe depression at birth: an Apgar score <3, umbilical artery blood pH <7.0, and seizures in the immediate postpartum period, appear to be at risk for long-term asphyxial injury.[39]

What should the anesthesiologist extract from all of this? The answer is relatively simple. Unless the life of either the mother or her fetus is judged to be in immediate jeopardy, careful consideration of the risks inherent in emergency induction of a general anesthetic must take precedence in decisions regarding anesthesia for cesarean section. In those instances in which the patient refuses a regional anesthetic but is at obvious increased risk (e.g., a micrognathic patient), or for example is so morbidly obese that attempts at regional anesthesia fail for technical reasons, then it is appropriate to invest the comparatively short additional time in securing the airway with the patient still awake. All evidence points to the likelihood of this being accomplished with minimal additional risk to the fetus, even in the face of nonreassuring fetal heart rate patterns.

Is Epidural Analgesia/Anesthesia an Appropriate Anesthetic Technique for the Patient With Severe Preeclampsia? How Aggressive Should You Be With Invasive Hemodynamic Monitoring?

Clinical Scenario 4

You are asked to render your opinion on the appropriateness of using continuous epidural analgesia for pain relief in a severely preeclamptic patient at 34 weeks' gestation. An oxytocin infusion is being used in an attempt to cause a vaginal delivery, while efforts to optimize her condition continue. On examination, the patient demonstrates significant facial and dependent edema, she has a blood pressure of 160/110 mm Hg, urine output has fallen to 10 mL/hour, and laboratory results indicate a hemoglobin of 10 g% and a platelet count of 105,000 mm^{-3}.

The benefits of effective pain relief from skillfully administered epidural analgesia in the patient with pregnancy-induced hypertension (PIH) are now well-recognized. Denervation of the adrenal glands and uterus, and the associated lowered levels of circulating catecholamines, result in improvement in uteroplacental and renal perfusion.[41, 42] Increases in urine output have been observed, together with a decreased incidence of eclampsia, and of seizures in the eclamptic.[43, 44] Hemodynamic stability is promoted with only moderate reductions (averaging only slightly greater than 20%) in blood pressure being the usual response.[45] Moreover, these benefits can be achieved without risk of further depressant effects in either the mother or newborn. In circumstances in which an instrumented (i.e., low forceps delivery or vacuum extraction) or even operative delivery is highly probable, continuous epidural anesthesia can be readily manipulated to suit the obstetrician's requirements.

In the past, opposition to the use of regional anesthesia in these patients was based on the belief that the risk of profound hypotension and associated placental hypoperfusion was too great.[46] It was theorized that the vasodilatation produced by sympathetic blockade, combined with the usual intravascular volume contraction of hypertensive states, would result in rapid cardiovascular collapse. Furthermore, there was concern that the resuscitative measures taken to treat these events would result in increased fetal and maternal morbidity. Experience over the past two decades has shown that typically only moderate declines in blood pressure occur with epidural analgesia and anesthesia, provided preparatory steps are taken to optimize the patient's volume status, aortocaval compression is avoided, and administration of local anesthetic is slow enough to allow compensatory mechanisms to evolve.

Our understanding of the cardiovascular pathophysiology of preeclampsia and eclampsia has been heightened by the application of invasive hemodynamic monitoring to the treatment of these afflicted parturients.[47] We are emerging from a period during which, in our zeal to optimize maternal antepartum cardiac output and thus fetal oxygen availability, we were often guilty of overhydrating mothers.[48] With mobilization of extravascular fluid after delivery, and perhaps some lessening of left ventricular function, these patients commonly decompensated and developed pulmonary edema. The general consensus now appears to be that monitoring of intravascular volume status via a central venous pressure catheter is probably adequate in the majority of patients. The current recommendation is that prehydration prior to initiating epidural analgesia should be aimed at raising the central venous pressure (CVP) to 2 to 4 cm H_2O only.[49] Debate over the relative merits of colloid vs. crystalloid solutions to accomplish this continue. Addition of plasma expanders such as 25% albumin to balanced salt solutions may allow volume expansion to proceed more expeditiously and may, by increasing colloid oncotic pressure, diminish the risk of pulmonary edema postpartum.[50] Since in most preeclamptic-eclamptic patients CVP will adequately reflect left ventricular function, use of a pulmonary artery catheter should probably be reserved for those patients demonstrating refractory oliguria, evidence of disparate ventricular function (e.g., pulmonary edema despite acceptable CVP readings), or biventricular decompensation.

Decisions regarding the appropriate level of hemodynamic monitoring to use in a particular patient must include consideration of the relative risk involved against the potential benefits. While most anesthesiologists would agree that the convenience and advantages of an indwelling arterial catheter in the severe preeclamptic patient far outweigh the small chance of complications, more caution is necessary in planning central venous access. Whenever feasible it is preferable to introduce a CVP catheter through a venous branch of the basilic system in the antecubital fossa. Even experienced anesthesiologists find placement of CVP lines via one of the great veins in the neck to be challenging in the preeclamptic and eclamptic patient. Frequently the vessels are difficult to secure because of the extreme degree of hypovolemia, but the patient is often restless and quite intolerant of the Trendelenberg position. The threat of significant complications is greatest, however, whenever there is a bleeding dyscrasia present. I have knowledge of a case in which attempted cannulation of the internal jugular vein in a severely preeclamptic patient was complicated by sudden and complete airway obstruction when a "seeker needle" was inadvertently placed into the carotid artery.

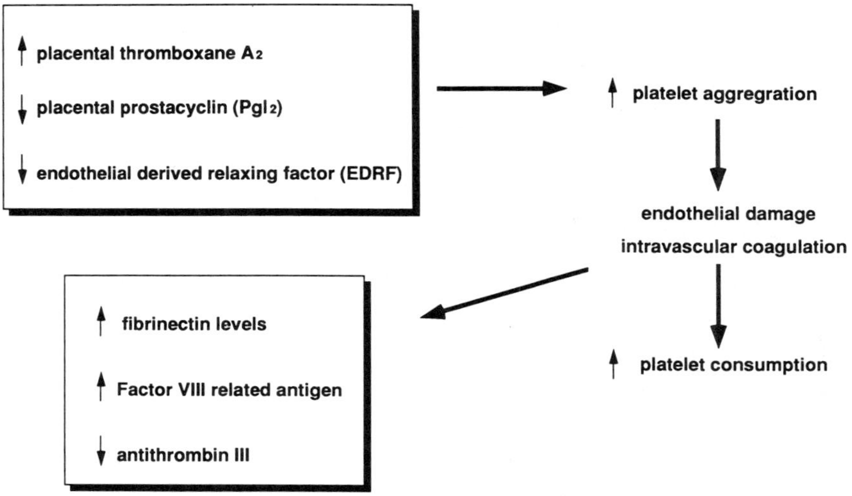

FIG 5.
Coagulation abnormalities in pregnancy-induced hypertension. Proposed mechanisms for increased platelet aggregation include a relative imbalance of thromboxane and prostacyclin, and decreased endothelial derived relaxing factor (EDRF). Endothelial damage and intravascular coagulation produce increased levels of fibrinectin and factor VIII antigen and decreased antithrombin III activity.

It is this same concern for the implications of impaired clotting that should also influence decisions about the propriety of epidural anesthesia in PIH. Practitioners remain understandably confused on the issue of when it is safe to proceed with regional anesthesia and when the risk of bleeding is prohibitive. In part this results from the wide spectrum of severity with which PIH disorders present and their sometimes fulminant evolution. Mild or early cases will often demonstrate a normal coagulation profile, but with increasing severity of PIH, thrombocytopenia, hemolysis, and disseminated intravascular coagulation may supervene. Figure 5 shows the proposed mechanism and hematologic sequelae of the abnormal platelet aggregation seen in PIH.

Accelerated platelet consumption and reduced platelet life span are commonly observed even early on in the disease process. The resultant thrombocytopenia does not necessarily correlate with disease severity or accurately reflect the patient's bleeding tendency.[51] Independent studies by Ramanathan et al.[52] and Schindler et al.[53] both indicated that good correlation between platelet count and template bleeding time (as an indicator of bleeding tendency) can only be expected when platelet counts fall below 100,000 mm^{-3}. In addition to quantitative platelet abnormalities, some investigators have described functional platelet disorders.[52, 54] This group of patients may show prolonged bleeding times, yet have platelet counts in the normal range.

Faced with this complex clinical picture, many anesthesiologists have opted to cover all bases and obtain both platelet counts and bleeding times in all patients with PIH who are candidates for regional anesthesia. (On a practical note, acute loading with magnesium, standard therapy in the patient with PIH, has been shown to transiently prolong bleeding times.[55]) Securing reliable information from standardized bleeding tests can however prove difficult, either because of lack of availability of the test during evening hours, or simply because of operator error. This has spurred others to search for additional signs indicating that a coagulopathy may be present. A recent advance in the laboratory detection of subclinical intravascular coagulation is a monoclonal assay for D-dimers,[56] D-dimers being plasmin degradation products of stable fibrin and thus evidence of in vivo clot dissolution. While early data do suggest a positive correlation between D-dimers and severity of PIH,[57] their presence does not definitively indicate a bleeding tendency.[53] In our institution, we have used thromboelastography (TEG) as a means of monitoring coagulation status in a patient with preeclampsia. We have found it both reliable and convenient, providing us with valuable information within 30 minutes, as opposed to the usual delays incurred in sending samples to a central laboratory.[58] TEG has also allowed us to be more logical with transfusion therapy by avoiding empiric treatment with platelet transfusion simply on the basis of some arbitrarily set numerical lower limit.

A recent report has reassuringly pointed out the rarity of spinal hematoma formation as a complication of epidural anesthesia even in the presence of significant thrombocytopenia.[59] This has added strength to the recommendation that a platelet count of greater than 100,000 mm^{-3} probably serves as an adequate screen for patients with PIH prior to regional anesthesia.[53, 60] Patients with counts lower than this or who are categorized as having severe PIH, and therefore at increased risk of platelet dysfunction, should undergo a bleeding time test.

We will undoubtedly be asked to provide anesthesia for increasing numbers of patients with PIH who have been receiving chronic low-dose aspirin therapy.[61] Aspirin, when given in low doses, has been shown to be capable of selectively inhibiting platelet thromboxane, the theorized culprit in the abnormal platelet activation of PIH. The results of early clinical studies hold promise that this therapy can be effective in preventing preeclampsia in selected cases. What effects, if any, such treatment may produce on platelet function remains to be answered. It would seem prudent then to obtain bleeding times in these patients also.

In summary, continuous epidural anesthesia can be safely used for both vaginal and abdominal delivery of even severely preeclamptic and eclamptic patients provided careful attention is paid to adequate evaluation and preparation. In the typical case example previously given, this patient would certainly be categorized as having severe PIH. She, in addition, should be suspected as suffering from a variant of PIH generally referred to as HELLP syndrome (Hemolysis, Elevated Liver enzymes, and Low Platelet count). Her low hemoglobin level is significant, and when put in the context of probable marked hypovolemia, might indicate either hemolysis or even a placental abruption. While efforts at rapid stabilization are proceeding, hematological studies including a platelet count, bleeding time, and liver function tests should be obtained. A pulmonary artery catheter should be placed if, after raising the CVP by 3 to 4 cm H_2O, no improvement in urine output is seen. Providing the patient does not show any evidence of a coagulopathy, circulating blood volume is assessed as adequate, and she is not excessively drowsy, she may still be considered a candidate for epidural analgesia. Should cesarean section become necessary, then again epidural anesthesia can be carefully titrated to provide suitable conditions for the obstetrician unless a recognized maternal or fetal problem precludes this. The risks of general anesthesia in this patient population should not be underestimated and include difficult or failed endotracheal intubation because of unsuspected laryngeal edema,[62] and transient but severe episodes of hypertension possibly resulting in intracranial bleeding or pulmonary edema.[63]

Summary

Obstetric anesthesia remains an incredibly challenging but potentially very rewarding field. A strong interdisciplinary approach is essential if outcome of mother and baby are to be optimum.

References

1. Gibbs CP et al: Obstetric anesthesia: A national survey. *Anesthesiology* 65:298–306, 1986.
2. Vacanti C: Chairman A.S.A. Consultation Program, personal communication.
3. Joint Commission on Accreditation of Healthcare Organizations: Surgical and anesthesia services. In *Accreditation manual for hospitals.* JCAHO, 1989, Chicago, pp 269–279.
4. American Society of Anesthesiologists, House of Delegates: *Guidelines for patient care in anesthesiology.* American Society of Anesthesiologists, 1985, Park Ridge, Ill.
5. American Academy of Pediatrics and American College of Obstetricians and Gynecologists: Personnel for perinatal care services. In *Guidelines for perinatal care,* ed 3. 1992, Elk Grove Village, Ill, p 74.
6. Levinson G, Shnider SM: Obstetric anesthesia coverage—A continuing problem. *Anesthesiology* 65:245–246, 1986.
7. Bernstein AH: *Avoiding medical malpractice.* Pluribus Press, 1987, Chicago.
8. McKay S, Mahan C: How can aspiration of vomitus in obstetrics best be prevented? *Birth* 15:222–229, 1988.
9. Elkington KW: At the water's edge: Where obstetrics and anesthesia meet. *Obstet Gynecol* 77:304–308, 1991.
10. Cohen S, Chestnut D: At the water's edge: Where obstetrics and anesthesia meet. *Obstet Gynecol* 77:965–966, 1991.
11. Abouleish E, Merriman T: In obstetrics: Keep the water colorless and clear. *Anesth Analg* 73:674, 1991.
12. O'Sullivan GM et al: Noninvasive measurement of gastric emptying in obstetric patients. *Anesth Analg* 66:505–511, 1987.

13. Rochat RW et al: Maternal mortality in the United States: Report from the maternal mortality collaborative. *Obstet Gynecol* 72:91–97, 1988.
14. Endler GC et al: Anesthesia-related maternal mortality in Michigan 1972 to 1984. *Am J Obstet Gynecol* 159:187–193, 1988.
15. May WJ, Greiss FC: Maternal mortality in North Carolina: A forty-year experience. *Am J Obstet Gynecol* 161:555–561, 1989.
16. Atrash HK, Koonin LM, Lawson HW: Maternal mortality in the United States, 1979–1986. *Obstet Gynecol* 76:1055–1060, 1990.
17. Turnbull AC et al: *Report on confidential enquiries into maternal deaths in England and Wales 1979–81*. Her Majesty's Stationary Office, 1986, London.
18. Gibbs CP, Rolbin SH, Norman P: Cause and prevention of maternal aspiration. *Anesthesiology* 61:111–112, 1984.
19. Chadwick HS et al: A comparison of obstetric and nonobstetric anesthesia malpractice claims. *Anesthesiology* 74:242–249, 1991.
20. American Society of Anesthesiologists, House of Delegates: *Standards for post-anesthesia care*. American Society of Anesthesiologists, 1990, Park Ridge, Ill.
21. Lyons G: Failed intubation. *Anaesthesia* 40:759–762, 1985.
22. Mallampati SR et al: A clinical sign to predict difficult tracheal intubation: A prospective study. *Can Anaesth Soc J* 32:429–434, 1985.
23. Cormack RS, Lehane J: Difficult tracheal intubation in obstetrics. *Anaesthesia* 39:1105–1111, 1984.
24. Samsoon GLT, Young JRB: Difficult tracheal intubation: A retrospective study. *Anaesthesia* 42:487–490, 1987.
25. Tunstall ME, Sheikh A: Failed intubation protocol: Oxygenation without aspiration. In *Clinics in anaesthesiology*, vol 4, no 1. WB Saunders Co, 1986, Eastbourne, England, pp 171–187.
26. Palmer SK, Gibbs CP: Risk management in obstetric anesthesia. In *International anesthesiology clinics*, vol 27, no 3. Little, Brown & Co, 1989, Boston, pp 188–199.
27. Marx GF, Luykx WM, Cohen S: Fetal-neonatal status following cesarean section for fetal distress. *Br J Anaesth* 56:1009–1012, 1984.
28. Havercamp AD et al: A controlled trial of the differential effects of intrapartum fetal monitoring. *Am J Obstet Gynecol* 134:399–412, 1979.
29. Low JA et al: Intrapartum fetal asphyxia: A preliminary report in regard to long-term morbidity. *Am J Obstet Gynecol* 130:525–529, 1978.
30. Paneth N, Stark RI: Cerebral palsy and mental retardation in relation to indicators of perinatal asphyxia. *Am J Obstet Gynecol* 147:960–966, 1983.
31. Nelson KB, Ellenberg JH: Antecedents of cerebral palsy. Multivariate analysis of risk. *N Engl J Med* 315:81–86, 1986.
32. Freeman JM, Nelson K: Intrapartum asphyxia and cerebral palsy. *Pediatrics* 82:240–249, 1988.
33. Shields JR, Schifrin BS: Perinatal antecedents of cerebral palsy. *Obstet Gynecol* 71:899–905, 1988.
34. Nelson K: What proportion of cerebral palsy is related to birth asphyxia? *J Pediatr* 112:572–574, 1988.
35. Blair E, Stanley FJ: Intrapartum asphyxia: A rare cause of cerebral palsy. *J Pediatr* 112:515–519, 1988.
36. Painter MJ et al: Fetal heart rate patterns during labor: Neurologic and cognitive development at six to nine years of age. *Am J Obstet Gynecol* 159:854–885, 1988.

37. Parer JT, Livingston EG: What is fetal distress? *Am J Obstet Gynecol* 162:1421–1427, 1990.
38. Low J: The role of blood gas and acid-base assessment in the diagnosis of intrapartum fetal asphyxia. *Am J Obstet Gynecol* 159:1235–1240, 1988.
39. Gilstrap LC et al: Diagnosis of birth asphyxia on the basis of fetal pH, Apgar score, and newborn cerebral dysfunction. *Am J Obstet Gynecol* 161:825–830, 1989.
40. Low JA, Muir DW, Pater EA: The association of intrapartum asphyxia in the mature fetus with newborn behavior. *Am J Obstet Gynecol* 163:1131–1135, 1990.
41. Abboud T et al: Sympathoadrenal activity, maternal, fetal and neonatal responses after epidural anesthesia in the preeclamptic patient. *Am J Obstet Gynecol* 144:915–918, 1982.
42. Jouppila P et al: Lumbar epidural analgesia to improve intervillous blood flow during labor in severe preeclampsia. *Obstet Gynecol* 59:158–161, 1982.
43. Bigler von R, Stamm O: Die periduralanasthesis zur Verhinderung des eklamptischen Anfalls und als Therapie des eklamptischen Comas. *Gynaecologia* 158:228–233, 1964.
44. Merrell DA, Koch MAT: Epidural anaesthesia as an anticonvulsant in the management of hypertensive and eclamptic patients in labour. *S Afr Med J* 58:875–877, 1980.
45. Moir DD, Victor-Rodrigues L, Willocks J: Extradural analgesia during labour in patients with preeclampsia. *J Obstet Gynaecol Br Commonw* 79:465–469, 1972.
46. Lindheimer MD, Katz AI: Hypertension in pregnancy. *N Engl J Med* 313:675–680, 1985.
47. Newsome LR, Bramwell RS, Curling PE: Severe preeclampsia: Hemodynamic effects of lumbar epidural anesthesia. *Anesth Analg* 65:31–36, 1986.
48. Benedetti TJ, Kates R, Williams V: Hemodynamic observations in severe preeclampsia complicated by pulmonary edema. *Am J Obstet Gynecol* 152:330–334, 1985.
49. Experts opine: *Surv Anesthesiol* 30:306–308, 1986.
50. Joyce TH, Loon M: Preeclampsia: Effect of albumin 25% infusion (abstract). *Anesthesiology* 55:313, 1981.
51. Sage DJ: Epidurals, spinals and bleeding disorders in pregnancy: A review. *Anaesth Intensive Care* 18:319–326, 1990.
52. Ramanathan J et al: Correlation between bleeding times and platelet counts in women with preeclampsia undergoing cesarean sections. *Anesthesiology* 71:188–191, 1989.
53. Schindler M et al: Thrombocytopenia and platelet functional defects in pre-eclampsia: Implications for regional anesthesia. *Anaesth Intensive Care* 18:169–174, 1990.
54. Kelton JG, Hunter DJS, Neame PB: A platelet function defect in pre-eclampsia. *Obstet Gynecol* 65:107–109, 1985.
55. Kelleher JF et al: Effect of intravenous magnesium sulphate on the bleeding time. Proceedings of the 19th Annual Meeting of the Society of Obstetric Anesthesia and Perinatology, Halifax, 1988, p 86.
56. Greensberg CS, Devine DV, McCrae CE: Measurement of plasma fibrin D-dimer levels with the use of a monoclonal antibody coupled to latex beads. *Am J Clin Pathol* 87:94–100, 1987.
57. Troffater KF et al: Use of the fibrin D-dimer in screening for coagulation abnormalities in pre-eclampsia. *Obstet Gynecol* 73:435–439, 1989.

58. Campbell C, Nahrwold ML: Is thromboelastography useful for the evaluation of coagulopathies in high risk parturients? (abstract). *Anesthesiology* 73:992, 1990.
59. Hew-Wing P, Rolbin EW, Amato D: Epidural anaesthesia and thrombocytopenia. *Anaesthesia* 44:775–777, 1989.
60. Barker P, Callander CC: Coagulation screening before epidural analgesia in pre-eclampsia. *Anaesthesia* 46:64–67, 1991.
61. Brown MA: Pregnancy-induced hypertension: Current concepts. *Anaesth Intensive Care* 17:185–197, 1989.
62. Heller PJ, Scheider EP, Marx GF: Pharyngolaryngeal edema as a presenting symptom in preeclampsia. *Obstet Gynecol* 62:523–524, 1983.
63. Hodgkinson R, Husain FJ, Hayash H: Systemic and pulmonary blood pressure during cesarean section in patients with gestational hypertension. *Can Anaesth Soc J* 27:389–394, 1980.

Mechanisms of Anesthetic Hepatotoxicity

Janet B. Clarke, Ph.D.

Research Associate in Anesthesiology, Department of Anesthesiology, College of Medicine, University of Arizona, Tucson, Arizona

Richard C. Lind, M.S.

Senior Research Specialist, Department of Anesthesiology, College of Medicine, University of Arizona, Tucson, Arizona

A. Jay Gandolfi, Ph.D.

Professor of Anesthesiology, Pharmacology, and Toxicology; Department of Anesthesiology, College of Medicine, University of Arizona, Tucson, Arizona

All volatile halogen-substituted inhalation anesthetics have, at one time or another, been associated with hepatic injury.[1] Halothane, though, has been the volatile anesthetic principally associated with this syndrome. The liver damage associated with halothane is wide, ranging from mild acute injury (20% of patients) to massive liver cell necrosis.[2] The severe injury occurs in 1:30,000 patients and is often fatal and always unexpected.[3] This has made the sporadic form of injury difficult to study and model. It is not clear if the liver injury exists as one continuous event or represents two different forms of halothane hepatotoxicity. The bulk of the investigative efforts has been directed toward the acute form of the injury as it allows better opportunities for laboratory studies. The acute form may be relevant to the latent, more severe injury since a significant portion of the patients who subsequently develop the fulminant necrosis were observed to have a previous mild reaction to halothane.[4] For many years, the liver injury following halothane anesthesia was contested; however, it is now accepted. Even now halothane hepatitis cannot be predicted, carries the prospect of lethality, and cannot be specifically treated.

The general use of halothane in the United States has been curtailed due to medicolegal problems. It does, though, remain in use in children. The two volatile anesthetics that replaced halothane have less hepatotoxic potential but have not been risk-free. Enflurane and isoflurane have both been linked to a low incidence of unexplained postoperative jaundice.[5–7] Many of these cases remain in contention, but their association with these anesthetics cannot be excluded. A detailed case report concerning isoflurane has many of the characteristics of halothane-associated liver injury.[8] Overall, halothane remains in significant use worldwide. In a recent survey in the United Kingdom, almost half of the anesthesias involving volatile anesthetics used halothane.[9]

Liver injury associated with halothane anesthesia continues to the present day. Due to the sporadic occurrence of volatile anesthetic-induced livery injury, the usual anecdotal case report, and the spectrum of morphological and clinical features, the correlation of the injury to anesthetic exposure is often ignored for a time.[10] However, a broader recognition and acceptance of the symptoms has expanded the "susceptible population."[11]

Clinical Features of Halothane Hepatotoxicity

Many advantages were attributed to halothane when it was first introduced into clinical use; however, these were counterbalanced when signs of minor hepatic damage began to appear.[12] The reports of fulminant hepatic hepatitis and liver necrosis that followed caused even greater concern.[13, 14] Eventually, the characteristics of the severe liver injury associated with halothane became apparent.[15] The classic patient was often an overweight woman who prior to anesthesia showed no signs or symptoms of hepatitis. Three days after halothane anesthesia, the patient would typically develop nausea, fever, circulating eosinophilia, and pain. This would be followed by a rapid degeneration into severe liver disease, with jaundice, greatly elevated liver enzymes, and hepatic coma. Death resulted in an estimated 15% to 50% of cases[16] with massive hepatic centrilobular necrosis found at autopsy.[17] At first, many of these cases were attributed to a number of other causes (i.e., viral hepatitis), which could not be excluded. A National Institutes of Health (NIH)-sponsored prospective study, however, established that for a number of cases no cause other than halothane could be discerned.[18] Numerous reviews have now summarized the case reports and studies concerning halothane hepatitis, which has become a recognized volatile anesthetic complication.[4]

Factors Predisposing Patients to Halothane Hepatitis

The numerous case reports have revealed several predisposing factors as increasing the risk of hepatotoxicity of halothane: multiple exposures, obesity, middle age, gender, and ethnic origin. When last examined, more than 80% of halothane hepatitis cases had more than one exposure to the agent.[10] The time for maximum susceptibility between these exposures is estimated to be 28 days.[2] A significant proportion of post-halothane anesthesia-associated hepatic complications have occurred in obese patients.[15] Since obesity has been shown to increase the biotransformation of volatile anesthetics, this may be a contributing factor.[19] At one time, case reports of halothane-induced liver injury in the young were rare; however, more case reports are now appearing.[20] The recognition of halothane hepatotoxicity in children is of concern because halothane remains a widely used pediatric anesthetic.[21] Regardless, middle-aged individuals remain the more likely target. Furthermore, middle-aged women are at greater risk than men, by approximately 2:1, for halothane hepatitis.[10] There is some indication that susceptibility to halothane-induced liver injury is a heritable characteristic.[22]

Proper diagnoses of halothane hepatitis are difficult due to its extremely sporadic nature. Its unpredictable appearance has made defining its characteristics and predisposing factors a protracted process. This further compounds the problem in the determination of the toxicological mechanisms with clinical and basic science approaches.

Premise of Halothane Hepatotoxicity Models

A critical step to establish the link between volatile anesthetics and liver injury has been the development of animal models (Fig 1). Since halothane was the first current major anesthetic linked to liver injury, early animal studies concentrated on it.[3] These studies occurred during the time when the hepatotoxicity of numerous chemicals was found to be associated with their biotransformation. The biotransformation of chemicals to reactive intermediates is now recognized as the major reason for their organ-specific toxicity.[23] Most of the animal models for halothane-induced liver injury were based on this premise. Due to the pharmacologic properties of halothane, its complex biotransformation, and its ability to produce products that bind to various macromolecules, a number of animal models have been developed through the years.

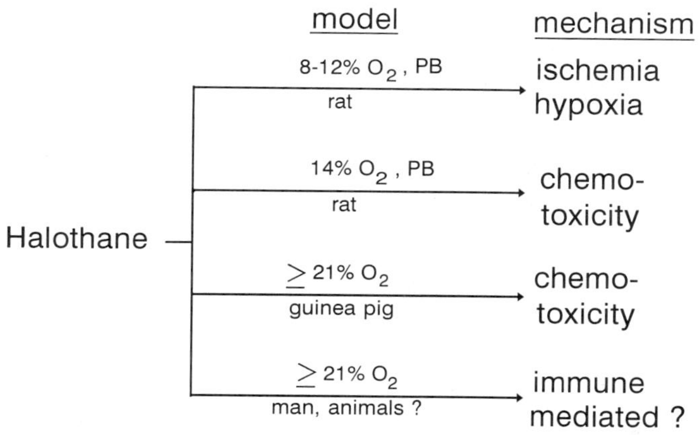

FIG 1.
General models and mechanisms of halothane hepatotoxicity.

General Mechanisms of Intoxication

Several mechanisms of hepatotoxicity for halothane have been proposed (see Fig 1). Due to its chemical structure, halothane can be biotransformed by both oxidative and reductive pathways (Fig 2).[11] The reductive biotransformation of halothane only occurs when there are elevated levels of hepatic cytochrome P-450 and under reduced oxygen tension (14% O_2). The resulting free radical product reacts primarily with hepatic phospholipids to produce a chemotoxic liver injury.[24] Due to the hypoxia required to cause halothane to be reductively metabolized, studies were performed in which the halothane exposure was conducted under a more severe hypoxia (8% to 12% O_2 inspired).[25, 26] Under these conditions liver injury was also produced; however, it was of a type caused more by ischemia and hypoxia and was not necessarily related to the anesthetic itself.[27, 28] Other halothane toxicity models that operate through an induced cellular hypoxia condition (triiodothyronine pretreatment) also have a ischemia/hypoxia mechanism.[29, 30] The predominant role of halothane biotransformation in all species is oxidative to its principal metabolite, trifluoroacetic acid.[31] In the process of producing trifluoroacetic acid an acetylating intermediate is produced that can attack liver tissue (principally protein) to again produce a chemotoxic liver injury.[32] Considerable recent efforts have been directed toward the possibility that halothane would be biotransformed to

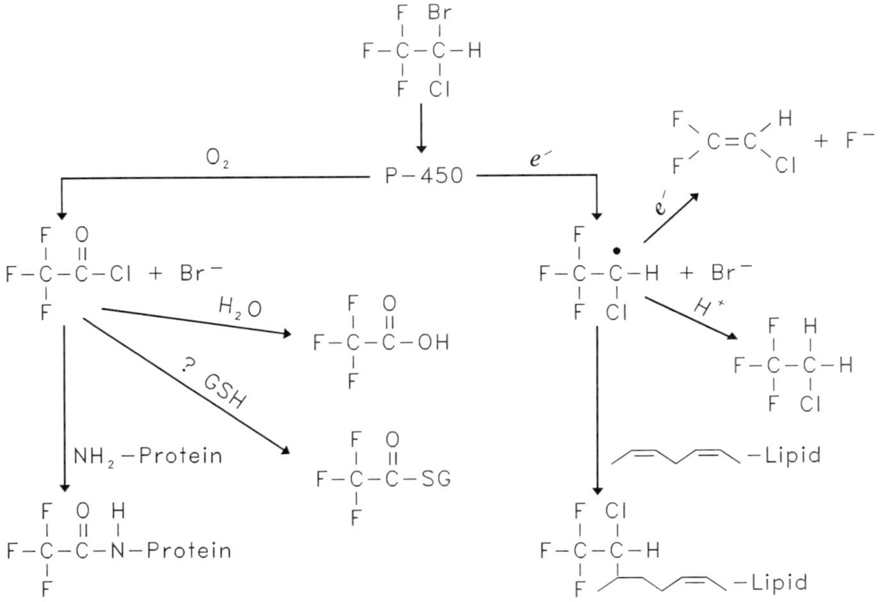

FIG 2.
Halothane biotransformation and interaction with macromolecules.

its oxidative intermediate, which would acylate liver proteins converting them into neoantigens that would have the potential to initiate an immune-mediated liver injury.[33]

Chemotoxic Models in the Rat

Once the oxidative and reductive biotransformation of halothane was clearly defined, rat halothane hepatotoxicity models were developed that manipulated the biotransformation of halothane through different pathways by stringent pretreatments or exposure conditions (Table 1).

PCB-Halothane Model

The first rat model for halothane-induced hepatic injury was based on the premise that halothane required bioactivation to be hepatotoxic.[34, 35] Rats were treated with polychlorinated biophenyls (PCB: Aroclor 1254) to dramatically increase hepatic biotransformation enzymes and then exposed to halothane in a 99% O_2 atmosphere. Although the rats developed a centrilobular hepatic necrosis, use of the model was limited since the PCB treatment alone caused significant liver injury.

Isoniazid-Halothane Model

Isoniazid is known to enhance the oxidative hepatic biotransformation of halothane. When Fisher 344 rats were pretreated with isoniazid before halothane exposure in room air (21% O_2), a centrilobular lesion was observed 24 hours after exposure.[36] Substantial resolution of the lesion occurred by 4 days after exposure. This model indicates that oxidative biotransformation of halothane in rats can produce a chemotoxic injury. With the advent of the guinea pig models which did not require any pretreatment, this model did not receive much additional attention.

Halothane-Hypoxia Model

Although the major route of biotransformation of halothane in all species is oxidative, it also has the chemical properties to undergo reductive biotransformation (see Fig 2). Reductive biotransformation of halothane forms free radical intermediates that can react covalently with liver macromolecules.[37] This form of biotransformation and covalent binding is similar to that observed with carbon tetrachloride.[1] Although capable of reductive biotransformation, halothane does not proceed readily by this pathway. To be metabolized reductively, the hepatic biotransformation enzymes (cytochrome P450) of the male rat had to be extensively induced with phenobarbital pretreatment and the halothane exposure carried out in a hypoxic (14% O_2) atmosphere.[24, 38] Even under these conditions, the quantity of reductive metabolites is minor (<1%) compared to the principal oxidative metabolite, trifluoroacetic acid. Even with all these manipulations, the male

TABLE 1.
Rat Models for Volatile Anesthetic-Induced Hepatotoxicity

Model	Conditions	Results	Year	Reference
PCB-halothane	Pretreatment with Aroclor 1254 followed by halothane exposure	Centrilobular lesion produced, but PCB alone also produced liver damage, confounding the interpretation of the halothane-induced lesion	1976 1977	34 35
Halothane-hypoxia	Pretreatment with phenobarbital followed by halothane exposure in 14% O_2 (hypoxic) atmosphere	Limited centrilobular lesion in males only that did not progress	1979 1979 1980	24 39 38
Severe hypoxia-halothane	Pretreatment with phenobarbital, halothane exposure in 8%–12% O_2 atmosphere	Immediate hypoxia-ischemia type lesoin that rapidly resolves, model not selective for halothane	1982 1983	25 26
Tri-iodothyronine-halothane	Pretreatment with T3 followed by halothane exposure in normoxia	Similar results as those seen with the severe-hypoxia model	1980 1983	29 30
Isoniazid-halothane	Isoniazid pretreatment followed by halothane exposure in normoxia	Centrilobular lesion but confounded by isoniazid toxicities	1987	36

rats only developed a limited centrilobular lesion that did not progress further and usually readily resolved.

Initially, it was thought that this model was relevant to the human situation since a small amount of reductive biotransformation of halothane was observed in patients.[39] This model and variations of it received considerable attention.[40, 41] As the model was further examined, though, concerns arose as to the true mechanism of injury and its clinical relevance.

Hypoxia-Based Models in the Rat

A number of investigators questioned the use of hypoxic exposures (14% O_2) in the halothane-hypoxia rat model. Subsequent studies found that all volatile anesthetics were hepatotoxic if rats were exposed to even greater (8% to 12% O_2) hypoxic atmospheres (see Table 1).[25] This caused investigators to conclude that the hepatotoxicity of anesthetics was due solely to hypoxic mechanisms since volatile anesthetics also reduced hepatic blood flow.[42] However, it should be pointed out that halothane was the only volatile anesthetic found to be hepatotoxic under less severe (14% O_2) hypoxic conditions.[26] Lind et al.[27, 28] were able to clarify this issue when they demonstrated that the hepatic injury produced under severe hypoxic conditions (8% to 12% O_2) was both qualitatively and temporally different from that produced in the halothane-hypoxia (14% O_2) model. The liver lesion in animals exposed to an anesthetic in a 10% O_2 atmosphere was representative of a hypoxia/ischemia lesion, which is characterized by an immediate hepatic injury of centrilobular watery vacuolization progressing to a frank panlobular coagulative necrosis by 6 hours. The liver pathology in the halothane hypoxia (14% O_2) model is normal after exposure and gradually progresses to a primarily hydropic vacuolization lesion in the centrilobular region over 24 hours. This is a time course followed by many other hepatic chemotoxicants.[43]

Hepatotoxicity was observed in rats pretreated with triiodothyronine prior to halothane exposure.[29, 30] Although these animals were exposed to halothane in nonhypoxic atmospheres ($\geq$21% O_2), triiodothyronine produces a hypermetabolic state in the centrilobular cell that causes a localized cellular hypoxia. When the cellular hypoxia is coupled with the reduced hepatic blood flow caused by the presence of halothane, a hypoxia/ischemia condition again occurred with the resultant lesion.

The liver lesion was not retained for any length of time in the hypoxia models. In many instances by 24 hours after exposure, there was considerable resolution of the lesion, which does not correspond to the hepatic injury seen clinically. Neither the severe hypoxia or triiodothyronine-based models received much subsequent attention.

Relevance of the Rat Models for Halothane Hepatotoxicity

In all the rat studies, stringent pretreatments and manipulations were required to produce a lesion with a limited degree of actual necrosis. Many of the pretreatments or conditions alone elicited morphological changes,[41] making the true histopathology associated with halothane-induced liver injury in rats difficult to interpret. Typically, the halothane-induced liver lesion in the rat appears within hours, quickly resolves, does not progress, and is usually limited to male rats.[41] Obviously, the appearance of this liver injury is in stark contrast to the clinical situation.[4, 10] In addition, both the incidence and type of liver pathology differed greatly between the rat models and that seen clinically. Thus the validity of the rat models as a representation of the human situation was questioned.[44]

Evolution of the Guinea Pig Halothane Hepatotoxicity Model

Most of the reservations with the rat models for halothane hepatotoxicity have been solved by utilizing the guinea pig as the model species.[45] The first evidence of halothane-induced hepatic injury in guinea pigs was presented by Hughes and Lang in 1972.[46] However, the unfortunate selection of only 1 hour of 1% halothane anesthesia combined with sampling times that were immediately after anesthesia and then 1 week later led to ambiguous results with no increases observed in serum activities of several hepatic enzymes. With the advent of rat models of halothane-associated hepatotoxicity, the potential guinea pigs held for halothane research remain unrealized until 1985 when Lunam et al. demonstrated consistent production of hepatic injury in naive colored Australian guinea pigs by lengthening the period of halothane anesthesia to 4 hours and collecting blood and liver samples daily (Table 2).[45] Approximately one third developed bridging centrilobular necrosis, another one third developed scattered small foci of necrosis while the remainder exhibited no damage. The use of a wide range (14% to 80%) of inspired oxygen concentrations during anesthesia had no effect on the incidence or severity of liver injury. Further work has shown that the commonly available albino Hartley guinea pig has an approximate 50% incidence of centrilobular necrosis following halothane exposure.[32, 47, 48] While early studies with these animals

TABLE 2.
Exposure Requirements for Production of Halothane-Induced Liver Injury in the Guinea Pig

Pretreatment	None
Halothane concentration	0.1%–1.0%
Oxygen concentration	14%–80%*
Exposure length	4 hr

*Can use up to 99% O_2 (unpublished results).

used a 21% inspired oxygen concentration during anesthesia, more recently 40% oxygen has been used to better mimic clinical administration of halothane. Another recent alteration to the model involves the use of subanesthetic concentrations of halothane (0.1% to 0.25%), which also produces centrilobular necrosis following a 4-hour exposure.[49]

Guinea Pig Lesion Characteristics

The lesion in halothane-exposed guinea pigs is acute and follows a time course similar to that typically observed with other organohalogen hepatotoxicants.[45, 50–52] Generally, development of fatty vacuoles within hepatocytes can be observed during the first 24 hours following halothane exposure.[45, 50, 51] By 48 hours, areas of necrotic hepatocytes, whether small foci scattered throughout the liver lobule or extensive areas in the centrilobular region, are readily apparent. This is followed by total infiltration of the necrotic areas by inflammatory cells over the next 24 to 48 hours.[51, 52] Often surviving hepatocytes throughout the liver present macrovesicular and microvesicular fat droplets, some of which can be observed 7 days after exposure by which time most or all of the necrosis is resolved.[45, 50] Plasma alanine aminotransferase (ALT) activity has been shown to be a good indicator of injury, reaching peak levels 48 to 72 hours after anesthesia and returning toward normal values by 96 hours.[45, 49, 50, 52] More recently, plasma isocitrate dehydrogenase activity has been presented as a better indicator of halothane liver injury in the guinea pig than ALT due to its greater sensitivity and its higher centrilobular/periportal activity ratio within the liver.[49]

Guinea Pig Susceptibility Factors

There are a variety of factors that appear to affect the incidence and severity of the injury (Table 3). Different strains of guinea pigs have been shown to have a wide variation in hepatotoxic response following halothane anes-

TABLE 3.
Susceptibility Factors for Halothane-Associated Liver Injury in Guinea Pigs and Humans

Factors	Guinea Pig	Human
Age/weight	×	×
Female gender	×	×
Heredity	×	×
Covalent binding to hepatic proteins	×	×
Degree of oxidative biotransformation	×	?
Hepatic glutathione content	×	?

thesia.[50] Further evidence for a heritable susceptibility factor was provided by a breeding study.[53] Offspring of guinea pigs that developed large increases in serum ALT activity following halothane anesthesia were found to be more vulnerable to halothane-induced hepatic injury than the offspring of resistant animals. Age and gender have also been shown to be an influence in colored strain 13 guinea pigs.[52] Older, heavier animals (>570 g) were more susceptible to injury and females more than males. Although the lesion that developed in these studies was acute in nature, it is intriguing to note parallels with factors considered to be involved with susceptibility to fulminant halothane hepatitis in humans. It is often regarded that obesity, middle age, and female gender are predisposing factors for hepatitis.[54] An apparent familial link in susceptibility has also been reported.[54] In addition, the pathology of liver injury typically observed in the guinea pig has been found to closely resemble that of nonfatal human halothane hepatitis.[55] The potentially fatal disease in humans is currently believed to be the result of an idiosyncratic immune reaction triggered by the alteration of native hepatic proteins into neoantigens by the reactive trifluoroacyl acid chloride intermediate generated by oxidative biotransformation of halothane, while current evidence indicates that the mechanism of the acute injury in guinea pigs involves direct damage to hepatocytes by the same metabolic intermediate.[32, 47, 54]

Mechanisms of Halothane Hepatotoxicity in the Guinea Pig

A series of studies have all pointed to a chemotoxic mechanism of halothane-associated hepatotoxicity in guinea pigs that involves biotransformation of halothane by the cytochrome P-450 enzyme system (see Fig 2).[32, 45, 47, 49] Pretreatment of colored Australian guinea pigs with the cytochrome P-450 inhibitor, SKF-525A, significantly reduced halothane biotransformation and resultant lesion severity.[45] Unfortunately, the use of SKF-525A in outbred Hartley guinea pigs led to severe complications following anesthesia that resulted in an inability to obtain toenail blood samples, hypothermia in the animals, and death from unknown causes of 50% of the treated animals within 48 hours. Conversely, enhancement of biotransformation via pretreatment with isoniazid potentiated injury; however, sensitivity of the guinea pigs to the inherent hepatotoxic nature of isoniazid made isolation of the mechanism of injury difficult.[48] Although the metabolism of halothane occurs primarily along the oxidative route, flux along each pathway can be altered by variations in inspired oxygen concentrations or by the use of the deuterated form of the drug (see Fig 2).[32, 45, 47] In the guinea pig, use of 14% oxygen during halothane anesthesia enhanced reductive biotransformation without affecting the degree of oxidative biotransformation or subsequent development of liver injury.[45] Lowering inspired oxygen to 10% or use of deuterated halothane inhibited oxidative halothane biotransformation and thus production of the reactive trifluoroacetyl acid chloride intermediate (see Fig 2).[32, 47] The result was large decreases in covalently bound reactive halothane biotransformation intermediates to hepatic proteins and an amelioration of the centrilobular lesion.[47] This reduction in lesion severity occurred even though the use of 10% inspired oxygen greatly enhanced flux along the reductive route with its generation of free radical intermediates and their covalent binding to intracellular lipids (see Fig 2).[47] Thus, it would appear that covalent binding to hepatic proteins by the oxidatively generated trifluoroacetyl acid chloride intermediate is the source of injury while the reductive pathway and lipid binding, which have been purported to be a mechanism of injury in rat models of halothane-associated hepatotoxicity,[54] are not critical factors for lesion development in the guinea pig.

Following halothane exposure, alterations in hepatic calcium homeostasis occur in a manner that is also indicative of a chemical-induced injury.[51] Prior to the development of necrosis (24 hours after halothane exposure), hepatic calcium content increases ninefold and microsomal calcium uptake is reduced by more than 50%. This is similar to changes that occur following administration of carbon tetrachloride in both rats and guinea pigs and may play a role in the cascade of events leading to cell death.[51]

Recently, further evidence was obtained that implicated the oxidative biotransformation of halothane as the culprit for the resultant liver injury in the guinea pig. A subanesthetic concentration (0.10%) of halothane caused centrilobular necrosis to develop following a 4-hour exposure.[49] Unfortunately, halothane has demonstrated a concentration-dependent inhibition of its own biotransformation, complicating comparisons of the extent of biotransformation and covalent binding between different concentrations.[56] At the end of a 4-hour exposure to 0.1% halothane, the extent of oxidative biotransformation and covalent binding to protein was several times greater than that obtained with a 1.0% exposure. However, in the hours following 1.0% exposure, extensive halothane biotransformation occurred as hepatic tissue concentrations decreased so that by 10 hours, the extent of biotransformation and binding was twice that obtained with 0.10%, which had not changed greatly. Thus, biotransformation of residual amounts of halothane that are slowly released from fat depots following anesthesia with high concentrations of the drug probably play an important role in the production of acute halothane-associated hepatic injury.

Fatal Halothane Hepatitis in Guinea Pigs

Although halothane is believed to become covalently bound to hepatic proteins via a trifluoroacetyl acid chloride intermediate and glutathione is a known protectant against damage caused by acid chloride intermediates,[57] halothane has yet to be shown to decrease hepatic glutathione concentrations.[24, 58, 59] However, the possibility exists that the trifluoroacetyl moiety is readily removed from glutathione, preventing a measurable loss of the protectant (see Fig 2). To determine if glutathione does play a role in the detoxification of halothane's oxidative biotransformation intermediate, studies were undertaken in which hepatic glutathione concentrations were depleted prior to halothane exposure.[60, 61] True to this proposed mechanism of action, glutathione depletion caused a significant enhancement in the covalent binding of halothane to hepatic protein but not to lipid. This was associated with a potentiation of the resultant injury whether subanesthetic (0.10%)[61] or anesthetic (1.0%)[60] concentrations of halothane were used. In fact, when glutathione-depleted guinea pigs were exposed to halothane concentrations of 0.25% to 1.0%, over one third of the animals became moribund or died 48 to 72 hours after exposure as a result of liver damage that ranged from submassive to massive in degree.[62] This breakthrough represents the first animal model to produce fatal halothane hepatitis. It also presents the possibility that some cases of human halothane hepatitis are due to the direct chemotoxic action of halothane biotransformation intermediates. Individuals who have ingested large amounts of acetaminophen-containing drugs or have had workplace or environmental exposure to glutathione-depleting chemicals could well be at risk for a more severe hepatic injury following halothane anesthesia. Having an animal model of fulminant halothane hepatitis in hand will now permit studies on mechanisms causing development of such severe injury, its prevention, and alleviation following onset. These findings may prove helpful in treating the patient with halothane hepatitis or avoiding the disease altogether.

Immune Mechanisms in Anesthetic Hepatotoxicity

A role for immune mechanisms in fulminant halothane hepatitis has been under investigation since the earliest clinical descriptions of rare reactions with the hallmarks of hypersensitivity. Liver damage as a result of halothane exposure can range from a mild acute form to an often fatal, rare fulminant hepatitis, and it is the latter that may be due to an aberrant immune response.[2, 4]

To confirm an immune-mediated toxic mechanism for any drug, two criteria must be fulfilled. The drug or its derivative must be shown to elicit a specific immune response and that response must be directly associated with toxicity in vivo. One of the most difficult scenarios to clarify where liver damage and an immune resonse are observed is a causal relationship. That is, to fulfill the second criterion, antibodies or specific immune cells should appear prior to and result in damage rather than be secondary to another form of toxic insult. Studies with halothane have clearly fulfilled the first criterion, immunogenicity, though there are gaps in this knowledge, notably in the cellular response. The second criterion, to delineate an immune-mediated toxicity in vivo, has proved the most difficult to demonstrate. Drug-induced hypersensitivity reactions of this type are the most difficult adverse drug reactions to reproduce in an animal model due to their rarity and inherent idiosyncracy.

The majority of drugs are far too small to be immunogenic but this can be overcome through conjugation to a macromolecular carrier, wherein the drug acts as a hapten. Thus the drug or drug metabolite must be capable of undergoing covalent reaction to have the potential to be immunogenic.[63] Biotransformation of halothane produces intermediates capable of combining with both lipids and proteins (reductive pathway) and proteins (oxidative pathway), the latter via trifluoroacetyl chloride that readily acylates proteins (see Fig 2). Proteins constitute the most likely carrier, since lipids are poor immunogens and this has been confirmed as the case for halothane. Once a response is induced, the mechanism by which toxicity might be mediated depends on the disposition of antibody and/or T cells and antigen. The basis for these interactions was described in simplified form as the type I to IV hypersensivity reactions.[64] Type I is termed anaphylactic hypersensitivity, which involves IgE antibodies activating mast cells to release vasoactive amines. Type II hypersensitivity reactions may be relevant to hepatitis. Antibodies are directed toward a cell surface antigen and can then mediate lysis through cytotoxic T cells or via activation of the complement system. Type III hypersensitivity is caused by the formation and deposition of antigen-antibody complexes. Finally, type IV or delayed hypersensitivity is mediated solely by antigen-specific T cells that can recognize antigen association with major histocompatibility complex (MHC) I on the surface of any targeted cell. Contact sensitivity is a classical example of this type of reaction, although it cannot be ruled out for immune-mediated halothane hepatitis. Thus the immunogenicity and immunotoxicity of halothane and other anesthetics will involve factors that are inherent both to the sensitizing drug and the host.

Evidence for a Hypersensitivity Reaction

Among the symptoms of patients with halothane hepatitis, fever, rash, eosinophilia, and arthralgias, are symptoms that suggest a hypersensitivity reaction.[4, 11] However, it is the association of halothane hepatitis with multiple exposures that is probably the strongest evidence for an immune mechanism. Walton et al.[15] found that 71 (95%) of 76 patients with halothane hepatitis had received halothane on more than one occasion; in a survey by Moult and Sherlock,[54] 24 (92%) of 26 patients had received multiple exposures. Furthermore, it was observed that in patients who mistakenly received subsequent halothane exposure, the onset of hepatitis occurred after an increasingly shorter latency period. A decreasing latent period is highly suggestive of the nature of a classical immune response where second (and subsequent) exposure would cause an expansion of preexisting memory immune cells.[66]

In support of the epidemiological data, laboratory analysis has shown, with indirect immunofluorescence, the presence of anti-liver/kidney microsome autoantibodies and in conjunction, antibodies directed against thyroid antigen.[67] The prevalence of these autoantibodies is significantly higher in patients with halothane hepatitis than in those with a known viral or other hepatic complication. These autoantibodies can also be detected in patients with autoimmune disorders such as chronic active hepatitis,[68] though they are not transient as is the case in patients with halothane hepatitis. The appearance of these antibodies has led to the suggestion that subjects prone to develop organ-specific autoimmunity may be more liable to develop halothane hepatitis. Though this may be an oversimplification, autoimmunity may play a role in potential mechanisms of halothane hepatitis. Other risk factors in halothane hepatitis patients are obesity, middle age, and female sex.[4, 11] Though these features are not necessarily pointers to immune involvement, the latter two are also prevalent in patients with certain organ-specific autoimmune diseases.[69]

Occasionally a clinical case of halothane hepatitis is reported that does not fit the previously highlighted characteristics of a hypersensitivity reaction. This includes where reexposure has not induced hepatitis or halothane hepatitis appears to have occurred after only one exposure. These incidences might be explained by incorrect diagnosis particularly in early cases due to hepatitis C viral infection and possibly through sensitization with trace amounts of anesthetic in equipment or cross-reaction with other anesthetics.[70] However, there may also be cases of severe hepatitis caused by a direct, chemical-induced injury as a result of metabolic idiosyncracy, for example in glutathione levels as discussed previously.[61] This direct toxicity may either act alone or be exacerbated by an immune response to lysed cell constituents. Possibly future directions of research will link metabolic and immunologic studies more closely.

The existence of an established hepatitis syndrome as a result of enflurance and isoflurane exposure is controversial, although several suspected cases have been reported.[5, 6] A recent report provided strong evidence of a hepatitis caused by isoflurane with many characteristics of halothane hepatitis notably female sex, obesity, multiple exposures, and the pathology of zone 3 necrosis.[8] No fever or eosinophilia was observed. It is possible that some cases may be a result of cross-reaction due to previous exposure to halothane and there is some preliminary animal data that support this.[70, 71] Theoretically, the related halogenated anesthetics have the potential to form the same hapten-protein adducts as halothane and thus be immunogenic.[70] However, the low rate of metabolism (0.2% for isoflurane and 2% for enflurane) in comparison to that of halothane[11] may mean that an immune response would be less likely due to insufficient haptenation of sensitive proteins.

Clinical Immune Response to Halothane

The demonstration of a specific drug-induced immune response is an essential requirement to implicate an immunotoxicological mechanism. The first studies of a drug-directed specific response induced by halothane examined cellular sensitivity. An immune response to the vast majority of antigens requires a T cell response, which stimulates B cells to produce specific antibodies (helper T cells) while other populations of T cells are themselves able to cause lysis (cytotoxic T cells). Paronetto and Popper[72] observed specific sensitization of lymphocytes to halothane, from patients with halothane hepatitis, in an in vitro transformation assay, though cellular sensitization could not be confirmed in subsequent studies.[73] Failure to detect a cellular response to halothane itself should not be unexpected due to its small size, well below what is thought to be the minimum size (approximately 10 kD) for an immunogen.[69] Furthermore, T cells, unlike antibodies, recognize short sequential peptides that must be presented in association with surface glycoproteins, coded for in the MHC.[74] Ironically, the earliest attempts to demonstrate an immune response chose the more difficult field of cellular sensitization and, to date, halothane-induced specific T cells have not unequivocally been detected in humans or animals sensitized to halothane.

Recent studies[75] have put forward a possible explanation for this difficulty in an attempt to measure drug-specific lymphocytes in patients with hepatitis resulting from various drugs (though no anesthetics). With a standard lymphocyte proliferation assay, only 21% of 42 patients had a positive response to the specific drug implicated in the hepatitis. However, additon of a prostaglandin inhibitor greatly enhanced positive identification of sensitized patients to 57%. Under normal circumstances, a mixture of lymphocytes are present that include suppressor cells activated by prostaglandins.[74] Thus it would appear that, in vitro, these suppressor cells were responsible for dampening the cellular response to the co-incubated drugs. This might also have been a factor in attempts to measure halothane-specific cell populations. However, in the studies described, the native drugs were used and presumably became covalently bound to protein in vitro during the 6-day incubation period. The low rate of metabolism for halothane may still cause the anesthetic itself in native form to be an unsuccessful stimulus.

Attempts in our laboratory to demonstrate cellular immunity to an alternative antigen, trifluoroacetyl (TFA)-rabbit serum albumin, have failed to demonstrate a specific response while suggesting a unique property of the TFA hapten moiety, that of a mitogen.[76] In these experiments, spleen cells from naive animals proliferated on exposure to TFA-albumin but not to the albumin alone.

The humoral response is generally more amenable to detection with various techniques and antibody studies with halothane have proved more successful. Mieli-Vergani[77] and Vergani [78] were the first to demonstrate that IgG antibodies were present in patient sera that could bind to whole hepatocytes from rabbits treated with halothane. The antibodies were specific to halothane-modified determinants and could mediate antibody-dependent cell-mediated toxicity in vitro (type II hypersensitivity mechanism). The antibodies were not present in sera from patients exposed to halothane with no ill effect or in patients with viral hepatic injury. An association between humoral immunity and toxicity was also suggested since raised levels of circulating immune complexes were detected in patients with halothane hepatitis and viral hepatitis and levels were elevated in few patients with acetaminophen-induced liver damage.[79, 80] The identification and nature of the proteins (antigens) recognized by the antibodies and more specifically which of these are involved in the initiation of a response (immunogens) is clearly important to delineate the early steps in the hypersensitivity reaction.

A novel application of the Western blot technique was used to investigate antibody specificity at the subcellular level.[81, 82] Antibodies in the sera of patients with halothane hepatitis recognized antigens mainly in the hepatic microsomal fraction of rats treated with halothane. Cross-reaction with these proteins (principally of 100, 76, 59, 57, and 54 kD) was related to oxidative metabolism to a TFA intermediate and the conjugation of the TFA moiety to protein. However the TFA hapten forms only part of the determinant recognized since incubation of sera with the hapten derivative N-ϵ-TFA-lysine did not entirely negate recognition.[83] An increasing number of these antigens formed in the rat liver and recognized by patient sera have now been identified.[84, 85] They include cytochrome P-450, which oxidizes halothane, proteins in proximity to this enzyme, and/or proteins in abundance in the endoplasmic reticulum. The appearance of the antigens recognized by patient sera change with time,[86] and induction with different hepatic cytochrome P-450 isoenzyme inducers alters the expression of different antigens and the level of expression and immunogenicity of the haptenated proteins may be influenced by half life and the repertoire of cytochrome P-450 enzymes present in an individual's liver. If made available to the immune system on the surface of the cell, the antigen(s) could act as targets to incur lysis. Which of these adducts are implicated as targets, or at an early stage in initiation of the immune response is not yet known.

The development of enzyme-linked immunosorbent assays has allowed screening of patient sera for antibodies with relative technical ease and rapidity. The earliest assay involved a homogenate of halothane-treated liver microsomes as an ex-vivo antigen,[87] and subsequently a synthetic conjugate of TFA-rabbit serum albumin has also been used.[88] It is evident that the specificity of the response in patients varies, since not all sera positive with the ex-vivo microsomal antigen are positive with the synthetic TFA antigen. This supports the previous observation that the TFA hapten does not comprise the whole antigenic determinant. Positive results have been obtained with sera from patients with chronic active hepatitis and to a lesser extent from those with primary biliary cirrhosis.[89] The presence of anti-TFA like antibodies in organ-specific autoimmune disease suggests that the TFA moiety may be able, unlike larger drug haptens, to mimic self determinants. Christen and colleagues[90] have detected proteins in hepatocytes from naive rats that cross-react with anti-TFA antibodies.

This should also underline the fact that a positive anti-TFA antibody result, while a powerful indicator in the diagnosis of halothane hepatitis, should be supported by elimination of the possibility of an autoimmune-type disease in the patient. An immune response specifically related to halothane can most readily be confirmed by analysis of both preexposure and postexposure serum samples.

Immune Response to Halothane in Animals

Further investigation of the mechanism of immunogenicity and potential toxicity of halothane must of necessity come from animal studies (Table 4).

TABLE 4.
Animal Models for Production of Antigens or Antibodies Following Halothane Exposure

Animal	Conditions	Results	Year	Reference
Rabbit	Multiple halothane, 2-hr, 2-wk intervals	Antibody and antigen production, no test for liver damage	1988	93
	Single 45-min exposure, 16 hr interval to sacrifice	Antigen production only	1988	97
Rat	Halothane, intraperitoneal (ip) injection, 12-hr.	Antigens only	1989	85
	Phenobarbital pretreatment, 4 hr; killed at 12 hr	Antigens only	1988	83
Guinea pig	TFA-albumin, intradermal	Cutaneous hypersensitivity and necrosis, no test for liver damage	1974	91
	Halothane, 4-hr, 2-wk intervals	Antibody, transient liver damage	1987	94
	S-ethylthiotrifluroacetate (SETFA) ip then halothane, 4-hr, 2-wk interval	Enhanced antibody, transient hepatotoxicity, leukocyte infiltration; confounded by SETFA toxicity	1990	105

These have concentrated on two different animal models: the rat, which has predominantly been used in studies of antigen formation; and the guinea pig, which has been used to investigate the immune response induced by halothane. Immunization of guinea pigs with synthetic conjugates of TFA and albumin or serum induced a delayed-type cutaneous reaction.[91] Skin sensitization in guinea pigs and in a phenobarbital-induced rat model could not be correlated with liver damage; however, in these early studies sensitization to TFA was measured indirectly with a relatively crude skin test. In conditions perhaps closer to those of the patient, multiple inhalation exposure of rabbits[92, 93] or guinea pigs[94] to halothane alone resulted in the induction of antibodies that cross-react with TFA-albumin. The anti-TFA antibodies thus induced are relatively low in titer in comparison with sera raised against TFA-albumin alone or in combination with halothane. Histological studies show that antigens cross-reactive with anti-TFA antibody are present in the centrilobular area of the liver in guinea pigs and rabbits exposed once or multiple times to halothane.[95] In support of experiments with human liver, appearance of antigen is related to oxidative metabolism since exposure to deuterated halothane reduced detection. The TFA antigens have also been detected following in vitro incubation of guinea pig liver slices with halothane, and this may represent a novel technique to investigate the mechanism of formation and subsequent manipulation of these antigens.[96]

In an attempt to develop an animal model of immune-mediated hepatitis, three different strains of guinea pigs were exposed to halothane and anti-TFA antibodies, and liver damage was monitored.[94] Animals were exposed to halothane up to four times and anti-TFA antibodies were induced, to differing degrees, in all strains. In strain 2 and Amana strain guinea pigs, peaks in anti-TFA antibody titer paralleled ALT levels. However, the relatively low and transitory elevations in ALT are consistent with mild liver damage rather than the severe fulminant hepatitis observed in patients.

In summary, halothane is immunogenic in the rabbit and the guinea pig. This is in contrast to humans where antibodies cross-reactive with TFA appear to be present only in patients with fulminant hepatitis. The anti-TFA antibody response so far induced in animals does not appear to mediate fulminant hepatic necrosis in vivo. Manipulation of the magnitude and type of response may be required to produce toxicity, and these problems highlight the need for an animal model of halothane hepatitis.

Potential Immunotoxic Mechanisms in Hepatitis

An aberrant, toxic immune response to halothane in patients may be the result of a large number of contributing and not necessarily mutually exclusive factors and may explain the difficulty in producing the same immune responses in animals. Broadly, areas of potential idiosyncrasy could include biotransformation and subsequent TFA protein adduct formation and the myriad of antibodies, T cells, cytokines, and complement that comprise the complex immune system.

Contrary to some earlier beliefs,[3, 41] idiosyncratic biotransformation of halothane may be insufficient alone to explain the delay in the appearance of liver damage in halothane hepatitis, the association with multiple exposures, and reduced latency period on reexposure. Formation of protein-reactive derivatives is of prime importance to immunogenicity; however, halothane-modified protein antigens can be detected in patients given halothane regardless of an anti-TFA response or hepatitis, suggesting that antigen formation is not the limiting step.[97] Changes in the balance between toxication and detoxication pathways, for example reduced glutathione levels, may alter the hapten density of TFA-labeled proteins or alter the portfolio of modified proteins so that sensitization occurs more readily. The route by which the halothane-modified proteins become exposed to the immune system may also affect the consequent reaction (Fig 3, lysed cell). As previously discussed, TFA-proteins may be released through lysis of hepatocytes via direct toxic mechanisms. The immune response would essentially be secondary to the initial damage and proceed via engulfment of the TFA-protein adduct by Kupffer cells. In this case, antigen would be presented with MHC II and result in T helper cells and subsequent B cell stimulation to produce antibodies (Fig 4).

Another hypothetical possibility is that the cell in which the TFA-protein adduct is formed presents the initiating signal (Fig 3, viable cell) and would most likely induce cytotoxic T cells in a mechanism similar to the immune response to viruses.

Thus, it is evident that a core consideration in any immune response is

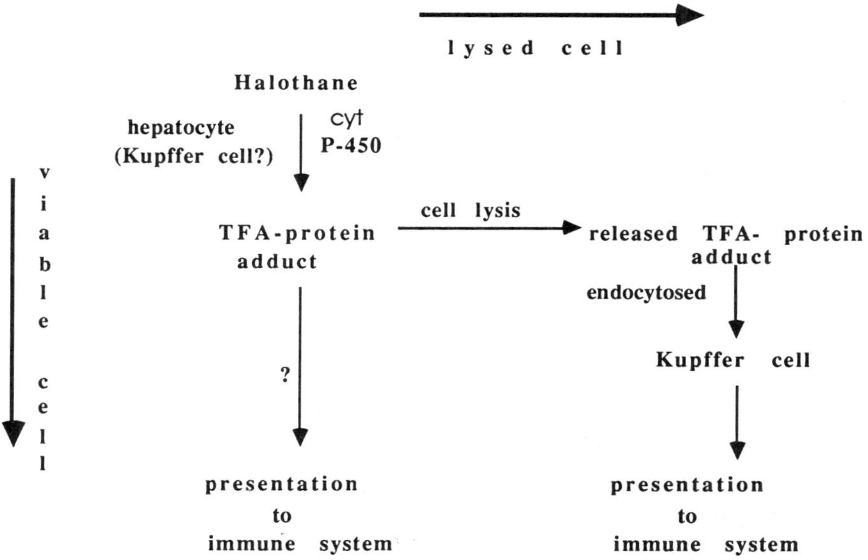

FIG 3.
Potential pathways of TFA-protein adduct presentation for initiation of an immune response.

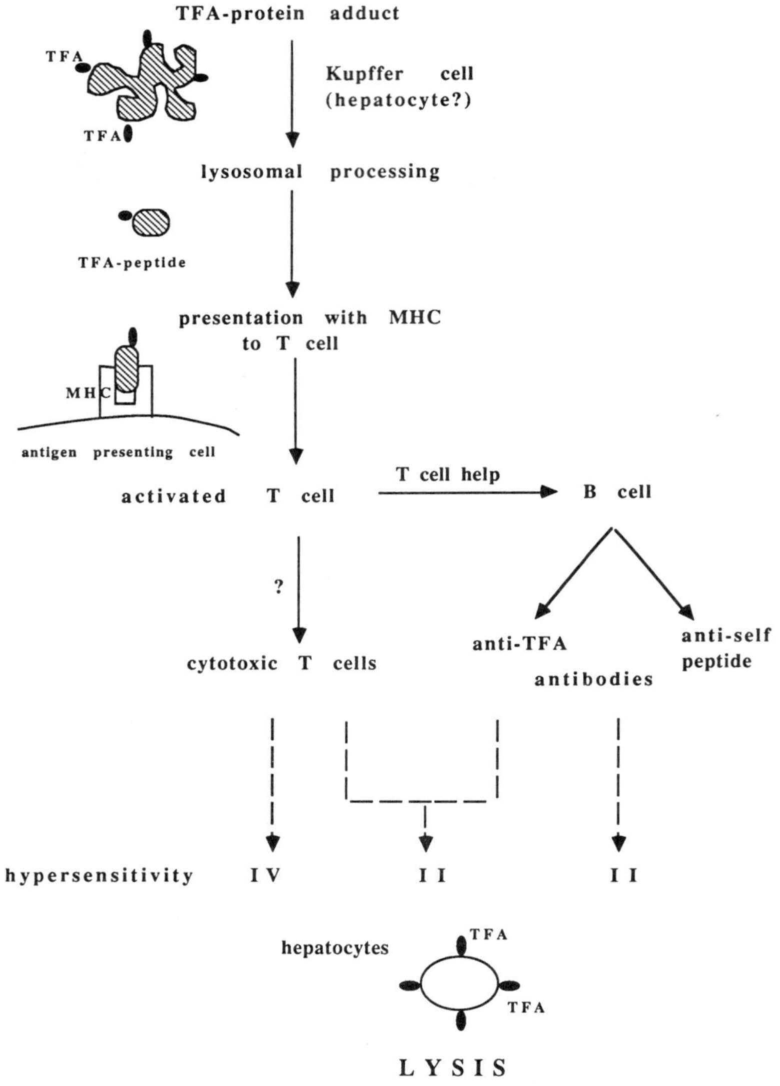

FIG 4.
Scheme to show the manner in which TFA-protein adducts could undergo processing and presentation to the immune system, and the resulting mechanism of liver damage.

the interaction between the T cell and the MHC-associated TFA-peptide.[74] Once appropriate proteins have been trifluoroacetylated or otherwise modified, presentation in association with MHC II glycoproteins on specific antigen-presenting cells is required for cell activation and subsequent antibody production/cellular sensitization. A genetic analysis of MHC genotypes in a group of Japanese patients[98] with halothane hepatitis found a significant correlation with the DR 2 MHC phenotype in those with jaundice, though other studies have failed to identify a common genetic restriction of this type.

Proteins that cross-react with anti-TFA antibodies have been detected in antigen-presenting immune (Kupffer) cells that express MHC II isolated from the liver of rats given halothane.[99] As briefly mentioned previously, T cells recognize short sequential peptides while antibodies interact with three-dimensional peptide structures. This is due to the fact that the protein antigens for cell recognition must first undergo intracellular digestion so that only peptide segments appear with the MHC on presentation to the T cell.[74] Antigen processing would thus most likely be required for the generation of an immune response from TFA-protein adducts (see Fig 4). Soluble antigen is digested within lysosomes or similar acidic subcellular compartments and this process can be inhibited by weak base amines.[100] This phenomenon was first investigated in antigen-presenting cells (to which Kupffer cells belong) but has since also been demonstrated in B cells. Both would present antigen with MHC II.

Less is known about the processing of protein synthesized within the cell that may subsequently be presented with MHC I to cytotoxic T cells. However, intracellular digestion is involved and may use a different route than that in the MHC II pathway since certain weak base amines have no inhibitory effect.[101] Probing pathways with inhibitors of intracellular antigen processing, such as chloroquine,[102] may uncover which antigens are important as immunogens.

Under normal circumstances, an immune response once achieved is regulated by feedback inhibition mechanisms possibly by the antiidiotype network and/or specific suppressor T cells that prevent any response from overamplification and potential tissue damage. One suggested mechanism for the bypass of normal regulatory control in autoimmunity is the activation of MHC II genes in cells that otherwise would not normally express it. Indeed, MHC II surface antigens have been detected on the surface of hepatocytes from patients with autoimmune, viral, and other liver diseases.[103] These cases include those of autoimmune chronic active hepatitis, a disease that can induce autoantibodies that cross-react with TFA-albumin.

Aside from the role of halothane (via the trifluoroacetyl chloride metabolite) as a target for the immune response, a number of studies have shown that halothane itself can have an inhibitory effect on the ability of lymphocytes to respond to other antigens and mitogens.[104] Obviously, inhibition of cells that should control anti-TFA and anti-self responses could exacerbate an otherwise potentially harmless response. Although regulatory alterations may not initiate tissue damage alone, they may enhance an otherwise benign response.

Hastings and colleagues[105] were able to demonstrate that the trifluoroacetyl moiety is highly immunogenic, and that the anti-TFA response on subsequent exposure to halothane was enhanced by immunization with TFA conjugated to autologous lymphocytes; to mycobacterial protein; or when treated with S-ethylthio-trifluoroacetate, which reacts directly with amino groups to produce trifluoroacetyl adducts. Thus, even in the presence of very high titers to anti-TFA antibodies, no liver damage in the guinea pigs could be detected. This may be a result of regulatory controls or differences in the type of immune response induced in comparison to the human immune response.

It would appear that a wide range of different variables both in metabolism and the immune system may be involved in an immune-mediated halothane, isoflurane, or enflurane hepatitis. Fortunately, the concurrent expression of the appropriate variables is rare. Many of the potential mechanisms of an aberrant response to halothane can be borrowed, at least in part, from those postulated in organ-specific autoimmune diseases and the advances with animal models in this area may be a route for this goal in halothane hepatitis. A working animal model of fulminant halothane hepatitis would both clarify the role(s) of direct and immune-mediated mechanisms in hepatic necrosis and may ultimately provide a means to predict which patients are most at risk in future anesthetic exposure.

Summary

Investigations concerning the mechanism of hepatotoxicity of volatile anesthetics have been protracted and convoluted. A variety of species have been used to develop models that are representative of the two forms of hepatic injuries seen clinically. At this time, the guinea pig is, without a doubt, the best model we have for the acute form of hepatic injury caused by halothane. The toxicity is initiated by the oxidative biotransformation of halothane to a trifluoroacetyl moiety that attacks liver proteins. The critical subcellular targets and mechanism of cell death from these toxic intermediates remain to be discerned, but the chemotoxic basis for this injury is unequivocal.

The latent, severe form of hepatic injury by volatile anesthetics has been more difficult to model in the laboratory; however, an immune response appears to either mediate or be associated with this response. Due to the numerous variables in metabolism and the immune system that probably need to be in place for an immune-mediated halothane hepatotoxicity to occur in a patient, the rarity of this occurrence can be understood. Development of an animal model for the immune-mediated toxicity must manipulate these same variables in the appropriate manner.

The hepatotoxicity of enflurane and isoflurane, though considerably less than that of halothane, is becoming increasingly documented by case reports. Clarification of the mechanism in halothane hepatitis will indicate the potential for current anesthetics, and those in development, to prevent similar adverse reactions.

References

1. Zimmerman HJ: Anesthetic agents. In *Hepatotoxicity: The adverse effects of drugs and other chemicals on the liver. New York, 1978, Appleton Century Croft, pp 370–394.*
2. Neuberger J, Williams R: Halothane anaesthesia and liver damage. *Br Med J* 289:1136–1139, 1984.
3. Brown BR, Gandolfi AJ: Adverse effects of volatile anesthetics. *Br J Anaesth* 59:14–23, 1987.
4. Ray DC, Drummond GB: Halothane hepatitis. *Br J Anaesth* 67:84–99, 1991.
5. Lewis JH, Zimmerman HJ, Ishak KG, Mullick FG: Enflurane hepatotoxicity. A clinicopathologic study of 24 cases. *Ann Int Med* 98:984–992, 1983.
6. Stoelting RK et al: Hepatic dysfunction after isoflurane anesthesia. *Anesth Analg* 66:147–153, 1987.
7. Carrigan TW, Straughen WJ: A report of hepatic necrosis and death following isoflurane anesthesia. *Anesthesiology* 67:581–583, 1987.
8. Brunt EM et al: Fulminant hepatic failure after repeated exposure to isoflurane anesthesia. A case report. *Hepatology* 13:1017–1021, 1991.
9. Lew JKL, Spence AA, Elton RA: Cross-sectional study of complications of inhalational anaesthesia in 16995 patients. *Anaesthesia* 46:810–815, 1991.
10. Benjamin SB et al: The morphologic spectrum of halothane-induced hepatic injury: Analysis of 77 cases. *Hepatology* 5:1163–1171, 1985.
11. Gandolfi AJ, Hubbard AK, Nunn JF: Viscerotoxicity of volatile anesthetics. In Stonehan MA et al, editors: *General anesthesia,* ed 5. New York, 1988, Butterworth, pp 88–95.
12. Wright R et al: Controlled prospective study of the effect on liver function of multiple exposure to halothane. *Lancet* i:814–820, 1975.
13. Temple RL, Cole RA, Gorens SW: Massive hepatic necrosis following general anesthesia. *Anesth Analg* 41:586–592, 1962.
14. Brody GL, Sweet RB: Halothane anesthesia as a possible cause of massive hepatic necrosis. *Anesthesiology* 24:29–37, 1963.
15. Walton B et al: Unexplained hepatitis following halothane. *Br Med J* 1:1171–1176, 1976.
16. Touloukian J, Kaplowitz N: Halothane-induced hepatic disease. *Semin Liver Dis* 1:134–142, 1981.
17. Slater EM et al: Postoperative hepatic necrosis. Its incidence and diagnostic value in association with the administration of halothane. *N Engl J Med* 270:983–987, 1964.
18. Bunker JP, et al, editors: National Halothane Study: A study of the possible association between halothane anesthesia and postoperative hepatic necrosis. U.S. Government Printing Office, 1969, Washington, D.C.
19. Bentley JB et al: Halothane metabolism in obese versus non-obese patients. *Anesthesiology* 57:94–97, 1982.
20. Walton B: Halothane hepatitis in children. *Anesthesiology* 41:575–578, 1986.
21. Hals J et al: Halothane-associated liver damage and renal failure in a young child. *Acta Anaesthesiol Scand* 30:651–655, 1986.
22. Cousins MJ, Plummer JL, Hall P: Risk factors for halothane hepatitis. *Aust NZ J Surg* 59:5–14, 1989.

23. Liebler DC, Sipes IG: Bioactivation: The role of metabolism in chemical toxicity. In Sullivan JB, Kreiger GR, editors: *Hazardous materials toxicology: Clinical principals of environmental health.* New York, 1992, Williams and Wilkens, pp 31–45.
24. McLain GE, Sipes IG, Brown BR: An animal model of halothane hepatotoxicity: Roles of enzyme induction and hypoxia. *Anesthesiology* 51:321–326, 1979.
25. Shingu K, Eger EI, Johnson BH: Hypoxia per se can produce hepatic damage without death in rats. *Anesth Analg* 61:820–823, 1982.
26. Shingu K et al: Hepatic injury induced by anesthetic agents in rats. *Anesth Analg* 62:140–145, 1983.
27. Lind RC et al: Comparison of the requirements for hepatic injury with halothane and enflurane in rats. *Anesth Analg* 64:955–963, 1985.
28. Lind RC, Gandolfi AJ, Brown BR: Are the requirements for hepatic injury with halothane and enflurane in rats really different? *Anesth Analg* 65:545–547, 1986.
29. Wood M et al: Halothane-induced hepatic necrosis in triiodothyronine-pretreated rats. *Anesthesiology* 52:470–476, 1980.
30. Smith AC et al: Characterization of hyperthyroidism enhancement of halothane-induced hepatotoxicity. *Biochem Pharmacol* 32:3531–3539, 1983.
31. Rehder K et al: Halothane biotransformation in man: A quantitative study. *Anesthesiology* 28:711–715, 1967.
32. Lind RC, Gandolfi AJ, Hall P de la M: The role of oxidative biotransformation of halothane in the guinea pig model of halothane-associated hepatotoxicity. *Anesthesiology* 70:649–653, 1989.
33. Hubbard AK, Roth TP, Gandolfi AJ: Immunological methods for investigating the mechanisms of halothane hepatotoxicity. Meeks, Bull, editors: *Hepatotoxicology* CRC Press, 1991, Boca Raton, Fla, pp 647–665.
34. Sipes IG, Brown BR Jr: An animal model of hepatotoxicity associated with halothane anesthesia. *Anesthesiology* 45:622–628, 1976.
35. Reynolds ES, Moslen MT: Halothane hepatotoxicity: Enhancement by polychlorinated biphenyl pretreatment. *Anesthesiology* 47:19–27, 1977.
36. Rice SA et al: Halothane hepatotoxicity in Fischer 344 rats pretreated with isoniazid. *Tox Appl Pharmacol* 87:411–419, 1987.
37. Widger LA, Gandolfi AJ, Van Dyke RA: Hypoxia and halothane metabolism in vivo: Release of inorganic fluoride and halothane metabolite binding to cellular constituents. *Anesthesiology* 44:197–201, 1976.
38. Jee RC et al: Factors influencing halothane hepatotoxicity in the rat hypoxic model. *Tox Appl Pharmacol* 52:267–277, 1980.
39. Cousins MJ et al: Hepatotoxicity and halothane metabolism in animal model with application for human toxicity. *Anaesth Intensive Care* 7:9–24, 1979.
40. Ross WT, Daggy BP, Cardell RR Jr: Hepatic necrosis caused by halothane and hypoxia in phenobarbital-treated rats. *Anesthesiology* 51:327–333, 1979.
41. Cousins MJ, Plummer JL, Hall P de la M: Toxicity of volatile anaesthetic agents. *Clin Anaes* 2:551–575, 1984.
42. Gelman S, Fowler KC, Smith LR: Regional blood flow during isoflurane and halothane anesthesia. Anesth Analg 63:557–565, 1984.
43. Zimmerman HJ: *Expressions of hepatotoxicity: The adverse effects of drugs and other chemicals on the liver.* Appleton Century Croft, 1978, New York, pp 167–197.

44. Gandolfi AJ, Brown BR: Hypoxia and halothane hepatotoxicity. *Anesthesiology* 62:859–861, 1983.
45. Lunam CA, Cousins MJ, Hall P de la M: Guinea-pig model of halothane-associated hepatotoxicity in the absence of enzyme induction and hypoxia. *J Pharmacol Exp Ther* 232:802–809, 1985.
46. Hughes HC, Lang CM: Hepatic necrosis produced by repeated administration of halothane to guinea pigs. *Anesthesiology* 36:466–471, 1972.
47. Lind RC, Gandolfi AJ, Hall P de la M: Covalent binding of oxidative biotransformation intermediates is associated with halothane hepatotoxicity in guinea pigs. *Anesthesiology* 73:1208–1213, 1990.
48. Lind RC, Gandolfi AJ: Isoniazid potentiation of a guinea pig model of halothane-associated hepatotoxicity. *J Appl Toxicol* 10:161–165, 1990.
49. Lind RC, Gandolfi AJ, Hall P de la M: Subanesthetic halothane is hepatotoxic in the guinea pig. *Anesth Analg* 74:559–563, 1992.
50. Lind RC et al: Halothane hepatotoxicity in guinea pigs. *Anesth Analg* 66:222–228, 1987.
51. Farrell GC et al: Altered hepatic calcium homeostasis in guinea pigs with halothane-induced hepatotoxicity. *J Pharmacol Exp Ther* 247:751–756, 1988.
52. Lind RC, Gandolfi AJ, Hall P de la M: Age and gender influence halothane-associated hepatotoxicity in strain 13 guinea pigs. *Anesthesiology* 71:878–884, 1989.
53. Lunam CA, Cousins MJ, Hall P de la M: Genetic predisposition to liver damage after halothane anesthesia in guinea pigs. *Anesth Analg* 65:1143–1148, 1986.
54. Farrell GC: Mechanisms of halothane-induced liver injury: Is it immune or metabolic idiosyncrasy? *J Gastroenterol Hepatol* 3:465–482, 1988.
55. Lunam CA, Hall P de la M, Cousins MJ: The pathology of halothane hepatotoxicity in a guinea-pig model: A comparison with human halothane hepatitis. *Br J Exp Pathol* 70:533–541, 1989.
56. Lind RC, Gandolfi AJ: Concentration dependent inhibition of halothane biotransformation and covalent binding in the guinea pig. *Toxicologist* 12:152, 1992.
57. Anders MW, Pohl LR: Halogenated alkanes. In Anders MW, editor: *Bioactivation of foreign compounds. Rochester, 1985, Academic, pp 283–315.*
58. Dale O, Nilsen OG: Glutathione and glutathione S-transferases in rat liver after inhalation of halothane and enflurane. *Toxicol Lett* 23:61–66, 1984.
59. Smith AC et al: Paradoxical effect of perturbation of intracellular levels of glutathione on halothane-induced hepatotoxicity in hyperthyroid rats. *Fundam Appl Toxicol* 4:221–230, 1984.
60. Lind RC, Gandolfi AJ: Glutathione depletion exacerbates halothane-associated hepatotoxicity in guinea pigs (abstract). *Anesthesiology* 73:398, 1990.
61. Lind RC, Gandolfi AJ, Hall PM: Glutathione depletion enhances covalent binding and hepatotoxicity of subanesthetic halothane in the guinea pig (abstract). *Hepatology* 14:160, 1991.
62. Lind RC, Gandolfi AJ, Hall P de la M: An animal model for fatal halothane hepatitis (abstract). *IUTOX*, 1992.
63. Landsteiner K: The specificity of serological reactions. Cambridge, 1945, Harvard University.
64. Gell PHG, Coombs RKA: Clinical aspects of immunology. Oxford, 1963, Blackwell Scientific.
65. Moult PJA, Sherlock S: Halothane related hepatitis. A clinical study of 26 cases. *Q J Med* 44:99–114, 1975.

66. Inman WHW, Mushin WW: Jaundice after repeated exposure to halothane: An analysis of reports to the Committee on Safety of Medicines. *Br Med J* 1:5–10, 1974.
67. Walton B et al: Absence of cellular hypersensitivity in patients with unexplained hepatitis following halothane. *Anesthesiology* 44:391–397, 1976.
68. Rizzetto M, Swana G, Doniach D: Microsomal antibodies in active chronic hepatitis and other disorders. *Clin Exp Immunol* 15:331–344, 1973.
69. Roitt I: *Essential immunology*, ed 7. Blackwell Scientific, 1991, Oxford, pp 309–313.
70. Christ DD et al: Enflurane metabolism produces covalently bound liver adducts recognized by antibodies from patients with halothane hepatitis. *Anesthesiology* 69:833–838, 1988.
71. Christ DD et al: Potential metabolic basis for enflurane hepatitis and the apparent cross-sensitization between enflurane and halothane. *Drug Metab Dispos* 16:135–140, 1988.
72. Paronetto F, Popper H: Lymphocyte stimulation induced by halothane in patients with hepatitis following exposure to halothane. *N Engl J Med* 283:277–280, 1970.
73. Walton B et al: Lymphocyte transformation: Absence of increased responses in alleged halothane jaundice. *JAMA* 225:494–498, 1973.
74. Grey HM, Sette A, Buus S: How T cells see antigen. *Sci Am* 261:56–64, 1989.
75. Victorino RMM, Maria VAJ, Pinto La: Evidence for prostaglandin-producing suppressor cells in drug-induced liver injury and implications in the diagnosis of drug sensitization. *Clin Exp Immunol* 87:132–137, 1992.
76. Hubbard AK, Roth TP, Gandolfi AJ: Elicitation of a cell-mediated immune response to a reactive intermediate of halothane. *Toxicologist* 8:12, 1988.
77. Mieli-Vergani G et al: Lymphocyte cytotoxicity to halothane altered hepatocytes in patients with severe hepatic necrosis following halothane anaesthesia. *J Clin Lab Immunol* 4:49–51, 1980.
78. Vergani D et al: Antibodies to the surface of halothane-altered rabbit hepatocytes in patients with severe halothane-associated hepatitis. *N Engl J Med* 303:66–71, 1980.
79. Williams BD et al: Circulating immune complexes after repeated halothane anaesthesia. *Br Med J* 2:159–162, 1977.
80. Canalese J et al:; Circulating immune complexes in patients with fulminant hepatic failure. *Gut* 22:845–848, 1981.
81. Kenna JG, Neuberger J, Williams R: Specific antibodies to halothane-induced liver antigens in halothane-associated hepatitis. *Br J Anaesth* 59:1286–1290, 1987.
82. Kenna JG, Neuberger J, Williams R: Identification by immunoblotting of three halothane-induced liver microsomal polypeptide antigens recognized by antibodies in sera from patients with halothane-associated hepatitis. *J Pharmacol Exp Ther* 242:733–740, 1987.
83. Kenna JG et al: Metabolic basis for a drug hypersensitivity: Antibodies in sera from patients with halothane hepatitis recognize liver neoantigens that contain the trifluoroacetyl group derived from halothane. *J Pharmacol Exp Ther* 245:1103–1109, 1988.
84. Satoh H et al: Immunochemical evidence of trifluoroacetylated cytochrome P-450 in the liver of halothane-treated rats. *Mol Pharmacol* 28:468–474, 1985.

85. Satoh H et al: Human anti-endoplasmic reticulum antibodies in sera of halothane hepatitis patients are directed against a trifluoroacetylated carboxylesterase. *Proc Natl Acad Sci* USA 86:322–326, 1989.
86. Kenna JG et al: Factors affecting the expression of trifluroacetylated liver microsomal protein neoantigens in rats treated with halothane. *Drug Metab Dispos* 18:788–793, 1990.
87. Kenna JG, Neuberger J, Williams R: An enzyme-linked immunosorbent assay for detection of antibodies against halothane-altered hepatocyte antigens. *J Immunol Methods* 75:3–14, 1984.
88. Hastings KL et al: Screening for antibodies associated with halothane hepatitis. *Br J Anaesth* 67:722–728, 1991.
89. Martin JL et al: Assays for the detection of antibodies directed against halothane-induced liver neoantigens in the sera of patients with halothane hepatitis (abstract). *Anesthesiology* 69:439, 1988.
90. Christen U, Burgin M, Gut J: Halothane metabolism: Immunochemical evidence for molecular mimicry of trifluoroacetylated liver protein adducts by constitutive polypeptides. *Mol Pharmacol* 40:390–400, 1991.
91. Mathieu A et al: Experimental immunity to a metabolite of halothane and fluoroxene. Cutaneous delayed-type hypersensitivity. *Anesthesiology* 40: 383–390, 1974.
92. Callis AH et al: Characterization of a halothane-induced humoral immune response in rabbits. *Clin Exp Immunol* 67:343–351, 1987.
93. Roth TP et al: Chronology of halothane-induced antigen expression in halothane-exposed rabbits. *Clin Exp Immunol* 72:330–336, 1988.
94. Siadat-Pajouh M et al: Generation of halothane-induced immune response in a guinea pig model of halothane hepatitis. *Anesth Analg* 66:1209–1214, 1987.
95. Hubbard AK et al: Localization of halothane-induced antigen in situ by specific anti-halothane metabolite antibodies. *Clin Exp Immunol* 76:422–427, 1989.
96. Brown AP, Hastings KL, Gandolfi AJ: Generation and detection of neoantigens in guinea pig liver slices incubated with halothane. *Int J Immunopharmacol* 13:429–435, 1991.
97. Kenna JG, Neuberger J, Williams R: Evidence for expression in human liver of halothane-induced neoantigens recognized by antibodies in serum from patients with halothane hepatitis. *Hepatology* 8:1635–1641, 1988.
98. Otsuka S et al: HLA antigens in patients with unexplained hepatitis following halothane anaesthesia. *Acta Anaesth Scand* 29:497–501, 1985.
99. Christen U, Burgin M, Gut J: Halothane metabolism: Kupffer cells carry and partially process trifluoroacetylated protein adducts. *Biochem Biophys Res Commun* 175:256–262, 1991.
100. Ziegler HK, Unanue ER: Decrease in macrophage antigen metabolism caused by ammonia and chloroquine is associated with inhibition of antigen presentation to T cells. *Proc Natl Acad Sci (USA)* 79:175–178, 1982.
101. Roitt I: *Essential immunology,* ed 7. 1991, Blackwell Scientific, pp 76–79.
102. Clarke JB, Chen ML, Gandolfi AJ: Effect of chloroquine on the formation of halothane-induced liver antigens in guinea pigs. A tool to investigate immune-mediated toxicity. *Toxicology* 12:44, 1992.
103. Lobo-Yeo A et al: Class I and class II major histocompatibility complex antigen expression on hepatocytes: A study in children with liver disease. *Hepatology* 12:224–232, 1990.

104. Bruce DL: Halothane inhibition of phytohemagglutinin-induced transformation of lymphocytes. *J Anesthesiol* 36:201–205, 1972.
105. Hastings KL et al: S-ethylthiotrifluoroacetate enhancement of the immune response to halothane in the guinea pig. *Adv Exp Med Biol* 283:739–744, 1991.

Acute Spinal Cord Ischemia: Implications for Anesthetic Management

Arthur M. Lam, M.D., F.R.C.P.C.

Professor of Anesthesiology and Neurologic Surgery, University of Washington School of Medicine, Attending Anesthesiologist, Harborview Medical Center, Seattle, Washington

Acute spinal cord ischemia is not a common occurrence in the perioperative setting, yet the consequence is of such a potentially devastasting nature that every effort should be made to diagnose, prevent, and/or treat this complication. Until recently, little or no specific treatment was available, but recent advances in our understanding of pathophysiology and pharmacotherapy have offered at least a glimpse of hope if not a definitive cure. In the perioperative period, acute spinal cord ischemia primarily occurs in one of two situations: (1) during a surgical procedure on the spinal cord and/or spinal column, which would include (a) decompression and stabilization of the patient with an acute spinal cord injury, (b) surgical repair or excision of other spinal cord lesions such as tumors or arteriovenous malformations, or (c) corrective procedure on the spinal column such as Harrington rod instrumentation; and (2) during thoracoabdominal aortic procedures, where cross-clamping of the thoracic or abdominal aorta is required. The initiating event of spinal cord ischemia differs in these conditions: the acutely injured patient suffers from traumatic impact, the patient with a spinal cord lesion may succumb to surgical retraction, the patient with scoliosis is subjected to mechanical distraction and deformation of the spinal cord, and the patient undergoing aortic reconstruction procedures endures spinal cord hypoperfusion secondary to aortic cross-clamping. However, once the ischemic process begins, the pathophysiology follows a common pathway leading to transient or permanent neurological dysfunction.

This article will review the normal anatomy and physiology of the spinal cord and the anesthetic implications of spinal cord ischemia, and the recent advances in pharmacological treatment. Emphasis wil be placed on the anesthetic management of the patient with acute spinal cord injury since this is the most frequent cause of spinal cord ischemia. Moreover, most of the considerations will also apply to surgical procedures on the spinal cord/column. Since the cause of spinal cord ischemia in thoracoabdominal procedures is different, the anesthetic implications will be discussed separately.

Normal Anatomy and Physiology of the Spinal Cord

Spinal Cord Circulation

The anterior 75% of the spinal cord is supplied by a single anterior spinal artery that arises from the vertebral arteries and runs longitudinally for the length of the spinal cord with important contributions from radicular vessels from the aorta via the intercostal arteries. The spinal cord segment between the radicular arteries receives its blood supply from above as well as below. The superior segment of the spinal cord, which includes the cervical spinal cord and the first two thoracic segments, has a relatively rich blood supply, with contributions from the subclavian artery as well the vertebral arteries. The mid-thoracic segment consisting of the first seven segments is characterized by a poor blood supply, with a contribution usually only from one afferent vessel arising from an intercostal artery. The most important of the radicular vessels is the artery of Adamkiewicz, which is the main blood supply for the thoracolumbar segment of the spinal cord. The site of entry of this large radicular vessel is variable; it joins the anterior spinal artery between T9 and T12 in 75% of the cases, between T5 and T8 in 15%, and between L1 and L2 in the other 10%. The two posterior spinal arteries, which arise from the posterior branch of the vertebral arteries and also receive contributions from radicular vessels, supply the posterior 25% of the spinal cord.[1] An illustration of the spinal cord circulation is shown in Figure 1.

Regulation of Spinal Cord Blood Flow

Although not as extensively studied as the cerebral circulation, and methodological problems virtually exclude the study of spinal cord circulation in humans, spinal cord blood flow appears to be regulated by the same factors as cerebral blood flow and the concept of cerebral perfusion pressure is equally applicable to the spinal cord; that is, spinal cord perfusion pressure = mean blood pressure−cerebrospinal fluid pressure. Between perfusion pressures of 50 and 130 mm Hg, there appears to be good autoregulation.[2–4] Similar to the cerebral circulation, hypercapnia increases spinal cord blood flow while hypocapnia decreases it.[3, 5] Both the range of autoregulation and the CO_2 reactivity appear to be less than that of the cerebral circulation. The absolute blood flow varies between species, but also appears to be less than the comparable cerebral circulation. The gray matter blood flow is about 60 mL/100 g/min and the white matter blood flow is about 10 mL/100 g/min in primates.[6] Interestingly, while systemic hypothermia decreases cerebral blood flow, presumably due to decreased metabolic demand, in the spinal cord it has been observed that

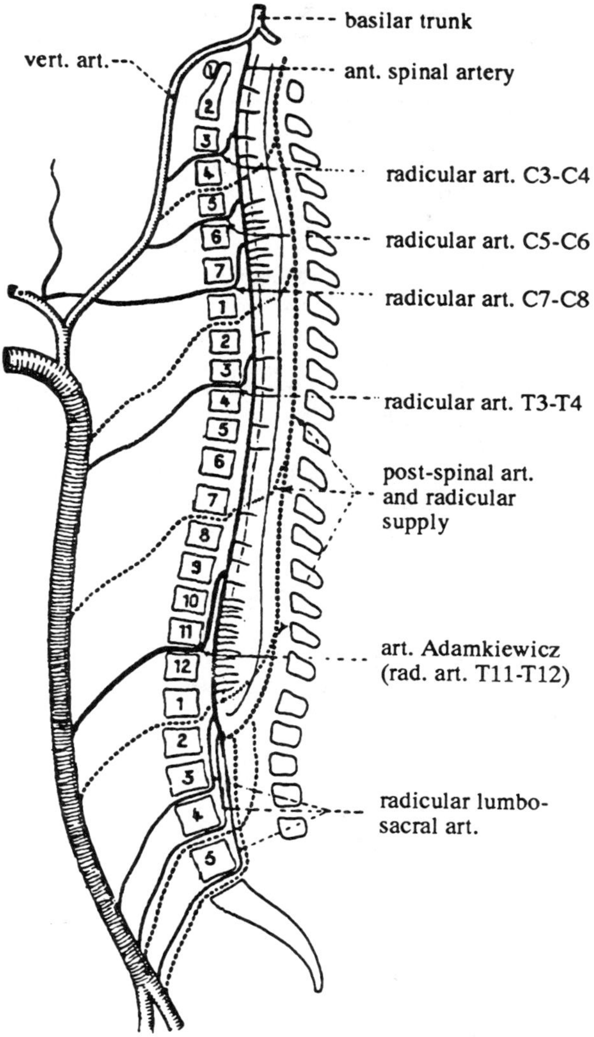

FIG 1.
Vascular supply of the spinal cord circulation, illustrating the contributions from the radicular arteries.

blood flow increases under these conditions (rectal temperature of 28° C).[7] This is thought to be secondary to loss of autoregulation coupled with increased systemic blood pressure during hypothermia. In contrast, local cooling of the spinal cord to 25° to 28° C decreases spinal cord blood flow.[8]

Importance of Ischemia in the Pathophysiology of Acute Spinal Cord Injury

Primary and Secondary Injury

Although trauma to the spinal cord often causes immediate and complete disruption of spinal cord function, anatomically the spinal cord itself is seldom transected. These observations, coupled with findings from experimental research, give rise to the concept of primary and secondary injury. The primary injury results from the original impact of force and compression against the spinal cord, resulting in damage to the small intramedullary vessels, causing hemorrhage in the central gray matter of the spinal cord, and perhaps vasospasm. Although the cause remains unclear, an immediate reduction of blood flow to the gray matter occurs, followed by a similar reduction in flow to the white matter.[6] The resultant ischemia triggers a biochemical cascade that may cause further spinal cord ischemia, which signals the onset of secondary injury leading to eventual infarction of the spinal cord with permanent loss of function.

The primary injury cannot be treated and can only be prevented, pri-

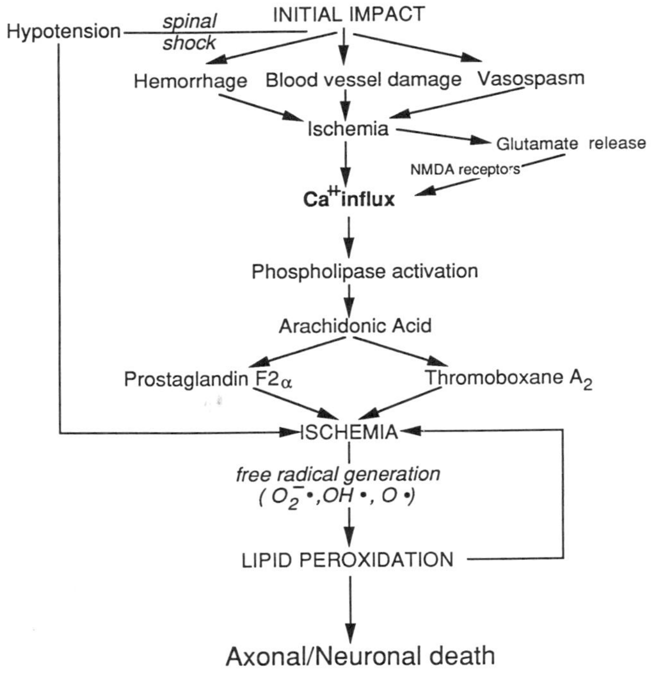

FIG 2.
Biochemical cascade initiated by the primary event with acute spinal injury leading to ultimate axonal/neuronal death. NMDA = N-methyl-D-aspartate

marily with implementation of educational programs.[9] Secondary injury occurs within minutes to hours following the primary injury[10] and is thought to involve a complex biochemical cascade. The initial injury causes hemorrhage, ischemia, release of excitotoxic amino acids (glutamates), and an intracellular influx of calcium ions. The binding of glutamate to N-methyl-D-aspartate (NMDA) opens the receptor-gated channels and leads to a further increase in calcium influx. The intracellular accumulation of calcium then leads to activation of phospholipase, and release of arachidonic acid and its metabolites of prostanoids and thromboxanes. These potent vasoconstrictors result in further ischemia and generation of free radicals, causing lipid peroxidation and eventual destruction of neurons and axons.[11, 12] A schematic summary of this event is shown in Figure 2. This reduction in blood flow has been found to be related to the severity of spinal cord injury, as well as a change in motor- and somatosensory-evoked potentials in experimental spinal cord ischemia in rats induced with epidural compression.[13] More recently, this reduction in blood flow during secondary injury has been positively correlated with functional deficits in experimental spinal cord injury in rats inflicted by the weight-drop method.[14]

Other pathophysiological changes include loss of autoregulation[15, 16] and perhaps impairment of CO_2 reactivity,[17] although the latter findings were made in a neoplastic spinal cord compression rather than a traumatic model. The loss of autoregulation coupled with spinal shock and hypotension also play a contributory role in the genesis of ischemia.

Reperfusion injury may also contribute to the spinal cord injury as the reactive hyperemia that follows restoration of circulation creates hyperoxia, which favors the further production of free radicals, accumulation of calcium, and destruction of the neuron.[18] The occurrence of this reperfusion injury is supported indirectly by experimental studies demonstrating that graded hypoxia following reperfusion after ischemia actually improves outcome.[19]

Experimental Spinal Cord Injury

There are primarily two models used in the study of pathophysiology and treatment of spinal cord injury: the block weight-drop method described by Allen,[20] and the extradural clip compression model developed by Rivlin and Tator.[21] As previously explained, the timing and mechanism of secondary injury in these models suggest that the ischemia is an important factor and that pharmacologic treatment may be possible in the immediate period after the initial injury. These aspects were recently reviewed by Tator and Fehlings.[22]

Pharmacologic Treatment

Drugs that have been found to be efficacious in experimental spinal injury models include calcium channel blockers,[23–29] naloxone,[30–32] thyrotropin-releasing hormone,[33–35] NMDA antagonists,[36] and corticosteroids.[37, 38]

Calcium Channel Blockers

As secondary injury may involve vasospasm and reduction in blood flow as well as intracellular accumulation of calcium ions, it is logical that calcium channel blockers be examined for their treatment potentials. The results, however, have been conflicting. Tator and his group found that nimodipine increases spinal cord blood flow following compression injury provided a vasopressor was administered to counteract its hypotensive effect.[23, 24] Subsequent study with the combination of dextran and nimodipine not only increase spinal cord blood flow but also improve axonal conduction as evidenced by somatosensory- and motor-evoked potentials.[25] However, other investigators have not been able to demonstrate either an increase in flow or an improvement in function.[26–28] Black et al. investigated another calcium channel blocker, nicardipine, and were also unable to substantiate any improvement in functional recovery.[29] The differences in the models and the timing of drop administration may have accounted for the discrepancy. Clearly more studies are required before any conclusion regarding the therapeutic effect of calcium channel blockers can be drawn.

Naloxone and Thyrotropin-Releasing Hormone

It has long been suggested that release of endogenous opioids may mediate some of the pathophysiological changes seen in spinal cord injury. Initial studies by Holaday and Faden showed that naloxone can reverse hypotension, hypoventilation, and hypothermia in feline spinal shock.[30] However, subsequent studies failed to demonstrate any consistent beneficial effect in the rat spinal cord trauma model.[31] Wallace and Tator were also unable to demonstrate any increase in spinal cord blood flow in the rat model.[32] Similarly, studies with thyrotropin-releasing hormone, which has a more potent antagonist effect than naloxone, yield conflicting results in different species and different spinal cord injury models.[33–35] In a multicenter clinical trial for acute spinal cord injury, naloxone was not found to be useful when compared to placebo (see later).

NMDA Antagonists

These compounds have been found to have cerebroprotective value in focal cerebral ischemia, and given the similarity between the spinal cord circulation and injury pattern to that of the brain, it is reasonable to expect beneficial effects. Indeed, a study with a neoplastic spinal cord compression model has demonstrated that MK-801 and ketamine (both NMDA antagonists) decreased the formation of cytotoxic edema, although no apparent improvement in function was evident.[36] More studies are required to delineate the efficacy of NMDA antagonists in spinal cord ischemia.

Corticosteroids

These have been the most extensively studied agents for the treatment of experimental spinal cord injury. There is good experimental evidence that high-dose glucocorticoid can improve post-injury spinal cord blood flow and reduce intracellular calcium influx.[38] In addition, it is a potent inhibitor of lipid peroxidation, an effect that may be its most important action.[39]

Nonpharmacologic Treatment

Local Hypothermia

Local spinal cord cooling to a temperature of 10° C as a therapy was first investigated by Albin et al. in 1968.[40] These investigators found that cooling the spinal cord 4 hours after trauma was effective in preventing the development of neurologic dysfunction in primates and postulated this may be due to reduction of metabolic rate and edema formation. The clinical application of this method, however, proves to be impractical since laminectomy is required to institute the cooling process. In cerebral ischemia it is now recognized that even mild hypothermia can have significant cerebroprotective effect,[41, 42] and that the mechanism has more to do with suppression of excitotoxic amino acid release and less with metabolic depression.[43] Thus there is a need to investigate the benefits of mild hypothermia on spinal cord injury.

Elevation of Systemic Blood Pressure

Since spinal cord ischemia can be further aggravated by systemic hypotension during the spinal shock phase, it is important to maintain normal perfusion pressure in the acute stage. Improvement in post-injury spinal cord blood flow has been demonstrated experimentally with the combination of volume expansion with dextran and nimodipine.[25] Excessive elevation of systemic blood pressure, however, may cause intramedullary hemorrhage and increase edema formation.[44]

Clinical Trial of Pharmacologic Agents

Methylprednisolone

The only treatment to date that has been shown to be effective clinically is high-dose corticosteroid. In a multicenter, randomized, placebo-controlled trial in acute spinal cord injury (National Acute Spinal Cord Injury Study or NASCIS II), 162 patients received methylprednisolone 30 mg/kg followed by a continuous infusion of 5.4 mg/kg/hr for the next 23 hours. At 6-week and 6-month follow-up, the outcome was found to be improved in patients with complete as well as incomplete lesions.[45] Improvements in sensory and motor function were noted. Similar results were observed at 1-year follow-up.[46] However, consistent with the mechanism of secondary injury, the drug must be given within 8 hours of injury to have any effect. In contrast, in the same study, 154 patients received naloxone 5.4 mg/kg followed by an infusion of 4 mg/kg/hr for 23 hours and no significant benefit was demonstrated. One hundred seventy-one patients received placebo bolus and infusion. Mortality and major morbidity were similar in all three groups. Thus all patients considered to be at risk of spinal cord ischemia should receive methylprednisolone according to the protocol reported in that study.

The neuroprotective effects of steroid were recently reviewed by Hall.[39] The protective effects of methylprednisolone are not dependent on steroid receptors and are probably mediated through inhibition of lipid peroxidation and improvement of spinal cord blood flow. Indeed, the glucocorticoid effect, by causing hyperglycemia, may have a negative protective effect by aggravating lactic acidosis during ischemia.[47] To circumvent these negative effects, compounds with the steroid nucleus but without glucocorticoid effects have been synthesized (21-aminosteroids). One compound, tirilazid (U-74006F) appears to be particularly promising in experimental head injury and cerebral ischemia[48–50] and is currently in phase II clinical trial. It is our clinical practice to treat all our patients at risk of spinal cord ischemia prophylactically according to the methylprednisolone protocol during the perioperative period.

Monosialotetrahexosylganglioside (GM-1)

Gangliosides are complex acidic glycosphingolipids found in high concentrations in the central nervous system cell membrane. In experimental neurologic injury, gangliosides have been found to promote healing and regeneration. In a clinical series of 34 patients with major motor deficits from acute spinal cord injury, the 16 patients assigned to receive GM-1 100 mg/day for a mean of 26 days had a significantly better recovery of motor function than the placebo group at the end of 1-year follow-up.[51] Although the number of patients enrolled in the clinical trial is small and the mechanism of improvement remains unclear, it is of some significance that GM-1 was administered at a mean time of 48 hours after the inital injury, well outside the therapeutic time window of 8 hours observed with methylprednisolone. This raises the interesting prospect of combination therapy to maximize the treatment effect. Unfortunately the results with GM-1 therapy in other clinical and experimental studies have not been consistenly favorable, and the compound has not been approved by the Food and Drug Administration (FDA) for clinical use.[51, 52]

Acute Spinal Cord Injury

As previously mentioned, the major considerations for the anesthesiologist regarding spinal cord ischemia is the anesthetic care of the patient with an acute spinal cord injury undergoing spinal cord/column procedures. The major anesthetic considerations of acute spinal cord injury are reviewed here. Treatment of patients undergoing thoracoabdominal aortic procedures will be reviewed in a subsequent section.

The incidence of spinal cord injuries in North America is estimated to be

15 to 50 per million population.[53, 54] In the United States, this means approximately 12,000 new cases per year with a mortality rate approaching 50% and a prevalence of 200,000.[53] Most victims are young (age 15 to 24)[54] and the survivors end up with debilitating neurologic deficits, although the development of regional spinal cord injury centers as well as improved treatments have reduced the incidence of complete lesions from 65% to 45%.[55] The major causes are motor vehicle accidents, falls, sports and recreational injuries, and other violent causes. Alcohol and recreational drug use are frequently contributing factors.

Mechanism and Classification of Spinal Cord Injury

Injuries in the cervical spine are generally caused by: (1) flexion, (2) flexion-rotation, (3) vertical compression (axial loading), (4) extension, (5) extension-rotation, and (6) lateral flexion.[56] The mechanism of injury in the thoracolumbar spine is similar except there is less mobility and injuries are more likely due to compression and rotational forces.

The three-column concept[57] of the structure of the vertebral column helps to clarify the mechanism of injury. The posterior column is formed by the posterior neural arch, spinous process, facetal articular processes, and their corresponding posterior ligamentous complex. The middle column consists of the posterior one third of the vertebral body and annulus fibrosus and the posterior longitudinal ligament. The anterior column comprises the anterior longitudinal ligament and the anterior two thirds of the vertebral body and annulus fibrosus. Flexion injury causes disruption of the posterior column and extension injury causes disruption of the anterior column. If two or more columns are disrupted, then acute spinal instability exists and predicts the possibility of late instability. Spinal cord injuries most frequently involve the lower cervical spine and the thoracolumbar junction, the former because of its mobility, and the latter because it is the junction between the rigid thoracic spine and the flexible lumbar spine.

The Pediatric and the Elderly Spine

Up until 10 years of age, the immature spine has increased physiological mobility due to ligamentous laxity, and incompletely ossified wedge-shaped vertebrae, affording some protection against spinal column injuries but at the same time increasing the incidence of spinal cord injury without radiographic abnormality.[58–60] The elderly patient, on the other hand, with the development of degenerative changes and osteophytes, and narrowing of the spinal canal, may develop spinal cord injury even with trivial trauma, and the injury may be missed.[61]

Spinal cord injuries can be complete with loss of all motor and sensory functions below the level of injury, or incomplete including the central cord syndrome, the Brown-Sequard syndrome, the anterior cord syndrome, and the posterior cord syndrome.

Systemic Effects of Acute Spinal Cord Injury

Cardiovascular System

The initial injury is associated with a sudden rise in blood pressure, bradycardia, and dysrhythmias due to intense sympathetic activation. This is followed within minutes by hypotension as the stage of spinal shock sets in with total loss of neuronal conduction, flaccid paralysis, and absence of tendon and plantar reflex responses below the level of lesion. This is characterized by a decrease in systemic vascular resistance, an increase in venous capacitance with venous pooling, and hypotension. Lesions above T5, because of the interruption of sympathetic outflow to the heart (T2 to T5) and unopposed parasympathetic tone, are frequently associated with severe bradycardia and hypotension. Cardiac dysfunction can also occur. Systemic hypovolemia from other causes may be missed since tachycardia is frequently absent. Untreated hypotension will further aggravate potential spinal cord ischemia. Spinal shock may last from hours to weeks, and with return of reflex activity below the level of lesion, somatic or visceral stimulation may result in massive sympathetic-mediated vasoconstriction below the level of lesion, causing systemic hypertension, bradycardia, and compensatory vasodilation above the level of the lesion.[62] This phenomenon of autonomic hyperreflexia is more prevalent in patients with lesions above T6 because of the inadequate compensatory vasodilatory response.[63] Interestingly enough, even in patients with high cervical cord lesions, the tachycardic response to hypercapnia and hypoxia remains intact, possibly mediated by vagal inhibition rather than sympathetic activation.[64]

Respiratory System

The extent of respiratory impairment depends on the level of the lesion. The diaphragm is innervated by C4 to C5, and lesions above this level cause total diaphragmatic paralysis and an inability to generate any significant tidal volume and account for a large number of the pre-hospital deaths. Patients with lesions below C6 have an intact diaphragm with variable loss of intercostal and abdominal muscle depending on the level of the lesion. There is a reduction in functional residual capacity, forced vital capacity, maximum inspiratory pressure, maximum expiratory pressure, and the presence of paradoxical breathing. The vital capacity is reduced to about 1,500 mL with acute cervical spinal cord injury, which usually improves with time to about 50% of normal. The reduction in tidal volume can reach 60% in these patients.[65, 66] The overall effect is severe hypoventilation with a high prevalence of hypoxemia and hypercapnia. Because of diaphragmtic mechanics, quadriplegic patients have a higher vital capacity in the supine position compared to the seated position.[65] The inability to cough and clear secretions leads to a high incidence of atelectasis and pneumonia in the acute period.[67] The initial surge of sympathetic activity with the injury can also cause neurogenic pulmonary edema, the mechanism of which is unclear but may be mediated by both hemodynamic and permeability factors.[68]

Gastrointestinal System

Paralytic ileus usually accompanies spinal shock and the abdominal distension may further compromise ventilation.

Genitourinary System

Acute distention of the urinary bladder also occurs. In the chronic phase, recurrent urinary tract infection with renal dysfunction is a major problem.

Temperature Regulation

With high cervical spinal cord lesions, patients become poikilothermic and maintenance of normal body temperature becomes difficult.

Associated Injuries

The incidence of head injuries in patients with cervical spinal cord lesions can be as high as 50%, while thoracolumbar spine injuries may be complicated by chest contusion, rib fractures, pelvic fracture, and other long bone fractures.

Anesthesiologist's Role

The anesthesiologist may encounter a patient with acute spinal cord injury during: (1) initial resuscitation in the emergency department, typically airway management; (2) administration of anesthesia for acute decompression/stabilization of the spinal cord to preserve or improve function; or (3) administration of anesthesia for surgical treatment of associated injuries.

Surgical Indications for Spinal Cord Injuries

While it is a surgical decision regarding the timing and advisability of operative treatment of spinal cord injury, understanding of the surgical concerns and indications improves the anesthetic management and facilitates the team approach.

Goal of Treatment of Spinal Cord Injuries

The treatment goals are: (1) to protect the spinal cord from further damage, (2) to maintain alignment of the bony structures to allow maximal recovery in incomplete lesions, and (3) to achieve stability of the bony column to allow rehabilitation.

Surgical Indications for Treatment During the Acute Phase

Surgical indications are: (1) decompression with or without fusion in a neurologically deteriorating patient—this includes complete as well as incomplete lesions; (2) reduction and stabilization when conservative management fails to achieve these objectives; and (3) surgical treatment

for other life-threatening conditions unrelated to the spinal cord injury.
In addition, although there is a continuous debate on the merit of surgical vs. conservative treatment in neurologically stable patients,[69–72] there is growing evidence that while surgical results are not better,[70, 71] the economic cost may be less than that of conservative management[70] and that early surgical decompression may indeed be beneficial,[73] at least in experimental studies.[72] Therefore, there may be a growing trend to operate on these patients early when they are least stable and the anesthetic management most difficult. On the other hand, because of the unstable conditions, neurologic deterioration has been noted in patients operated on within 5 days of injury.[74]

Anesthetic Management

A high index of suspicion of spinal cord injury should always be maintained in all multiply injured patients and head-injured patients (up to 10% may have spinal injury), particularly in the pediatric and the geriatric groups. Until proved otherwise, all patients suspected to have spinal injuries should be immediately immobilized. Collars should be used for all patients suspected to have cervical injuries since they not only immobilize but serve as reminders of the possibility of neck injury.

Airway Management in Patients Suspected To Have Cervical Injuries

The goal here is to establish tracheal intubation without causing further injury to the spinal cord. The considerations are valid for both complete and incomplete lesions, because manipulations can aggravate even complete lesions resulting in ascending deterioration. This difficult issue was recently reviewed in depth by Crosby and Lui,[75] and Hastings and Marks.[76] The optimal method depends on the patient's conditions, the level of cooperation, and the skill of the anesthesiologist. An adequate history and physical examination are essential before approaching this problem. This difficult topic can be clarified by these facts: (1) the patient's condition may not allow postponement of intubation until an x-ray is taken; (2) a negative cross-table lateral x-ray (CTLX) does not rule out all cervical injuries, although a combination of CTLX, the open mouth view, and the anteroposterior view would suffice[77]; (3) the flat board immobilization maintains a neutral position for the altanto-occipital joint in 90% of the cases[78]; (4) collars, whether soft or rigid, do not completely eliminate movement of the neck during intubation,[79] although the rigid collar is more effective; (5) manual in-line traction (MILT) is more effective in immobilizing the neck during intubation[79]; (6) MILT may cause excessive distraction in C1 to C2 fractures[80]; and (7) oral intubation under general anesthesia with MILT has an extremely safe record[81, 82] comparable to that of intubation with an alert patient.[83, 84]

Recommendations

Elective Intubation in an Awake Patient Without Hypoxia or Hypercapnia.—Obtain necessary x-rays to clear the spine and treat the patient as if he had a spinal cord injury if clinically indicated. Computed tomography scans are necessary in equivocal cases and magnetic resonance imaging may play an increasing role.[85] In a cooperative patient, awake intubations are recommended, and in the absence of head injury, fiberoptic intubation, either oral or nasal, should be performed. Blind nasal intubation is an acceptable alternative. In my institution, awake fiberoptic nasal intubation with topical anesthesia with translaryngeal nerve block (omitted in patients with a full stomach) is the preferred technique. Nasal intubation, however, should not be performed in any patient suspected to have a basal skull fracture or facial fracture involving the sinuses.

Emergency Intubation in an Unconscious or Uncooperative Patient.—Under these circumstances, fiberoptic intubation has no place and oral intubation should be achieved with general anesthesia with rapid sequence technique and MILT. Anesthesia induction can be achieved with etomidate or thiopental, but the patient's unstable cardiovascular status (spinal shock) must be taken into consideration. Vigorous fluid resuscitation should be initiated simultaneously. Hyperkalemia from denervation sensitivity[86] does not occur until 48 hours after injury, and succinylcholine therefore remains the muscle relaxant of choice in the acute setting but should not be used in subsequent anesthetic situations. Any concern about a potential rise in intracranial pressure is outweighed by the benefits of expedient establishment of airway with prompt reversal of hypoxemia and hypercapnia. In difficult cases, transtracheal ventilation of emergency cricothyroidotomy may be necessary.

Maintenance of Anesthesia

The main goal here is to maintain adequate spinal cord perfusion to prevent further damage. Again in the acute stage this consideration applies equally to complete lesions and incomplete lesions since in both instances deterioration as well as improvement can occur. Because of loss of autoregulation, spinal cord perfusion becomes dependent on systemic perfusion, and systemic hypotension may cause further secondary injury. On the other hand, hypertension may cause hemorrhage and increase edema formation.[16, 44] Since spinal cord blood flow as yet cannot be monitored and has not been measured intraoperatively, maintenance of normal systemic perfusion and gas exchange are the prime objectives. No one anesthetic technique has been shown to be superior. On an experimental basis, all anesthetic drugs that decrease metabolism appear to have a protective effect.[87] However, results are not always consistent,[87, 88] and a recent study suggests that halothane is superior to barbiturates.[89] At the moment, these studies must be considered inconclusive, and therefore an anesthetic regimen that can best fulfil the outlined objectives in any given patient is the best technique. Because of the cardiovascular lability, all drugs should be given slowly by titration of effect. Bradycardia is a frequent occurrence in patients with cervical spinal cord injuries and atropine is the drug of choice. Inotropic agents may also be required to maintain the circulation (see section on Monitoring).

Theoretically, since the spinal cord circulation is similar to the cerebral circulation, hyperventilation may help to decompress the spinal cord. This efficacy, however, has not been substantiated in experimental studies.[90] Moreover, hyperventilation may decrease perfusion and cause ischemia. Therefore, normocapnia or mild hypocapnia is recommended.

Monitoring.—In addition to the standard monitoring that now includes pulse oximetry and end-tidal capnometry, in acutely quadriplegic patients, direct intraarterial pressure monitoring and the insertion of a pulmonary artery catheter are advised because of cardiovascular instability and an unpredictable response to fluid challenge and the risk of pulmonary edema.[91] MacKenzie also recommends that hypotension should be treated with fluid and inotropic agents rather than direct vasoconstrictors because of the presence of cardiac dysfunction.[91]

Other Considerations

Hyperglycemia

There is growing experimental evidence to indicate that hyperglycemia aggravates ischemic injury in the central nervous system, presumably on the basis of occurrence of lactic acidosis with abundant supply of glucose and similar observations have been made in experimental spinal cord ischemia.[92, 93] Moreover, the influence of glucose appears to be a dose-related phenomenon; not only does hyperglycemia extend the injury, but moderate hypoglycemia induced by insulin has protective value against experimental spinal cord ischemia compared to normoglycemia.[93] Glucose-containing solutions therefore should not be used intraoperatively, and serum glucose above 200 mg% should probably be treated with insulin. On the other hand, severe hypoglycemia alone can cause injury, therefore overaggressive management of serum glucose is not warranted.

Spinal Cord Monitoring

In patients who had suffered vertebral column injuries but no neurologic deficits or in patients undergoing Harrington rod instrumentation for idiopathic scoliosis, spinal cord monitoring has become almost mandatory, if only from a legal point of view. In all intact patients with cervical injuries, we always perform awake intubations and do not administer general anesthesia until the patient is in final position for surgery and normal movement of all four extremities is documented. Intraoperatively, somatosensory-evoked potential (SSEP) is routinely monitored. Depending on the site of the lesion, either posterior tibial/femoral nerve or both posterior tibial and median nerve/ulnar nerve monitoring are instituted. Although the interpretation of SSEP changes remains imprecise and critics remain,[94] there is little doubt that its use is gaining acceptance.[95, 96] Excellent correlation between spinal cord blood flow and SSEP amplitude has been demonstrated in experimental studies.[13] Clinically, its value in the Harrington rod instrumentation procedure, which is associated with a risk of paraplegia of 1%, is also well established.[97, 98] SSEP can be recorded from scalp electrodes, from the epidural space, or directly from the spinal cord.[97, 98] In the most recent series reported on 1,168 patients undergoing Harrington Rod instrumentation for scoliosis, Forbes et al. found that the criterion of 50% reduction in amplitude correctly predicted all postoperative neurologic deficits and there were no false-negative results, although there was an incidence of 4.4% false-positive results.[99] There was a technical failure rate of 2.2%, many of them involving patients with preexisting peripheral neurologic disorders. Epidural recording electrodes were used in this particular study. The authors concluded that epidural recording of SSEP is far more sensitive than the wake-up test and that it is sufficiently reliable and reproducible that it should be used in all cases of spinal corrective surgery where there is a significant risk of neurologic complication. Other investigators have expressed the concern that SSEP monitors the dorsal column function only and theoretically motor paralysis can occur despite unchanged SSEP signals, and a small series of six cases have been reported.[100] Another false-negative result during anterior spinal fusion has also been reported.[101] Fortunately, such an occurrence appears to be an exceedingly rare event, and in each of the six cases reported, there was a plausible explanation for the findings.[102] The other major limitation concerns patients with incomplete lesions and abnormal preoperative SSEP, where interpretation of intraoperative changes are all but impossible, accounting for the technical failures in Forbes's series.

The SSEP signal is susceptible to anesthetic influence and inhaled anesthetics in high doses can abolish these responses. Nitrous oxide, however, is no less depressant compared to an equipotent dose of an inhaled anesthetic. The recommended anesthetic regimen for intraoperative monitoring of SSEP is therefore continuous intravenous infusion of a narcotic (fentanyl of sufentanil) supplemented with low-dose inhaled anesthetic (isoflurane or halothane) or with nitrous oxide.[103] The combination of nitrous oxide and an inhaled anesthetic should be avoided. In cases in which an epidural electrode can be placed, the choice of anesthetic becomes a minor matter since epidural recordings are much more resistant to anesthetic influence than cortical recordings.

Motor Evoked Potential

To complement SSEP monitoring of spinal cord integrity, recent advances have made it possible to record motor-evoked potentials (MEP) with either electrical or magnetic depolarization of the motor cortex and record from a peripheral nerve or the electromyographic response in a muscle.[104–106] This complements SSEP and allows simultaneous monitoring of both anterior and posterior column functions. Some investigators have suggested that MEP may be more sensitive to spinal cord ischemia.[107] Unfortunately, motor-evoked potentials are even more sensitive to anesthetic influence and despite early enthusiasm,[104] its clinical application remains in doubt. Magnetic MEPs, in particular, are extremely sensitive to anesthetic influence and are frequently unrecordable intraoperatively. Transcranial electrical MEPs appear to be more robust than magnetic MEP, although it can also be abolished by low-dose isoflurane.[105, 108] Propofol-nitrous oxide anesthesia has been suggested as a suitable anesthetic technique for intraoperative recording of electrical MEP although the inspired nitrous oxide concentration must not exceed 50%.[109, 110] In addition, to record MEP from the muscles, adequate neuromuscular function is necessary, consequently muscle relaxants must be either eliminated or administered in subparalytic doses.

As an alternative to SEEP and MEP, the wake-up test may be used.[111] This technique, however, is limited by technical difficulty, potential patient discomfort, as well as its nature of being a one-time evaluation only. A false-negative result with the wake-up test has also been reported.[112]

Use of Induced Hypotension

Induced hypotension is frequently used during fusion procedures on the spine to reduce blood loss and improve operating conditions[113, 114] and is appropriate in patients with stable complete lesions. However, in patients with incomplete lesions or intact but marginally perfused spinal cords, the reduction in blood flow during hypotension may cause ischemia in the spinal cord and therefore may be relatively contraindicated. Such occurrences have been demonstrated in experimental studies where induced hypotension is superimposed on spinal traction.[115, 116] In the feline model,[115] spinal SSEP amplitude decreased with induced hypotension and in the canine model, spinal cord blood flow decreased with hypotension.[116] This underscores the importance of monitoring intraoperative neurologic functions during these procedures where induced hypotension is planned since manipulation of blood pressure can sometimes reverse neurologic deterioration.[117] In addition, intracranial pressure in patients with head injury may increase with induced hypotension and should be monitored if this technique is used in patients with a recent history of head trauma. It should also be noted that the efficacy of this technique to reduce blood loss has not been substantiated by some investigators.[118, 119]

Spinal Cord Ischemia in Thoracoabdominal Aortic Procedures

Pathophysiology

Because the spinal cord arteries depend on the radicular arteries for blood supply and there is little anastomosis between the anterior and posterior spinal arteries, the spinal cord is vulnerable to cross-clamping of the aorta. This risk is dependent on many factors including the site of cross-clamping,

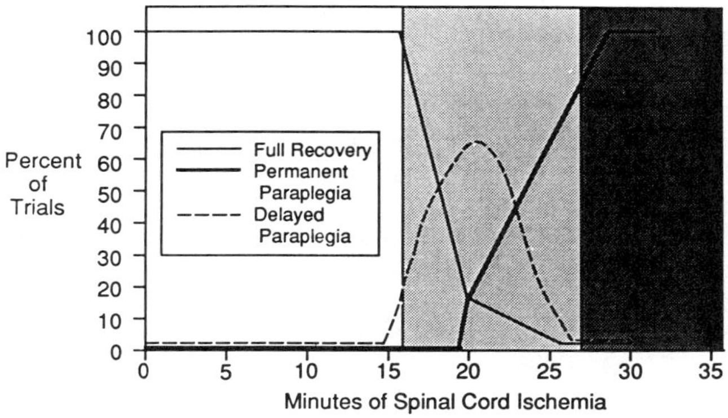

FIG 3.
Schematic graph illustrating the relationship of ultimate neurologic outcome in relation to duration of spinal cord ischemia. (Reproduced from Moore WM, Hollier LH: *Ann Surg* 213:427–432, 1991. Used by permission.)

the duration of the clamping, the adequacy of existing collateral circulation (e.g., longstanding aortic coarctation), and anatomical variations. In some patients, the spinal cord arteries are not even continuous in nature, thus depending completely on the segmental supply from the radicular arteries. Ischemia thus occurs from lack of blood supply from above, lack of segmental contribution, or from lack of distal perfusion because of inadequate collateral circulation. The risk of paraplegia thus varies from less than 1% in coarctation repair and abdominal aneurysmectomy[120] to between 5% and 45% in thoracic-abdominal aneurysm resection.[121]

Although the final common pathway of spinal cord ischemia is similar to that which occurs during procedures on the spinal cord/column, the mechanism and experimental model used is different. The clinical situation can be closely simulated with an animal model. Both dogs and rabbits have been studied extensively to investigate the appropriate monitor and strategy to prevent the occurrence of this complication. In an elegant experiment with awake rabbits, Moore has clarified the cause and the influence of time on onset of paraplegia. The animals subjected to an aortic occlusion time of less than 16 minutes always recovered with no neurologic deficits, whereas almost all animals subjected to 27 or more minutes of occlusion developed permanent paraplegia. Interestingly, between 17 and 26 minutes of occlusion, 91% of the animals initially recovered, but 58% went on to develop delayed paraplegia (Fig 3).[122] They also observed that the motor deficit always occurs before sensory deficits and the latter always return before the former. These results suggest that the cross-clamp is one of the most important determining factors of outcome and that the anterior spinal cord is more vulnerable than the posterior spinal cord in this ischemic model.

Spinal Cord Monitoring

Because spinal cord perfusion is unpredictable during cross-clamping of the aorta, it is highly desirable to have an objective means of measuring the severity of spinal cord ischemia so that surgical management can be altered to prevent the occurrence of paraparesis or paraplegia. The use of SSEP for this purpose was introduced in 1982.[120, 123] Subsequent studies, both experimental[124–126] and clinical,[127, 128] have demonstrated the efficacy of SSEP monitoring. Cunningham et al. found that in 33 patients undergoing surgery on the descending thoracic or thoracoabdominal aorta, the loss of SSEP for more than 30 minutes was associated with a 71.2% incidence of paraplegia whereas no neurologic deficit was noted in patients in whom SSEP loss was either prevented or limited in duration to 30 minutes.[127] However, Crawford et al. reported a false-positive rate of 67% and a false-negative rate of 13% for the loss of SSEPs in predicting neurologic deficits.[128] These results suggest that SSEP is a highly sensitive, but not very specific, monitor for spinal cord ischemia during aortic cross-clamping. These are similar to results obtained during monitoring for spinal cord/column procedures. Despite its low specificity, SSEP monitors adequacy of spinal cord perfusion and allows consideration of surgical therapy such as insertion of shunt, atria-femoral bypass, or reimplantation of intercostal vessels to improve perfusion.[129]

Motor evoked potential monitoring also has been investigated during aortic cross-clamping. In a porcine experiment, Svensson reported MEP to be a sensitive indicator of paralysis.[130] In contrast, Elmore et al. found MEP to be a poorer predictor of paraplegia/paraparesis than SSEP; loss of SSEP had a sensitivity of 95% and a specificity of 67%, while MEP had a high specificity of 100% but a low sensitivity of 46%.[131] These results suggest that MEP and SSEP complement each other in terms of enhancing both sensitivity and specificity. More correlative studies are needed to ascertain the clinical efficacy of MEP monitoring.

Anesthetic Considerations

Proximal and Distal Perfusion Pressure

Blood pressure distal to the cross-clamp provides a measurement of adequacy of collateral circulation and an indirect estimate of spinal cord perfusion. On the other hand, proximal blood pressure represents the afterload strain on the heart, which may become excessive during cross-clamping. It is therefore important to monitor both proximal and distal blood pressure and attempt to maintain both pressures as near normal as possible.

Cerebrospinal Fluid Drainage

Based on electrophysiological monitoring, factors that have been identified as contributory to the exacerbation of spinal cord ischemia include proximal hypertension causing a reflex increase in cerebrospinal fluid (CSF) pressure, distal hypotension and postoperative hypotension. Because spinal cord perfusion pressure (SCPP) is equal to the difference between systemic blood pressure and CSF pressure, Blaisdell and Cooley first proposed CSF drainage to maximize SCPP in 1961.[132] More recent experimental[124] and clinical studies[133] supports its efficacy, and some surgeons advocate routine spinal fluid drainage to improve SCPP. However, in the only prospective, randomized clinical trial carried out to date, no significant improvement in outcome with CSF drainage could be established.[134] This clinical trial, unlike canine experiments, showed that CSF drainage did not prevent the occurrence of paraplegia or paraparesis.[134] While the efficacy of CSF drainage remains unproven and may not be necessary with routine institution of bypass, no significant complications associated with it have been reported. Therefore, in patients with low distal perfusion pressure who exhibit deterioration of SSEP, it is entirely prudent to attempt to improve SCPP by draining CSF. Experimentally, various combinations of hypothermia, CSF drainage, intrathecal papaverine, and superoxide dismutase administration have been found to be superior to the use of one treatment modality.[135–137] The clinical utility of such combination therapy, however, remains to be established.

Use of a Vasodilator for Proximal Hypertension

For treatment of proximal hypertension, vasodilators such as sodium nitroprusside may cause an increase in CSF pressure while decreasing distal perfusion pressure by shunting blood away from the collateral circulation (steal). The reduction in distal pressure coupled with a concurrent increase in CSF pressure can lead to a severe reduction in SCPP, leading to significant spinal cord ischemia and development of paraplegia as demontrated by Marini et al.[138] Although anesthetic induction does not alter CSF pressure or the reflex increase in CSF pressure in response to aortic cross-clamping, one report suggests that isoflurane used to control systemic blood pressure causes a greater decrease in SCPP than sodium nitroprusside.[139] In any event, vasodilators, when deemed necessary, must be used judiciously and with extreme caution.

Postoperative Hypotension

Delayed paraplegia is one of the complications of spinal cord hypoperfusion, and postoperative hypotension has been identified as one of the factors.[129] It is therefore important to monitor the patient well into the postoperative period and treat hypovolemia promptly to prevent this complication.

Pharmacological Treatment

To date the only proven treatment available is high-dose methylprednisolone. Although the improvement, as reported in the NASCIS II, is modest, it is nevertheless important and should be considered if the patient is deemed to be at risk of spinal cord ischemia.

Optimal anesthetic management therefore consists of careful monitoring and control of proximal as well as distal perfusion pressure, judicious use of vasodilator when necessary, and careful fluid management in the perioperative period. Maintaining a hematocrit of about 30% to 35% ensures an optimal oxygen-carrying capacity. Somatosensory evoked potential, when available, is a useful adjunct to gauge the adequacy of spinal cord perfusion. Unfortunately, this is not applicable in emergency procedures, which are also associated with a higher risk of postoperative paraplegia.

Summary

Although acute spinal cord ischemia is a rare event, it is a major consideration in patients with spinal cord injuries and is a constant threat in patients undergoing thoracoabdominal aortic procedures. They represent a complex problem and an anesthetic challenge, and optimal anesthetic management depends on a thorough understanding of the pathophysiology and pharmacology involved.

References

1. Connolly JE: Prevention of paraplegia secondary to operations on the aorta. *J Cardiovasc Surg* 27:410–417, 1986.
2. Kobrine AI, Doyle TF, Rizzoli HV: Spinal cord blood flow as affected by changes in systemic arterial blood pressure. *J Neurosurg* 44:12–15, 1976.
3. Marcus ML et al: Regulation of total and regional spinal cord blood flow. *Circ Res* 41:128–134, 1977.
4. Hickey R et al: Autoregulation of spinal cord blood flow: Is the cord a microcosm of the brain? *Stroke* 17:1183–1189, 1986.
5. Smith AL, Pender JW, Alexander SC: Effects of P_{CO_2} on spinal cord blood flow. *Am J Physiol* 216:1158–1163, 1969.
6. Sandler AN, Tator CH: Effect of acute spinal cord compression injury on regional spinal cord blood flow in primates. *J Neurosurg* 45:660–676, 1976.
7. Sakamoto T, Monafo WW: The effect of hypothermia on regional spinal cord blood flow in rats. *J Neurosurg* 70:780–784, 1989.
8. Sakamoto T, Monafo WW: Regional spinal cord blood flow during local cooling. *Neurosurgery* 26:958–962, 1990.
9. Neuwelt EA et al: Oregon head and spinal cord injury prevention program and evaluation. *Neurosurgery* 24:453–458, 1989.
10. Senter HJ, Venes JL: Altered blood flow and secondary injury in experimental spinal cord trauma. *J Neurosurg* 49:569–578, 1978.
11. Hall ED, Wolf DL: A pharmacological analysis of the pathophysiological mechanisms of posttraumatic spinal cord ischemia. *J Neurosurg* 64:951–961, 1986.
12. Janssen L, Hansebout RR: Pathogenesis of spinal cord injury and newer treatments—a review. *Spine* 14:23–32, 1989.
13. Fehlings MG, Tator CH, Linden RD: The relationships among the severity of spinal cord injury, motor and somatosensory evoked potentials and spinal cord blood flow. *Electroencephalogr Clin Neurophysiol* 74:241–259, 1989.
14. Holtz A, Nystrom B, Gerdin B: Relation between spinal cord blood flow and functional recovery after blocking weight-induced spinal cord injury in rats. *Neurosurgery* 26:952–957, 1990.

15. Senter HJ, Venes JL: Loss of autoregulation and posttraumatic ischemia following experimental spinal cord trauma. *J Neurosurg* 50:198–206, 1979.
16. Guha A, Tator CH, Rochon J: Spinal cord blood flow and systemic blood pressure after experimental spinal cord injury in rats. *Stroke* 20:372–377, 1992.
17. Kato A et al: Circulatory disturbance of the spinal cord with epidural neoplasm in rats. *J Neurosurg* 63:260–265, 1985.
18. Chavko M et al: Blood flow and electrolytes in spinal cord ischemia. *Exp Neurol* 112:299–303, 1991.
19. Danielisova V et al: Postischemic hypoxia improves metabolic and functional recovery of the spinal cord. *Neurology* 40:1125–1129, 1990.
20. Allen AR: Surgery of experimental lesion of spinal cord equivalent to crush injury of fracture dislocation of spinal column: A preliminary report. *JAMA* 57:878–880, 1911.
21. Rivlin AS, Tator CH: Effect of duration of acute spinal cord compression in a new acute cord injury model in the rat. *Surg Neurol* 10:39–43, 1978.
22. Tator CH, Fehlings MG: Review of the secondary injury theory of acute spinal cord trauma with emphasis on vascular mechanisms. *J Neurosurg* 75:15–26, 1992.
23. Guha A, Tator CH, Piper I: Effect of a calcium channel blocker on posttraumatic spinal cord blood flow. *J Neurosurg* 66:423–430, 1989.
24. Guha A et al: Improvement in post-traumatic spinal cord blood flow with a combination of a calcium channel blocker and a vasopressor. *J Trauma* 29:1440–1447, 1989.
25. Fehlings MG, Tator CH, Linden RD: The effect of nimodipine and dextran on axonal function and blood flow following experimental spinal cord injury. *J Neurosurg* 71:403–416, 1989.
26. Faden AI, Jacobs TP, Smith MT: Evaluation of the calcium channel antagonist nimodipine in experimental spinal cord ischemia. *J Neurosurg* 60:797–799, 1984.
27. Ford RW, Malm DN: Failure of nimodipine to reverse acute experimental spinal cord injury. *Cent Nerv Syst Trauma* 2:9–17, 1985.
28. Holtz A, Nystrom B, Gerdin B: Spinal cord injury in rats: Inability of nimodipine or anti-neutrophil serum to improve spinal cord blood flow or neurologic status. *Acta Neurol Scand* 79:460–467, 1989.
29. Black P et al: Experimental spinal cord injury: Effect of a calcium channel antagonist (Nicardipine). *Neurosurgery* 22:61–66, 1988.
30. Holaday JW, Faden AI: Naloxone acts at central opiate to reverse hypotension, hypothermia and hypoventilation in spinal shock. *Brain Res* 189:295–299, 1980.
31. Long JB et al: Endogenous opioids in spinal cord injury: A critical evaluation. *Cent Nerv Trauma* 3:295–315, 1986.
32. Wallace MC, Tator CH: Failure of naloxone to improve spinal cord blood flow and cardiac output after spinal cord injury. *Neurosurgery* 18:428–432, 1986.
33. Faden AI, Vink R, McIntosh TK: Thyrotropin-releasing hormone and central nervous system trauma. *Ann N Y Acad Sci* 553:380–384, 1989.
34. Faden AI, Jacobs TP, Holaday JW: Thyrotropin-releasing hormone improves neurologic recovery after spinal trauma in cats. *N Engl J Med* 305:1063–1067, 1981.
35. Holtz A, Nyström B, Gerdin B: Blocking weight-induced spinal cord injury in

rats: effects of TRH or naloxone on motor function recovery and spinal cord blood flow. *Acta Neurol Scand* 80:215–220, 1989.
36. Siegal T et al: Experimental neoplastic spinal cord compression: Effect of ketamine and MK-801 on edema and prostaglandins. *Neurosurgery* 26:963–966, 1990.
37. Hall ED, Braughler JM: Glucocorticoid mechanisms in acute spinal cord injury: A review and therapeutic rationale. *Surg Neurol* 18:320–327, 1982.
38. Young W, Flamm ES: Effect of high-dose corticosteroid therapy on blood flow, evoked potentials, and extracellular calcium in experimental spinal injury. *J Neurosurg* 57:667–673, 1982.
39. Hall ED: The neuroprotective pharmacology of methylprednisolone. *J Neurosurg* 76:13–22, 1992.
40. Albin MS et al: Study of functional recovery produced by delayed localized cooling after spinal cord injury in primates. *J Neurosurg* 29:113–120, 1968.
41. Busto R et al: The importance of brain temperature in cerebral ischemic injury. *Stroke* 20:1113–1114, 1989.
42. Minamisawa H et al: The influence of mild body and brain hypothermia on ischemic brain damage. *J Cereb Blood Flow Metab* 10:365–374, 1990.
43. Busto R et al: Effect of mild hypothermia on ischemia-induced release of neurotransmitters and free fatty acids in rat brain. *Stroke* 20:904–910, 1989.
44. Rawe SE, Lee WA, Pweor PI Jr: The histopathology of experimental spinal cord trauma. The effect of systemic blood pressure. *J Neurosurg* 48:1002–1007, 1978.
45. Bracken MB et al: A randomized, controlled trial of methylprednisolone or naloxone in the treatment of acute spinal-cord injury. *N Engl J Med* 322:1405–1411, 1990.
46. Bracken MB et al: Methylprednisolone or naloxone treatment after acute spinal cord injury: 1-year follow-up data. Results of the second National Acute Spinal Cord Injury Study. *J Neurosurg* 76:23–31, 1992.
47. Koide T, Wieloch T, Siesjo BK: Chronic dexamethasone pretreatment aggravates ischemic brain damage by inducing hyperglycemia. *J Cereb Blood Flow Metab* 5:251–252, 1985.
48. Hall ED et al: Effects of the 21-aminosteroid U74006F on experimental head injury in mice. *J Neurosurg* 68:456–461, 1988.
49. Lesiuk H et al: Effect of U74006F on forebrain ischemia in rats. *Stroke* 22:896–901, 1991.
50. Perkins WJ et al: Pretreatment with U74006F improves neurologic outcome following complete cerebral ischemia in dogs. *Stroke* 22:902–909, 1991.
51. Geisler FH, Dorsey FC, Coleman WP: Recovery of motor function after spinal-cord injury—a randomized placebo-controlled trial with GM-1 ganglioside. *N Engl J Med* 324:1829–1838, 1991.
52. Rodden FA, Wiegandt H, Bauer BL: Gangliosides: The relevance of current research to neurosurgery. *J Neurosurg* 74:606–619, 1991.
53. Griffin MR et al: Traumatic spinal cord injury in Olmsted county, Minnesota, 1935–1981. *Am J Epidemiol* 121:884–895, 1985.
54. Kraus JF: Injury to the head and spinal cord—the epidemiological relevance of the medical literature published from 1960 to 1978. *J Neurosurg* 53:3–10, 1980.
55. Tator CH: Acute management of spinal cord injury. *Br J Surg* 77:485–486, 1990.
56. Harris JH Jr, Edeiken-Monroe B, Kopaniky DR: A practical classification of acute cervical spine injuries. *Orthop Clin North Am* 17:15–30, 1986.

57. Denis F: The three column spine and its significance in the classification of acute thoracolumbar spinal injuries. *Spine* 8:817–831, 1983.
58. Pang D, Wilberger JE: Spinal cord injury without radiographic abnormalities in children. *J Neurosurg* 57:114–129, 1982.
59. Pollack IF, Pang D, Sclabassi R: Recurrent spinal cord injury without radiographic abnormalities in children. *J Neurosurg* 69:177–182, 1988.
60. Hadley MN et al: Pediatric spinal trauma—review of 122 cases of spinal cord and vertebral column injuries. *J Neurosurg* 68:18–24, 1988.
61. Johnston RA: Management of old people with neck trauma—injury to the cervical cord is common but may be overlooked. *Br Med J* 299:633–634, 1989.
62. Desmond J: Paraplegia: Problems confronting the anaesthesiologist. *Can Anaesth Soc J* 17:435–451, 1970.
63. Schonwald G, Fish KJ, Perkash I: Cardiovascular complications during anesthesia in chronic spinal cord injured patients. *Anesthesiology* 55:550–558, 1981.
64. Pokorski M et al: Cardiac responses to hypoxia and hypercapnia in spinal man. *Eur Heart J* 11:611–618, 1990.
65. Mansel JK, Norman JR: Respiratory complications and management of spinal cord injuries. *Chest* 97:1446–1452, 1990.
66. Ledsome JR, Sharp JM: Pulmonary function in acute cervical cord injury. *Am Rev Respir Dis* 124:41–44, 1981.
67. Fishburn MJ, Marino RJ, Ditunno JF: Atelectasis and pneumonia in acute spinal cord injury. *Arch Phys Med Rehabil* 71:197–200, 1990.
68. Malik AB: Mechanisms of neurogenic pulmonary edema. *Circ Res* 57:1–18, 1985.
69. Wilmot CB, Hall KM: Evaluation of the acute management of tetraplegia: Conservative versus surgical treatment. *Paraplegia* 24:148–153, 1986.
70. Murphy KP et al: Cervical fractures and spinal cord injury: Outcome of surgical and nonsurgical management. *Mayo Clin Proc* 65:949–959, 1990.
71. Tator CH et al: Comparison of surgical and conservative management in 208 patients with acute spinal cord injury. *Can J Neurol Sci* 14:60–69, 1987.
72. Guha A et al: Decompression of the spinal cord improves recovery after acute experimental spinal cord compression injury. *Paraplegia* 25:324–339, 1987.
73. Levi L et al: Anterior decompression in cervical spine trauma: does the timing of surgery affect the outcome? *Neurosurgery* 29:216–222, 1991.
74. Marshall LF et al: Deterioration following spinal cord injury—a multicenter study. *J Neurosurg* 66:400–404, 1987.
75. Crosby ET, Lui A: The adult cervical spine: Implications for airway management. *Can J Anaesth* 37:77–93, 1990.
76. Hastings RH, Marks JD: Airway management of trauma patients with potential cervical spine injuries. *Anesth Analg* 73:471–482, 1991.
77. MacDonald RL et al: Diagnosis of cervical spine injury in motor vehicle crash victims: How many x-rays are enough? *J Trauma* 30:392–397, 1990.
78. Schriger DL et al: Spinal immobilization on a flat backboard: Does it result in neutral position of the cervical spine? *Ann Emerg Med* 20:878–881, 1991.
79. Majernick TG et al: Cervical spine movement during orotracheal intubation. *Ann Emerg Med* 15:417–420, 1986.
80. Bivins HG et al: The effect of axial traction during orotracheal intubation of the trauma victim with an unstable cervical spine. *Ann Emerg Med* 17:25–29, 1988.

81. Grande CM, Barton CR, Stene JK: Appropriate techniques for airway management of emergency patients with suspected spinal cord injury. *Anesth Analg* 67:714–715, 1988.
82. Rhee KJ et al: Oral intubation in the multiply injured patient: The risk of exacerbating spinal cord damage. *Ann Emerg Med* 19:511–514, 1990.
83. Suderam VS, Crosby ET, Lui A: Elective oral tracheal intubation in cervical spine-injured adults. *Can J Anaesth* 38:785–789, 1991.
84. Meschino A et al: The safety of awake tracheal intubation in cervical spine injury. *Can J Anaesth* 35:131–132, 1988.
85. Flanders AE et al: Acute cervical spine trauma: Correlation of MR imaging findings with degree of neurologic deficit. *Radiology* 177:23–33, 1990.
86. Gronert GA, Theye R: Pathophysiology of hyperkalemia induced by succinylcholine. *Anesthesiology* 43:89–99, 1975.
87. Cole DJ et al: Halothane, fentanyl/nitrous oxide, and spinal lidocaine protect against spinal cord injury in the rat. *Anesthesiology* 70:967–972, 1989.
88. Robertson CS et al: Protection against experimental ischemic spinal cord injury. *J Neurosurg* 64:633–642, 1986.
89. Salzman SK et al: Anesthesia influences the outcome from experimental spinal cord injury. *Brain Res* 521:33–39, 1990.
90. Ford RWJ, Malm DN: Therapeutic trial of hypercarbia and hypocarbia in acute experimental spinal cord injury. *J Neurosurg* 61:925–930, 1984.
91. MacKenzie CF et al: Assessment of cardiac and respiratory function during surgery on patients with acute quadriplegia. *J Neurosurg* 62:843–849, 1985.
92. Drummond JC, Moore SS: The influence of dextrose administration on neurologic outcome after temporary spinal cord ischemia in the rabbit. *Anesthesiology* 70:64–70, 1989.
93. Robertson CS, Grossman RG: Protection against spinal cord ischemia with insulin-induced hypoglycemia. *J Neurosurg* 67:739–744, 1987.
94. Aminoff MJ: Intraoperative monitoring by evoked potentials for spinal cord surgery: The cons. *Electroencephalogr Clin Neurophysiol* 73:378–380, 1989.
95. Schramm J: Spinal cord monitoring: Current status and new developments. *Centr Nerv Syst Trauma* 2:207–227, 1985.
96. Daube JR: Intraoperative monitoring by evoked potentials for spinal cord surgery: The pros. *Electroencephalogr Clin Neurophysiol* 73:374–377, 1989.
97. Roy EP III et al: Intraoperative somatosensory evoked potential monitoring in scoliosis. *Clin Orthop Relat Res* 229:94–102, 1988.
98. Whittle IR, Johnston IH, Besser M: Recording of spinal somatosensory evoked potentials for intraoperative spinal cord monitoring. *J Neurosurg* 64:601–612, 1986.
99. Forbes HJ et al: Spinal cord monitoring in scoliosis surgery. *J Bone Joint Surg* 73:487–491, 1991.
100. Lesser RP et al: Postoperative neurological deficits may occur despite unchanged intraoperative somatosensory evoked potentials. *Ann Neurol* 19:22–25, 1986.
101. Ben-David B, Haller G, Taylor P: Anterior spinal fusion complicated by paraplegia: A case report of a false-negative somatosensory evoked potential. *Spine* 12:536–539, 1987.
102. Friedman WA, Grundy BL: Are the sensory evoked potentials useful in the operating room? Monitoring of sensory evoked potentials is highly reliable and helpful in the operating room. *J Clin Monit* 3:38–40, 1987.

103. Lam AM: Monitoring neurologic evoked responses. *American society of anesthesiology annual refresher course.* Philadelphia, 1989, Lippincott.
104. Edmonds HL Jr et al: Transcranial magnetic motor evoked potentials (tcMMEP) for functional monitoring of motor pathways during scoliosis surgery. *Spine* 14:683–685, 1989.
105. Zentner J, Kiss I, Ebner A: Influence of anesthetics–nitrous oxide in particular–on electromyographic response evoked by transcranial electrical stimulation of the cortex. *Neurosurgery* 24:253–256, 1989.
106. Zentner J, Ebner A: Nitrous oxide suppresses the electromyographic response evoked by electrical stimulation of the motor cortex. *Neurosurgery* 24:60–63, 1989.
107. Tator CH, Linden RD, Fehlings MG: Current status and future prospects for the neurosurgical management of acute spinal cord injuries. *Paraplegia* 25:250–253, 1987.
108. Kalkman CJ, Drummond JC, Ribberink AA: Low concentrations of isoflurane abolish motor evoked responses to transcranial electrical stimulation during nitrous oxide/opioid anesthesia in humans. *Anesth Analg* 73:410–415, 1991.
109. Jellinek D et al: Effects of nitrous oxide on motor evoked potentials recorded from skeletal muscle in patients under total anesthesia with intravenously administered propofol. *Neurosurgery* 29:558–562, 1991.
110. Jellinek D, Jewkes D, Symon L: Noninvasive intraoperative monitoring of motor evoked potentials under propofol anesthesia: Effects of spinal surgery on the amplitude and latency of motor evoked potentials. *Neurosurgery* 29:551–557, 1991.
111. Waldman J et al: Wake-up technique to avoid neurologic sequelae during Harrington Rod procedure: A case report. *Anesth Analg* 66:1039–1042, 1987.
112. Diaz JH, Lockhart CM: Postoperative quadriplegia after spinal fusion for scoliosis with intraoperative awakening. *Anesth Analg* 1039–1041, 1987.
113. Lawhon SM et al: Controlled hypotensive anesthesia during spinal surgery. *Spine* 9:450–453, 1984.
114. Malcolm-Smith NA, McMaster MJ: The use of induced hypotension to control bleeding during posterior fusion for scoliosis. *J Bone Joint Surg* 65:255–258, 1983.
115. Yeoman PM et al: Influence of induced hypotension and spinal distraction on feline spinal somatosensory evoked potentials. *Br J Anaesth* 63:315–320, 1989.
116. Kling TF Jr et al: The influence of trimethaphan(arfonad)-induced hypotension with and without spine distraction on canine spinal cord blood flow. *Spine* 11:219–224, 1986.
117. Grundy BL, Nash CL, Brown RH: Arterial pressure manipulation alters spinal cord function during correction of scoliosis. *Anesthesiology* 54:249–253, 1981.
118. Lennon RL et al: The effects of intraoperative blood salvage and induced hypotension on transfusion requirements during spinal surgical procedures. *Mayo Clin Proc* 62:1090–1094, 1987.
119. Grundy BL, Nash CL Jr, Brown RH: Deliberate hypotension for spinal fusion: Prospective randomized study with evoked potential monitoring. *Can Anaesth Soc J* 29:452–461, 1982.
120. Laschinger JC et al: Detection and prevention of intraoperative spinal cord

ischemia after cross-clamping of the thoracic aorta: use of somatosensory evoked potentials. *Surgery* 92:1109–1117, 1982.
121. Crawford ES et al: Thoracoabdominal aortic aneurysms: Preoperative and intraoperative factors determining immediate and long-term results of operations in 605 patients. *J Vasc Surg* 3:389–404, 1986.
122. Moore WM, Hollier LH: The influence of severity of spinal cord ischemia in the etiology of delayed-onset paraplegia. *Ann Surg* 213:427–432, 1991.
123. Cunningham JN et al: Measurement of spinal cord ischemia during operations upon the thoracic aorta. *Ann Surg* 196:285–296, 1982.
124. Grubbs PE Jr et al: Somatosensory evoked potentials and spinal cord perfusion pressure are significant predictors of postoperative neurologic dysfunction. *Surgery* 104:216–223, 1988.
125. Laschinger JC et al: Monitoring of somatosensory evoked potentials during surgical procedures on the thoracoabdominal aorta. I. Relationship of aortic cross-clamp duration, changes in somatosensory evoked potentials, and incidence of neurologic dysfunction. *J Thorac Cardiovasc Surg* 94:260–265, 1987.
126. Kaplan BJ et al: Somatosensory evoked potential monitoring of spinal cord ischemia during aortic operations. *Neurosurgery* 19:82–90, 1986.
127. Cunningham JN Jr, Laschinger JC, Sencer FC: Monitoring of somatosensory evoked potentials during surgical procedures on the thoracoabdominal aorta. IV. Clinical observations and results. *J Thorac Cardiovasc Surg* 94:275–285, 1987.
128. Crawford ES et al: The impact of distal aortic perfusion and somatosensory evoked potential monitoring on prevention of paraplegia after aortic aneurysm operation. *J Thorac Cardiovasc Surg* 95:357–367, 1988.
129. Laschinger JC, Izumoto H, Kouchoukos NT: Evolving concepts in prevention of spinal cord injury during operations on the descending thoracic and thoracoabdominal aorta. *Ann Thorac Surg* 44:667–674, 1987.
130. Svensson LG et al: Influence of preservation or perfusion of intraoperatively identified spinal cord blood supply on spinal motor evoked potentials and paraplegia after aortic surgery. *J Vasc Surg* 13:355–365, 1991.
131. Elmore JR et al: Failure of motor evoked potentials to predict neurologic outcome in experimental thoracic aortic occlusion. *J Vasc Surg* 14:131–139, 1991.
132. Blaisdell FW, Cooley DA: The mechanism of paraplegia after temporary thoracic aortic occlusion and its relationship to spinal fluid pressure. *Surgery* 51:351–355, 1961.
133. McCullough JL, Hollier LH, Nugent M: Paraplegia after thoracic aortic occlusion: Influence of cerebrospinal fluid drainage. *J Vasc Surg* 7:153–160, 1988.
134. Crawford ES et al: A prospective randomized study of cerebrospinal fluid drainage to prevent paraplegia after high-risk surgery on the thoracoabdominal aorta. *J Vasc Surg* 13:36–45, 1991.
135. Kirshner DL et al: Spinal cord ischemia: An evaluation of pharmacologic agents in minimizing paraplegia after aortic occlusion. *J Vasc Surg* 9:305–308, 1989.
136. Svensson LG et al: Crossclamping of the thoracic aorta: Influence of aortic shunts, papaverine, calcium channel blocker, allopurinol, and superoxide dismutase on spinal cord blood flow and paraplegia in baboons. *Ann Surg* 204:38–42, 1986.
137. Granke K et al: Longitudinal study of cerebral spinal fluid drainage in poly-

ethylene glycol-conjugated superoxide dismutase in paraplegia associated with thoracic aortic cross-clamping. *J Vasc Surg* 13:615–621, 1991.

138. Marini CP et al: Effect of sodium nitroprusside on spinal cord perfusion and paraplegia during aortic cross-clamping. *Ann Thorac Surg* 47:379–383, 1989.
139. Grum DF, Svensson LG: Changes in cerebrospinal fluid pressure and spinal cord perfusion pressure prior to cross-clamping of the thoracic aorta in humans. *J Cardiothorac Vasc Anesth* 5:331–336, 1991.

End-Tidal Carbon Dioxide Monitoring During Cardiopulmonary Resuscitation

Jay L. Falk, M.D.

Director, Emergency Medicine Residency Program, Orlando Regional Medical Center, Orlando, Florida

End-tidal CO_2 ($ETCO_2$) monitoring has emerged as a valuable noninvasive clinical tool in the setting of cardiopulmonary arrest.[1–6] Measurement of $ETCO_2$ may provide the clinician with the earliest evidence of return of spontaneous circulation (ROSC).[1, 2] It may also contribute to the clinician's ability to prognosticate outcome from resuscitative maneuvers.[5, 6] Some investigators have suggested using $ETCO_2$ as a guide to either using more aggressive maneuvers such as open chest massage or abandoning resuscitative efforts.[7] $ETCO_2$ monitoring can be used to verify intratracheal endotracheal tube position during cardiopulmonary arrest.[8, 9] Recent data suggest that $ETCO_2$ monitoring may also be useful during shock states.[10–13]

To properly utilize this newly available tool, one must be familiar with both the technology and techniques of end-tidal CO_2 monitoring as well as the physiology and pathophysiology involved in carbon dioxide excretion. These issues form the basis of this report.

Physiology of End Tidal CO_2

Expired CO_2 is determined by the body's CO_2 production and the relationship between minute ventilation (V) and pulmonary perfusion (Q) (Table 1). When the circulatory status is normal and pulmonary perfusion is in the usual physiologic ranges, $ETCO_2$ is determined primarily by the minute ventilation, since CO_2 production tends to remain constant over short periods of time. For these reasons, pulmonary physicians have traditionally used $ETCO_2$ as an approximation of arterial P_{CO_2} or minute ventilation.[14] The determinants of $ETCO_2$ are altered under conditions of severely decreased pulmonary perfusion, as seen when cardiac output is very low. This occurs clinically in shock states and during cardiac arrest and resuscitation.[1, 10–13, 15, 16] In this setting, the $ETCO_2$ is determined primarily by the level of pulmonary blood flow (cardiac output) as opposed to the

TABLE 1.
Physiology of $ETCO_2$*

Determinants of $ETCO_2$
$\dot{V}CO_2$
$\dot{V}/\dot{Q}$
Normal circulation
$ETCO_2 \propto$ minute ventilation
Low flow states
$ETCO_2 \propto$ pulmonary blood flow

*$ETCO_2$ is determined by the relationship between carbon dioxide production ($\dot{V}CO_2$) and ventilation perfusion ratio ($\dot{V}/\dot{Q}$).

minute ventilation. Under conditions of very low pulmonary blood flow, little carbon dioxide is delivered from tissues to the pulmonary circuit and therefore, exhalation of CO_2 gas is minimized.

Weil and colleagues demonstrated a linear correlation between $ETCO_2$ and cardiac output at the very low flows seen in a porcine model of closed chest massage.[16] These observations were subsequently confirmed by Gudipati et al.[15] Ornato and colleagues methodically studied the relationship between cardiac output and $ETCO_2$ during fixed minute ventilation and controlled hemorrhage in sheep.[12] At low flows, $ETCO_2$ varied with cardiac output, while at normal or high flows it did not. The relative impact of varying minute ventilation under conditions of very low blood flow on $ETCO_2$ is currently unknown and is the focus of our current laboratory investigations.

End Tidal CO_2 During Cardiopulmonary Resuscitation

During experimental studies in the porcine cardiopulmonary resuscitation laboratory of Weil, a veno-arterial CO_2 gradient during circulatory arrest was detected.[18] Subsequent clinical studies in our intensive care units verified the presence of this venoarterial CO_2 gradient in patients. Thus, acid-base status during cardiac arrest and resuscitation included the presence of respiratory alkalosis on the arterial side while simultaneously acidosis resulting from hypercarbia was present in mixed venous (pulmonary artery) blood.[17, 18] We hypothesized that this veno-arterial CO_2 gradient resulted from the abrupt decrease in pulmonary blood flow following circulatory arrest so that CO_2 clearance was critically reduced.[16] Concomitant with decreases in pulmonary perfusion, the volume of carbon dioxide gas presented to alveoli for exhalation would decrease, resulting in a low $ETCO_2$. A way of conceptualizing this is that the entire minute ventilation of the lung under conditions of no flow becomes physiologic dead space ventilation and therefore expired CO_2 approaches zero.

This hypothesis was subsequently verified in the porcine laboratory in a model of ventricular fibrillation during which continuous thermodilution cardiac output indicated a very close correlation between pulmonary blood flow (cardiac output) and $ETCO_2$.[15, 16] Indeed, during these experiments it became clear that $ETCO_2$ had potential utility as a noninvasive measurement of the blood flow generated by precordial compressions during cardiopulmonary resuscitation (CPR). Furthermore, $ETCO_2$ during closed chest massage seemed to differentiate between animals successfully resuscitated (1.7% ± 0.2%) and those that failed to achieve ROSC (0.5% ± 0.1%, $P < .001$). Finally, $ETCO_2$ was noted to increase immediately in response to successful defibrillation.[15]

Canine studies by Sanders and colleagues subsequently elucidated the correlation of $ETCO_2$ during closed chest massage with coronary perfusion pressure.[5, 19] Coronary perfusion pressure during CPR has long been known to be an important determinant of ROSC.[5, 20–22] Accordingly, these observations lent a strong theoretical basis to earlier empiric observations indicating $ETCO_2$ during CPR could prognosticate outcome from cardiac arrest.[15] Further canine experiments by Kern et al. confirmed the relationship between $ETCO_2$, coronary perfusion pressure, and ROSC.[23]

We studied the $ETCO_2$ during cardiac arrest in a group of ten patients in our critical care unit during 13 episodes of cardiopulmonary arrest.[1] At the time of circulatory arrest, $ETCO_2$ fell precipitously within 1 minute to 0.4% ± 0.4%. During closed chest massage, ETCO2 increased along with the pulmonary blood flow. Cardiac output could not be measured in this setting. Changes in $ETCO_2$ did correlate with changes in the arterial-venous oxygen saturation difference, suggesting that $ETCO_2$ was, in fact, highly influenced by cardiac output. Injection of bicarbonate resulted in a transient increase in the expired CO_2 from 0.8% ± 0.5% to 2.1% ± 1.4%. This effect dissipated within 2 minutes. From these clinical studies we concluded that: (1) $ETCO_2$ is an accurate noninvasive monitor of the effectiveness (cardiac output) of closed chest massage during cardiopulmonary resuscitation in patients, (2) that $ETCO_2$ is transiently affected by the injection of sodium bicarbonate buffer, and (3) that $ETCO_2$ allows for the earliest noninvasive identification of return of spontaneous circulation, since in every patient in whom spontaneous circulation was re-established there was an abrupt and dramatic increase in the expired CO_2.

These early clinical studies[1–4] created substantial interest in $ETCO_2$ as a clinically usable noninvasive monitor during CPR. It was hoped that $ETCO_2$ could help distinguish patients likely to be resuscitated from those who were not. In the study by Falk et al.,[1] patients achieving ROSC had higher $ETCO_2$ values than those who did not but because of the small sample size, these data did not reach statistical significance. It was also hoped that clinical CPR efforts could be guided by $ETCO_2$ values so that more effective resuscitative techniques could be used.

$ETCO_2$ and Prognosis During Experimental and Clinical Resuscitation

In several experimental models it has been demonstrated that $ETCO_2$ was higher during closed or open cardiac massage in animals who could be resuscitated than in those who could not. Gudipati et al. identified significant differences ($P < .007$) between resuscitated and nonresuscitated animals at 1,3,5,9, and 11 minutes of CPR.[15] Sanders et al. likewise showed significant differences in $ETCO_2$ ($P < .01$) between surviving and nonsurviving canines each minute during 15 minutes of closed chest massage.[19] In studies by Kern et al., who used a similar canine CPR model, $ETCO_2$ did not help distinguish between survivors and nonsurvivors until 11 minutes had elapsed.[23] In this study, $ETCO_2$ was near 7.0 mm Hg in both groups at the onset of CPR but fell to levels below 4.0 mm Hg in the nonresuscitated group after 11 minutes. Duggal et al. demonstrated that survivability during porcine CPR decreased over time despite the fact that viable levels of coronary perfusion pressures and $ETCO_2$ were maintained.[24]

Clinical studies have examined this issue as well. Sanders and colleagues observed higher $ETCO_2$ values (15 ± 4 mm Hg vs. 7 ± 5 mm Hg; $P < .001$) in nine resuscitated patients than those in 26 patients who failed to respond to resuscitative efforts.[5] No patient with an $ETCO_2$ less than 10 mm Hg was successfully resuscitated; however, six patients with $ETCO_2$ greater than 10 mm Hg could not be resuscitated. One of these patients had an $ETCO_2$ greater than 20 mm Hg. Just as in the experimental study of Kern et al., as time progressed during the resuscitative effort, $ETCO_2$ seemed to help distinguish survivors from nonsurvivors more effectively (Fig 1). The authors acknowledge some limitations of the study, including the lack of controlled minute ventilation. Data obtained within 5 minutes of sodium bicarbonate injection were discarded to avoid this potentially confounding variable.

Callaham and Barton prospectively studied 55 patients who were experiencing cardiac arrest.[6] $ETCO_2$ was higher at the start of resuscitation in patients who subsequently developed a pulse than in those who did not (19 ± 14 mm Hg vs. 5 ± 4 mm Hg; $P < .0001$). With 15 mm Hg as the standard, eventual return of pulse could be predicted with a sensitivity of 71%, a specificity of 98%, a positive predictive value of 91%, and a negative predictive value of 91%.

In examining the totality of experimental and human data available on the predictive value of $ETCO_2$ during cariodpulmonary resuscitation, it seems clear that if resuscitative efforts have been ongoing for more than 10 to 15 minutes and the $ETCO_2$ is less than 10 to 15 mm Hg (1.4% to 2.0%), return of spontaneous circulation is highly unlikely. Early in CPR, $ETCO_2$ seems less able to help predict which patients will develop a pulse. Accordingly, at this juncture, $ETCO_2$ may be used as only one piece of the total clinical picture when making decisions regarding whether or not to continue or terminate resuscitative efforts. Small sample size and large vari-

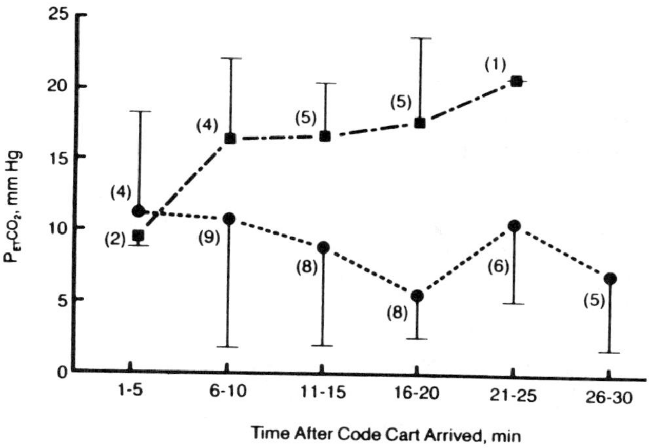

FIG 1.
Average end tidal partial pressure of carbon dioxide (P_{ETCO_2}) for 5-minute intervals during the 30 minutes following the arrival of the cardiac arrest code cart. The number of patients for which a reading was obtained in each 5-minute interval is shown in parenthesis. *Solid squares* = resuscitated patients; *solid circles* = nonresuscitated patients; and *vertical lines*, standard deviations. (From Sanders AB et al: *JAMA* 262:1347–1351, 1989. Used by permission.)

ability make precise application of the available data to individual patients a problem.

Several investigators have argued that since $ETCO_2$ correlates with cardiac output[15, 16] and coronary perfusion pressures[19] during closed chest massage, interventions aimed at increasing the effectiveness of pumping that result in higher $ETCO_2$ levels should be undertaken and will improve outcome from cardiac arrest.[25–27] Ward demonstrated that interposed abdominal compression CPR resulted in higher $ETCO_2$ levels ($P < .001$) than standard CPR in patients.[25] Outcomes were not different between the groups, but the study design involved patients at the end of the resuscitative effort. The authors suggested that their technique was superior to standard CPR because it resulted in higher $ETCO_2$ values. Similar arguments were implied in reports assessing optimum compression rates[26] and force[27] during closed chest massage. While there is a logical theoretic basis for the assertion that CPR techniques resulting in higher $ETCO_2$ may result in improved outcomes, this theory has never been tested experimentally or clinically. To do so would require prospective interventions during CPR aimed at achieving a predetermined $ETCO_2$ level. Outcome in this experimental group could then be compared to outcome in a standard protocol group. To date, these studies have not been performed. Recommendations that interventions to increase $ETCO_2$ during human resuscitation be attempted are currently based on the relationship between $ETCO_2$, cardiac output, coronary perfusion pressure, and observations that patients with low $ETCO_2$ at the end of a resuscitative effort cannot be revived.[7] They are not based on studies demonstrating improved outcome when such interventions are attempted.

Confounding Factors

Several factors may influence the $ETCO_2$ during resuscitation other than the level of pulmonary blood flow generated during chest compressions. The precise impact of changes in minute ventilation at fixed low pulmonary blood flow rates has never been evaluated. In experimental models of low flow rate and fixed minute ventilation, $ETCO_2$ varies with flow.[12, 15, 16] It would seem that very large changes in ventilation would be required to substantially influence $ETCO_2$ levels at pulmonary blood flow rates seen during CPR. We are currently examining this issue in a porcine mode.

Injection of sodium bicarbonate results in the generation of CO_2. We demonstrated transient increases in $ETCO_2$ after bicarbonate injection during CPR in patients[1] (Fig 2). This effect dissipated within 2 minutes. Other investigators have made similar observations.[5]

High-dose epinephrine has recently received attention as a potentially beneficial intervention during CPR based on its ability to increase coronary and cerebral perfusion pressure.[28–31] Several groups have reported that after high-dose epinephrine administration, $ETCO_2$ may decrease coincident with a demonstrated increase in coronary perfusion pressure.[32–36] This effect may result from decreased total blood flow following high-dose epinephrine administration due to increased afterload[32, 35, 36] or from increased pulmonary shunting following high-dose epinephrine administration.[34] These observations must be taken into account if $ETCO_2$ is to be used in the clinical arena as a prognostic indicator during CPR.

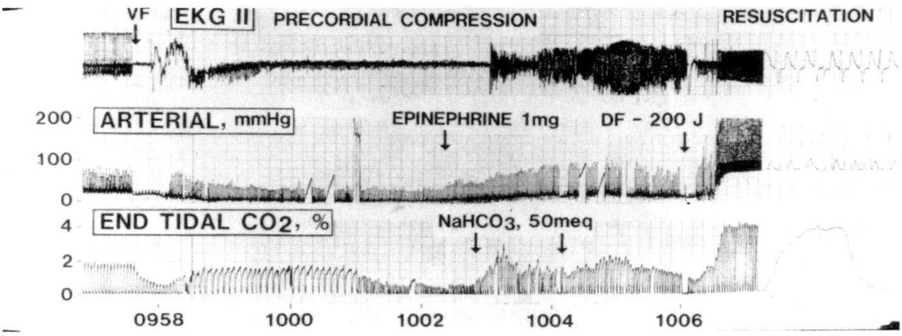

FIG 2.
Serial changes in the $ETCO_2$ in a patient just prior to and immediately after cardiac arrest, during precordial compression, and after defibrillation and resuscitation. The transient increase in $ETCO_2$ after the administration of sodium bicarbonate is demonstrated. The original tracing has been modified because of space limitations. (Adapted from Falk JL, Rackow EC, Weil MH: *N Engl J Med* 318:607–611, 1988. Used by permission.)

Monitoring

Techniques for monitoring expired carbon dioxide in the operating room, recovery room, and intensive care unit include the use of mass spectrometry and infrared absorption systems, which have been extensively reviewed in the anesthesia literature.[14] Portable infrared CO_2 monitors can be used successfully in the emergency department or on in-hospital resuscitation carts. They retain the advantage of providing capnographic waveform data but are technically more difficult to use in an emergency setting[8, 9, 37–42] than the more recently available colorimetric or miniaturized qualitative infrared devices. These devices are truly portable, require no warm-up time or calibration, and perform well even in the pre-hospital setting.[38–42]

The colorimetric device (EZ Cap, Nelcor) employs a chemically treated foam indicator contained in a plastic housing that functions as an endotracheal tube elbow adapter. The color of the foam adapter changes when it is exposed to exhaled carbon dioxide. The device is purple when the CO_2 concentration is less than 0.5% (A range), tan at CO_2 concentrations of 0.5% to 2.0% (B range), and yellow at CO_2 concentrations greater than 2.0% (C range).[9, 40] Jones demonstrated that observers could consistently detect a color change with the device at mean CO_2 concentrations of 0.54% (4.1 mm Hg). The minimum range for color change perception was 0.25% to 0.60% (1.9 to 4.6 mm Hg).[42]

The colorimetric device provides semiquantitative $ETCO_2$ data on a breath-by-breath basis. It is relatively insensitive in the ranges commonly encountered during cardiopulmonary resuscitation that may discriminate patients likely to achieve ROSC from those unlikely to do so.[1, 5, 6] It does appear sensitive enough to verify intratracheal tube placement during CPR in the majority of patients (see later).[8, 9, 37, 42] However, the lack of waveform limits its utility in this setting.[43] A miniaturized infrared qualitative CO_2 detector (Minicap III, Mine Safety Appliances Company, Pittsburgh) has recently become commercially available. It is a solid state, infrared spectrophotometer with mainstream optical bench requiring no warm-up or calibration. It detects CO_2 concentrations above 0.5% and is clinically usable.[38] It too suffers from the lack of waveform and is even less quantitative than the colorimetric device.

$ETCO_2$ as a Monitor During Circulatory Shock

Recently there has been an increased awareness that circulatory shock consists not only of failure of oxygen delivery, but also of failure of carbon dioxide excretion.[44] The veno-arterial carbon dioxide gradient reported during circulatory arrest and resuscitation[24, 45] is simply a most dramatic example of a pathophysiology at work in other forms of circulatory failure.[46–49] Hamalgyi and colleagues reported the presence of a veno-arterial CO_2 gradient and venous hypercapnia in a canine model of hemorrhagic shock.[46] Benjamin et al. confirmed these observations.[47] Androgue and colleagues reiterated these observations in patients with varying degrees of circulatory failure.[48] Patients with normal circulation had normal veno-arterial CO_2 gradients (<6.0 mm Hg). Patients with severe circulatory failure had veno-arterial CO_2 gradients of 24 mm Hg. Patients in circulatory arrest had veno-arterial gradients of 49 mm Hg. Others have made similar observations in patients with sepsis and septic shock.[49]

Venous hypercarbia during cardiac arrest has been demonstrated to result from decreased pulmonary perfusion and CO_2 excretion by the lungs as evidenced by very low levels of $ETCO_2$.[1, 15, 17] Similar pathophysiology is likely in the hypoperfusion states seen during circulatory shock. Tang et al. showed a close correlation between mean aortic pressure and $ETCO_2$ in a rodent hemorrhagic shock model.[10] Sun and colleagues made similar observations in a rodent model of anaphylactic shock.[11]

$ETCO_2$ monitoring has not been used widely to monitor patients in circulatory shock. It is likely that severe circulatory compromise and obvious hemodynamic instability would be present along with any aberration in $ETCO_2$. We have become interested in the potential utility of $ETCO_2$ monitoring during resuscitation of severely compromised trauma victims. These patients are almost always intubated, but in the early minutes of resuscitation, traditional methods of assessing circulatory status are difficult to use. Auscultated blood pressures are unreliable in patients with low output, vasoconstricted states.[50] However, immediate placement of intra-arterial lines takes time and personnel, both of which are in short supply in this setting. Many of these victims require massive fluid resuscitation but are at risk of serious complications resulting from fluid overload. This is especially relevant in patients with concomitant shock and closed head injury or pulmonary contusion. Currently, there are only very limited parameters to guide fluid therapy in this setting.

We reported a case in which $ETCO_2$ monitoring was used in a patient with head trauma, severe hemorrhagic shock, and central circulatory collapse (Fig 3).[13] $ETCO_2$ increased from 10 mm Hg to 25 mm Hg during the first several minutes of aggressive fluid resuscitation. This occurred while minute ventilation was held as constant as possible with bagged ventilation. Along with the rise in $ETCO_2$ improvement in hemodynamic parameters was apparent. Additional studies to determine the correlation of $ETCO_2$ with other hemodynamic and cardiorespiratory parameters are in progress. It is hoped that these efforts may result in the ability to use $ETCO_2$ as a noninvasive monitor of perfusion in this setting.

Clinical Applications

While any technology must be used in the context of sound, traditional clinical judgement,[51] $ETCO_2$ has emerged as the gold standard for verifying proper endotracheal tube placement in the clinical setting.[52–59] Tradi-

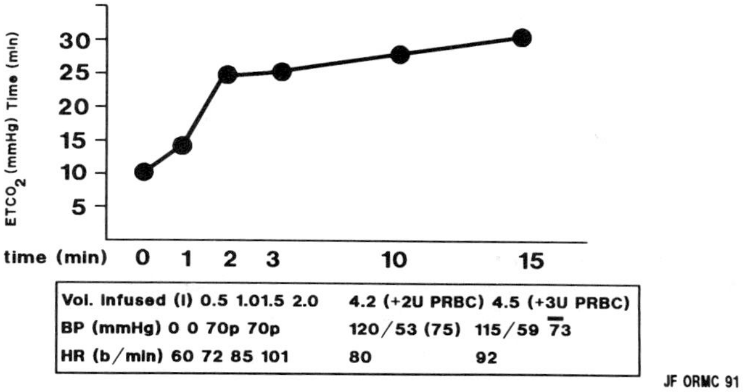

FIG 3.
The response of $ETCO_2$ to fluid resuscitation in a patient with central hemodynamic collapse following acute traumatic hemorrhagic shock. The $ETCO_2$ increased from very low levels on presentation in response to aggressive fluid resuscitation in this severely traumatized patient. This response appears to correspond to increases in total systemic flow and the hemodynamic parameters delineated in the figure. (Adapted from Falk JL, O'Brien JF, Kerr R: *Crit Care Clin* 8:323–340, 1992. Used by permission.)

tional methods of assessing tube placement are subjective and fraught with potential error.[54] Missed endotracheal intubation may have disastrous consequences for both the patient and the health care provider. Missed endotracheal intubation is recognized as a clinical problem that is not uncommon in the prehospital and emergency medicine settings.[55] Even in the best prehospital systems, the incidence of recognized esophageal intubation has been reported to be 2%.[60] The true incidence of unrecognized esophageal intubation in the prehospital and emergency department setting is unknown but is likely to be considerably higher.[9] Therefore, techniques that minimize the incidence of missed endotracheal intubation represent an important advance in the practice of emergency medicine.[55] In 1990, the American Society of Anesthesiology recognized $ETCO_2$ monitoring as the standard of care for determining endotracheal tube placement in the operating room.[56] Given that emergency intubations outside the operating room occur in an environment that is far less optimum, it would seem even more compelling that objective assessment to verify endotracheal tube placement be employed. Accordingly, many centers have adopted the practice of verifying all endotracheal tube placements done either in the prehospital or in-hospital setting with the use of expired CO_2 monitoring.

Due to the low levels of $ETCO_2$ that may be encountered during cardiac arrest, this circumstance presents a special challenge in utilizing $ETCO_2$ for verification of tube position. When using an infrared CO_2 absorption technique, the waveform of the capnogram will indicate that proper endotracheal tube placement has been achieved irrespective of the level of circulation or the level of $ETCO_2$.[43] That is to say, even under conditions of very low flow and during cardiopulmonary resuscitation, the capnogram will indicate a normal albeit low amplitude single-breath capnogram.[1]

In the setting of cardiopulmonary arrest, the colorimetric technique for determining $ETCO_2$ may fail to indicate whether the patient is appropriately intubated. Accordingly, Ornato et al. performed a multicenter trial testing the colorimetric device in the prehospital setting[8] (Fig 4). In 79 victims of prehospital cardiac arrest in whom the colorimetric device was used, a color change was noted among 55 (70%) of the patients, all of whom ultimately were determined to have been properly intubated. Of the 24 patients (30%) in whom no color change was achieved during circulatory arrest, 17 (70%) were determined to be intubated intratracheally. However, there were seven (29%) esophageal intubations in this group. Therefore, during cardiac arrest approximately two thirds of the time a color change will be noted on the colorimetric device despite the absence of spontaneous circulation and the low level of expired CO_2. In this group, appreciation of a color change was 100% specific for intratracheal tube placement. However, among one third of the patients in whom no color change occurs, the clinician is forced to rely on clinical assessment to determine endotracheal tube placement since the lack of color change in this patient group may represent either lack of adequate circulation or missed endotracheal intubation. Similar data confirming these conclusions have been reported.[9, 40, 41]

It should be noted that the presence of CO_2-containing gas in the stomach could potentially create some confusion regarding endotracheal tube position in patients with esophageal intubations.[61] Carbon dioxide gas is contained in carbonated beverages including beer and may be present in

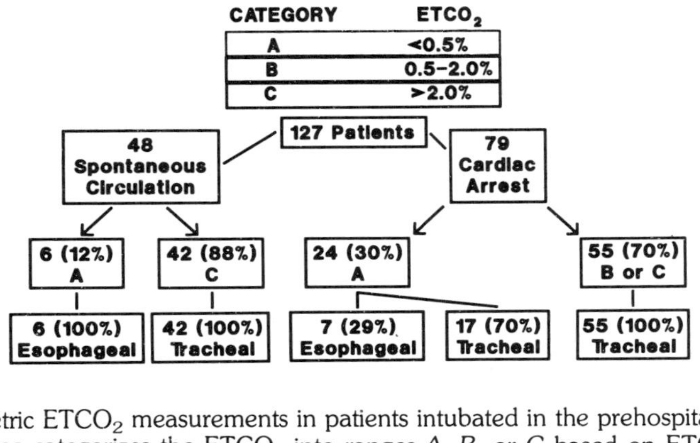

FIG 4.
Colorimetric $ETCO_2$ measurements in patients intubated in the prehospital setting. The device categorizes the $ETCO_2$ into ranges *A*, *B*, or *C* based on $ETCO_2$% as shown. In the patients intubated during cardiac arrest, *B* or *C* range reading occurred 70% of the time and was 100% specific for tracheal location of the endotracheal tube. Among the 30% of arrested patients who remained in the *A* range (no color change) approximately one third were improperly intubated. (Adapted from Ornato JP et al: *Am Emerg Med* 19:452, 1990.)

large quantities in certain patients.[62] If infrared capnography is being used, the clinician should recognize expulsion of CO_2 from the stomach in a pattern not typical of an exhaled breath, resulting in the detection of esophageal intubation. If the colorimetric device is being used, a color change indicating the presence of CO_2 may theoretically occur during ventilation of the esophagus under these circumstances. Heller and colleagues could not produce a color change with the colorimetric device when animals that had been given large intragastic quantities of carbonated beverages were intubated in the sophagus. In clinical studies, this consideration did not reduce the accuracy of the device.[64] In any case, the majority of CO_2 ought to be expelled from the stomach within a very short time. Accordingly, the current recommendation is that six ventilations be performed and the color change be determined after the sixth ventilation, which should give adequate time to wash out any gastric or esophageal CO_2.

Conclusion

$ETCO_2$ is an exceedingly useful tool for the verification of intratracheal endotracheal tube placement in the prehospital, emergency department, and operative settings and for guiding resuscitative efforts during cardiopulmonary resuscitation. It is the earliest, reliable noninvasive indicator of return of spontaneous circulation during CPR. In the future, the noninvasive monitoring of $ETCO_2$ during resuscitation from hemorrhagic shock may also prove to be of considerable value.

References

1. Falk JL, Rackow EC, Weil MH: End tidal carbon dioxide concentration during cardiopulmonary resuscitation. *N Engl J Med* 318:607–611, 1988.
2. Garnett RA et al: End tidal carbon dioxide monitoring during cardiopulmonary resuscitation. *JAMA* 257:512–515, 1987.
3. Kalenda Z: the capnogram as a guide to the efficacy of cardiac massage. *Resuscitation* 6:259–262, 1978.
4. Smalhout B, Kalenda Z: *An atlas of capnography,* vol 1. Zeist, Netherlands, 1975, Kerckebosch, p 28.
5. Sanders AB et al: End tidal carbon dioxide monitoring during cardiopulmonary resuscitation. A prognostic indicator for survival. JAMA 262:1347–1351, 1989.
6. Callaham M, Barton C: Prediction of outcome of cardiopulmonary resuscitation from end tidal carbon dioxide concentration. *Crit Care Med* 18:358–362, 1990.
7. Weil MH, Gazmuri RJ, Rackow EC: Immediate resuscitation. *Crit Care Med* 18:455, 1990.
8. Ornato JP et al: Multicenter study of end tidal carbon dioxide in the prehospital setting. *Ann Emerg Med, vol 19.* 4:452, 1990.
9. MacLeod BA et al: Verification of endotracheal tube placement with colorimetric end trial CO_2 detection. *Ann Emerg Med* 20:267–270, 1991.

10. Tang W et al: $ETCO_2$ as a hemodynamic determinant of hemorrhagic shock in the rat. *Chest* 100:134, 1991.
11. Sun S et al: End tidal PCO_2 and arterial PCO_2 indicate severity of perfusion failure during anaphylactic shock. *Clin Res* 39:422, 1991.
12. Ornato JP, Garnett AR, Glauser FL: Relationship between cardiac output and the end tidal carbon dioxide tension. *Ann Emerg Med* 19:1104–1106, 1990.
13. Falk JL, O'Brien J, Kerr R: Fluid resuscitation in traumatic hemorrhagic shock. *Crit Care Clin* 8:323–340, 1992.
14. Moon RE, Camporesi EM: Respiratory monitoring. In Miller RD, editor: *Anesthesia,* ed 3. New York, 1990, Churchill Levingston, pp 1124–1163
15. Gudipati CV et al: Expired carbon dioxide: A noninvasive monitor of cardiopulmonary resuscitation. *Circulation* 77:234–239, 1988.
16. Weil MH et al: Cardiac output and end tidal carbon dioxide. *Crit Care Med* 13:907–909, 1985.
17. Grundler W, Weil MH, Rackow EC: Arteriovenous carbon dioxide and pH gradients during cardiac arrest. *Circulation* 74:1071–1074, 1986.
18. Weil MH et al: Difference in acid base state between venous and arterial blood during cardiopulmonary resuscitation. *N Engl J Med* 315:153–156, 1986.
19. Sanders AB et al: Expired PCO_2 as an index of coronary perfusion pressure. *Am J Emerg Med* 3:147–149, 1985.
20. Redding JJ, Pearson JW: Evaluation of drugs for cardiac resuscitation. *Anesthesiology* 24:203–207, 1963.
21. Niemann JT et al: Coronary perfusion pressure during experimental cardiopulmonary resuscitation. *Ann Emerg Med* 11:127–131, 1982.
22. Sanders AB, Ewy GA, Taft TV: Prognostic and therapeutic importance of the aortic diastolic pressure in resuscitation from cardiac arrest. *Crit Care Med* 12:871–873, 1984.
23. Kern KB et al: Changes in expired end tidal carbon dioxide during cardiopulmonary resuscitation in dogs: A prognostic guide for resuscitation efforts. *J Am Coll Cardiol* 13:1184–1189, 1989.
24. Duggal C et al: Effect of duration of cardiac arrest on coronary perfusion pressure and end tidal CO_2 as predictors of resuscitability. *Crit Care Med* 18:222, 1990.
25. Ward K et al: A comparison of interpored abdominal compression CPR and standard CPR by monitoring end tidal PCO_2. *Ann Emerg Med* 18:831–837, 1989.
26. Ornato JP et al: Effect of cardiopulmonary resuscitation compression rate on end tidal carbon dioxide concentration and arterial pressure in man. *Crit Care Med* 16:241–245, 1988.
27. Ornato JP et al: The effect of applied chest compression force on systemic arterial pressure and end tidal carbon dioxide concentration during CPR in human beings. *Ann Emerg Med* 18:732–737, 1989.
28. Brown CG et al: Comparative effect of graded doses of epinephrine on regional blood flow during CPR in a swine model. *Ann Emerg Med* 15:1138–1144, 1986.
29. Brown CG et al: The effect of graded doses of epinephrine on regional myocardial blood flow during cardiopulmonary resuscitation in swine. *Circulation* 75:491–497, 1987.
30. Brown CG et al: The effect of high dose phenylephrine versus epinephrine on cerebral blood flow during CPR. *Ann Emerg Med* 16:743–748, 1987.
31. Lindner KH, Ahnefeld FW, Bowdler IM: Comparison of different doses of epi-

nephrine on myocardial perfusion and resuscitation success during cardiopulmonary resuscitation in a pig model. *Am J Emerg Med* 9:27–31, 1991.
32. Martin GB et al: Effect of epinephrine on end tidal carbon dioxide monitoring during CPR. *Ann Emerg Med* 19:396–398, 1990.
33. Paradis NA et al: The effect of standard and high dose epinephrine on coronary perfusion pressure during prolonged cardiopulmonary resuscitation. *JAMA* 265:1139–1144, 1991.
34. Tang W et al: Pulmonary ventilation/perfusion defects induced by epinephrine during cardiopulmonary resuscitation. *Circulation* 84:2101–2107, 1991.
35. Chase PB et al: The effect of high and low dose epinephrine on myocardial perfusion, cardiac output and end tidal carbon dioxide during prolonged CPR. *Ann Emerg Med* 19:466–467, 1990.
36. Paradis NA et al: Increases in coronary perfusion pressure after high dose epinephrine result in decreases in end tidal CO_2 during CPR in human beings. *Ann Emerg Med* 19:491, 1990.
37. Raemer DB, Calalang I: Accuracy of end tidal carbon dioxide tension analyzers. *J Clin Monit* 7:195–208, 1991.
38. Vukmir RB, Heller MB, Stein KL: Confirmation of endotracheal tube placement: A miniaturized infrared qualitative CO_2 detector. *Ann Emerg Med* 20:726–729, 1991.
39. Varon AJ, Morrina J, Civetta JM: Clinical utility of a colorimetric end tidal CO_2 detector in cardiopulmonary resuscitation and emergency intubation. *J Clin Monit* 7:289–293, 1991.
40. Anton WR et al: A disposable end tidal CO_2 detector to verify endotracheal intubation. *Ann Emerg Med* 20:271–275, 1991.
41. Goldberg JJ et al: Colorimetric end tidal carbon dioxide monitoring for tracheal intubation. *Anesth Analg* 70:191–194, 1990.
42. Jones BR, Dorsey MJ: Sensitivity of a disposable end tidal carbon dioxide detector. *J Clin Monit* 7:268–270, 1991.
43. Sayah AJ, Peacock WF, Overton DT: End tidal CO_2 measurement in the detection of esophageal intubation during cardiac arrest. *Ann Emerg Med* 19:857–860, 1990.
44. Johnson BA, Weil MH: Redefining ischemia due to circulatory failure as dual defects of oxygen deficits and of carbon dioxide excesses. *Crit Care Med* 19:1432–1438, 1991.
45. Weil MH et al: Difference in acid-base state between venous and arterial blood during cardiopulmonary resuscitation. *N Engl J Med* 315:153–156, 1986.
46. Halmaggi DFJ, Kennedy M, Varga D: Hidden hypercapnia in hemorrhagic hypotension. *Anesthesiology* 33:594–601, 1970.
47. Benjamin E et al: Venous hypercarbia in canine hemorrhagic shock. *Crit Care Med* 15:516–518, 1987.
48. Adrogue HJ et al: Assessing acid base status in circulatory failure. Differences between arterial and central venous blood. *N Engl J Med* 320:1312–1316, 1989.
49. Mecher CE et al: Venous hypercarbia associated with severe sepsis and systemic hypoperfusion. *Crit Care Med* 18:585–589, 1990.
50. Cohn JN: Blood pressure measurement in shock: Mechanisms of inaccuracy of auscultatory and palpatory methods. *JAMA* 199:118–122, 1967.
51. Kharatian A: Capnography: Never forget the false positives! *Anesth Analg* 73:509–510, 1991.
52. Linko K, Paloheimo M, Tammisto T: Capnography for detection of accidental esophageal intubation. *Acta Anaesth Scand* 27:199–202, 1983.

53. Murray IP, Modell JH: Early detection of endotracheal tube accidents by monitoring carbon dioxide concentration in respiratory gas. *Anesthesiology* 59:344–346, 1983.
54. Birmingham PK, Cheney FW, Ward RJ: Esophageal intubation: A review of detection techniques. *Anesth Analg* 65:886–891, 1986.
55. Sanders AB: Capnometry in emergency medicine. *Ann Emerg Med* 18:1287–1290, 1989.
56. Eichhorn JH: Standard of care continues as key issue into the 1990's. *Am Soc Anesthesiol Newsletter* 54:10–13, 1990.
57. Stirt JA: Endotracheal tube misplacement. *Anaesth Intensive Care* 10:274–276, 1982.
58. Pollard BJ, Junius F: Accidental intubation of the esophagus. *Anaesth Intensive Care* 8:183–186, 1980.
59. Abarbanell NR: Esophageal placement of an endotracheal tube by paramedics. *Am J Emerg Med* 6:178–179, 1988.
60. Stewart RD, Paris PM, Winter PM: Field endotracheal intubation by paramedic personnel. *Chest* 85:341–345, 1984.
61. Garnett AR, Gervin CA, Gervin AS: Capnograph waveforms in eosphageal intubation: Effect of carbonated beverages. *Ann Emerg Med* 18:387–390, 1989.
62. Zbinden S, Schupfer G: Detection of esophageal intubation: the cola complication. *Anesthesia* 44:81, 1989.
63. Heller MB et al: Aeromedicine and trauma arrest: a question of perspective [editorial]. *Ann Emerg Med* 18:1375, 1989.
64. Gerard J et al: Verification of endotracheal intubation using a disposable end tidal CO_2 detector. *Prehospital Disaster Med* 4:74, 1989.

Pathophysiology of Asthma and Implications for Management in the Perioperative Period

Karen S. Lindeman, M.D.

Assistant Professor, Department of Anesthesiology/Critical Care Medicine, The Johns Hopkins Medical Institutions, Baltimore, Maryland

Asthma presents an increasingly significant health risk to susceptible patients and provides a difficult challenge for anesthesiologists involved in their perioperative treatment. Morbidity and mortality from asthma have risen over the past few years. From 1980 to 1987, the prevalence of asthma in the United States increased 29% and the hospitalization discharge rate increased threefold.[1] During the same period, mortality rates increased 31%. Although the reasons underlying this increase are unknown, anesthesiologists must be prepared to treat more of these patients. A better understanding of the pathophysiology of asthma will lead to improvements in the perioperative treatment of the patient with asthma.

Asthma is marked by three characteristics: (1) reversible airway obstruction, (2) airway inflammation, and (3) airway hyperresponsiveness.[2] Although each of these characteristics can exist separately, interactions typically occur.

Obstruction to airflow accounts for the clinical manifestations of wheezing, dyspnea, and cough. Mechanisms of airway obstruction include contraction of airway smooth muscle, airway edema, and accumulation of mucus in the airway.

Airway inflammation is thought to modulate the course of asthma both by initiating airway obstruction and by contributing to airway hyperresponsiveness. These effects may occur through activation of inflammatory cells and release of inflammatory mediators, through tissue damage and alterations in airway permeability, or through chronic airway wall thickening.

Airway hyperresponsiveness is manifested by exaggerated responses to a variety of bronchoconstrictor stimuli. Bronchoprovocation testing can be performed with nonspecific challenges, such as histamine, methacholine, hypoosmotic solutions, or cold air.[3] The extent of airway hyperresponsiveness correlates with the clinical severity of asthma and the need for medical therapy.[4]

Pathophysiology

The basic defect leading to the clinical syndrome of asthma is unknown. At least four major mechanisms have been considered: (1) increased contraction or impaired relaxation of airway smooth muscle, (2) neural imbalance, (3) airway inflammation, and (4) alterations in epithelial cell function.

Airway Smooth Muscle

Airway smooth muscle contraction is thought to be largely responsible for the airway obstruction that occurs during an acute episode of bronchospasm in the operating room. A significant amount of research has focused on airway smooth muscle hyperresponsiveness as a mechanism of asthma. Studies in both human subjects[5–10] and in the Basenji-greyhound (BG) dog model of asthma[11] attempted to correlate in vivo and in vitro airway hyperresponsiveness. None of these studies demonstrated significant relationships between in vivo responses to histamine or cholinergic agonists and in vitro airway smooth muscle responses to these stimuli. In fact, some studies[7, 11] demonstrated negative in vivo/in vitro correlations. One explanation for these findings is that the sites of airway hyperresponsiveness in vivo were distinct from the airway sections (primarily trachea) tested in vitro.[12] Alternatively, increased airway smooth muscle contractile responses are not the cause of asthma, and, perhaps, diminished responses represent a chronic adaptive response.

Like enhanced responsiveness to contractile stimuli, a reduction in responsiveness to relaxant stimuli can contribute to airway obstruction and asthma. Tracheal smooth muscle from patients with asthma, when compared to that from healthy patients, demonstrated impaired relaxation in response to isoproterenol.[7, 13] Similarly, trachealis muscle from BG dogs showed impaired isoproterenol relaxation when compared to trachealis muscle from allergic[14] or nonallergic[11] control dogs. This phenomenon was active in vivo as well. β-Adrenergic agonists were not as effective in attenuating airway constriction from cholinergic stimuli in BG dogs when compared to dogs that lacked airway hyperresponsiveness.[15] In addition, this reduction in β-adrenergic responsiveness affected small, peripheral airways[16] as well as larger, central airways. Since airway tone most likely reflects the balance between contracting and relaxing influences, a reduction in sensitivity to β-adrenergic agonists could contribute significantly to airway obstruction and airway hyperresponsiveness.

Nervous System

External to airway smooth muscle, the autonomic nervous system provides both contraction and dilation input to the airways. The parasympathetic nervous system influences airway tone via efferent cholinergic nerves that arise in the vagal nuclei of the brain stem. These nerves synapse at ganglia in the airway wall and activate postganglionic fibers to release acetylcholine. Acetylcholine contracts the airway by stimulating muscarinic receptors on airway smooth muscle. Acetylcholine also activates autoreceptors, which are muscarinic receptors on the nerve ending itself.[17] Several subclasses of muscarinic (M) receptors have been characterized. M1 receptors are located at the parasympathetic ganglia.[18] Muscarinic receptors on airway smooth muscle are thought to consist primarily of the M2 and M3 class (Fig 1). Stimulation of neuronal M2 autoreceptors on postganglionic parasympathetic nerves inhibits further release of acetylcholine from the nerve terminals.

For many years, exaggerated cholinergic efferent activity was considered to be a primary mechanism of asthma; however, the failure of anticholinergic agents to reverse asthmatic bronchospasm, coupled with more recent evidence of the importance of nonvagally mediated mechanisms, indicates a limited role of exaggerated cholinergic reflexes in the pathogenesis of asthma. In contrast, this is an important mechanism inducing bronchospasm during anesthesia.

One additional proposed mechanism of airway hyperresponsiveness is dysfunction of the M2 receptors, leading to excessive release of acetylcholine.[19] Although the role of this mechanism in asthma is uncertain, a functional impairment of these receptors has been well-established in a guinea pig model of viral infection.[20] Thus, the airway hyperresponsiveness seen clinically for about 6 weeks after an upper respiratory tract infection[21]

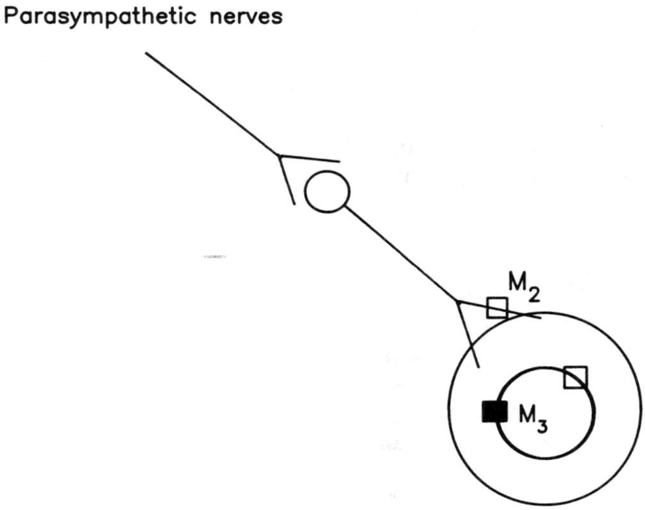

FIG 1.
Location of muscarinic receptors in parasympathetic nerves innervating the lung. Stimulation of M_2 and M_3 receptors on airway smooth muscle stimulates contraction. Stimulation of M_2 autoreceptors on parasympathetic nerves inhibits further release of acetylcholine.

could result from temporary dysfunction of muscarinic (M2) receptors. Similarly, a more permanent dysfunction of these receptors could lead to chronic airway hyperresponsiveness and asthma.

The sympathetic nervous system acts primarily to reduce airway tone. Human airway smooth muscle contains β-adrenergic receptors, but, in contrast to pulmonary vascular smooth muscle, sympathetic innervation is, at best, sparse.[22] Sympathetic efferent activity occurs primarily through release of catecholamines, which activate β_2-adrenergic receptors on airway smooth muscle. Because of the lack of sympathetic innervation to the airways, most theories suggesting a reduction in β-adrenergic sensitivity in asthma have centered on the smooth muscle, rather than the nerves.[23]

The α-adrenergic system plays a relatively less important role in the pathophysiology of asthma.[24, 25] Although α_1-adrenergic receptors are present in the lung and may produce airway constriction after stimulation, most evidence does not support the presence of enhanced α_1-adrenergic activity in asthmatic subjects.[25] Stimulation of α_2-adrenoceptors appears to dilate airways,[26] although this effect is small in magnitude.

In addition to efferent cholinergic and adrenergic neural pathways, recent work demonstrates the presence of nonadrenergic, noncholinergic (NANC) neural efferents to the airways.[27–29] This system supplies both excitatory (constricting) and inhibitory (dilating) input to the airways. Although the neurotransmitters released from these nerves have not been identified completely, the most likely candidates are neuropeptides (Table 1). Vasoactive intestinal peptide is thought to be one of the more important inhibitory peptides.[30] Potentially, an imbalance of the NANC system leading to a relative decrease in inhibitory input could contribute to airway hyperresponsiveness and asthma; however, the current evidence does not support a significant role for this mechanism in the pathophysiology of asthma. Although one group reported that vasoactive intestinal peptide staining was reduced in the lungs of a small group of patients with asthma,[31] patients with mild asthma showed no defect in NANC inhibitory pathways.[32]

TABLE 1.
Airway Neuropeptides

Inhibitory	Excitatory
Vasoactive intestinal peptide	Substance P
Peptide histidine methionine	Neurokinin A
	Calcitonin gene-related peptide
	Cholecystokinin octapeptide
	Neuropeptide Y

One additional group of nerves may influence bronchomotor tone and airway responsiveness. These nerves are the afferent sensory nerves located in the airway wall and epithelium. Stimulation of these C-fibers is thought to cause release of a large group of constricting neuropeptides, including substance P. The importance of these nerves in the mechanism of asthma has not been determined yet.

Airway Inflammation

A growing body of evidence supports the importance of inflammation as a modulating influence in asthma. A considerable number of studies document the presence of inflammation in the airways of some patients with asthma.[33] In this situation, airway edema occurs, and a variety of inflammatory cells infiltrate the airways.[34] These cells are involved in a number of complex events, including release of mediators of inflammation.[35] Mediators of inflammation have many effects, including provoking airway smooth muscle contraction, stimulating directed migration of other inflammatory cells, altering neural control of airway tone, increasing mucosal permeability, and disrupting airway epithelium (Fig 2). Furthermore, edema and cellular infiltration alone can obstruct airways and alter airway geometry to increase responsiveness.[36]

Inflammatory cells that infiltrate the airways include neutrophils, mast cells, and eosinophils. These cells primarily infiltrate the airway mucosa. The most important inflammatory mediators produced by these cells are histamine, leukotrienes, platelet activating factor, prostaglandins, throm-

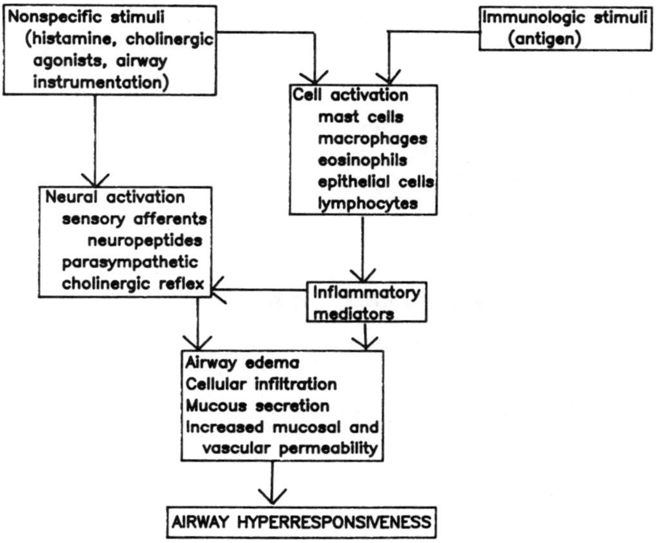

FIG 2.
Interaction between factors contributing to airway hyperresponsiveness.

boxanes, and serotonin. These mediators, in addition to directly contracting airway smooth muscle, alter reactivity by modifying neural control in both afferent and efferent nerves. In efferent nerves, these effects occur at the level of parasympathetic ganglia, at postganglionic presynaptic nerve terminals, and at postsynaptic sites.[37]

The precise role of inflammation in asthma is controversial. Although a majority of patients with asthma show inflammatory changes in the airways, these findings are not universal. Thus, while inflammation is considered an important modulating influence, it does not appear to be the only factor responsible for producing asthma.

Airway Epithelium

Disruption of the airway epithelium can contribute to airway hyperresponsiveness and asthma in a number of ways. The epithelium serves as a barrier to noxious stimuli. In patients with asthma, these ciliated epithelial cells appear to be destroyed in certain locations within the airways.[38] This increased access of constrictor stimuli to airway mucosa could increase airway hyperresponsiveness in patients with asthma.

In the past, the epithelium was considered to do little more than protect the airway mucosa from noxious stimuli. More recently, evidence has accumulated to implicate the epithelium in a more active role, including in the production of substances that constrict or dilate the airways.[39–41] A relative decrease in the production of dilating factors or increase in the production of constricting factors could contribute to airway hyperresponsiveness.

Another way in which the epithelium regulates airway tone is through the presence of enzymes that degrade constricting factors. A group of enzymes known as neutral endopeptidases are responsible for degrading neuropeptides, including substance P. Neutral endopeptidases are found in high concentration in epithelial cells.[42] With destruction of the epithelium, loss of these enzymes may potentiate the effects of constricting neuropeptides. In addition, destruction of the epithelium may expose afferent sensory nerve endings to irritant stimuli, resulting in increased release of neuropeptides. Inflammation may exacerbate these problems by increasing epithelial permeability,[43] which could also increase exposure of afferent sensory nerves. Furthermore, the whole cascade may be amplified by the ability of neuropeptides to stimulate neurogenic inflammation.[44] Although these processes appear to play a significant role in airway hyperresponsiveness following viral infection,[45] their role in asthma remains uncertain.

Anesthetic Management

Preoperative Assessment

The medical history of patients with asthma often reveals the characteristic triad of symptoms: wheezing, dyspnea, and cough (Table 2). A general as-

TABLE 2.
Symptoms/Signs of Severe Asthma

History	
	Chest tightness
	Cough
	Breathlessness
Physical examination	
	Tachypnea >30 breaths/min
	Paradoxical pulse >20 mm Hg
	Use of accessory respiratory muscles
	Wheezing
Laboratory findings	
	O_2 saturation <90%
	P_{CO_2} > 40 mm Hg
	$FEV_{1.0}$ < 30%–50% baseline*

*$FEV_{1.0}$ = forced expiratory volume in 1 second.

sessment of these symptoms should include frequency and severity of episodes, triggering agents, and time of most recent exacerbation. Patients at higher risk are those with increased frequency of attacks and severe attacks requiring hospitalization with admission to an intensive care unit. Current and past pharmacologic therapy should also be known.

Physical examination is directed to the pulmonary system. Tachypnea, an exaggerated (>20 mm Hg) pulsus paradoxus, and the use of accessory respiratory muscles suggest a severe ongoing asthmatic attack. Auscultation of the chest may be normal or may reveal wheezing and/or a prolonged expiratory phase. During marked bronchospasm, wheezing may not be audible because of severe reductions in air movement.

Laboratory tests most frequently include chest roentgenograms, arterial blood gas tensions, and pulmonary function tests. Chest roentgenograms are not particularly useful for diagnosing the presence of asthma or for assessing the severity of the disease.[46] However, chest roentgenograms can assist with the diagnosis of superimposed conditions, such as pneumonia, which can exacerbate symptoms of asthma. During an asthmatic attack, hyperinflation often is evident. Chest roentgenograms are also helpful in determining the presence of complications of asthma, such as pneumothorax, atelectasis, or heart failure, all of which may be amenable to therapy in the preoperative period.

In the absence of an acute asthmatic attack, arterial blood gas tensions add little to a routine preoperative evaluation. These tests typically show hypoxemia and respiratory alkalosis during an asthmatic attack. The predominant cause for a reduction in arterial oxygen tension is mismatching of ventilation and perfusion. The reduction in arterial carbon dioxide tension results from alveolar hyperventilation. With more severe or prolonged airway obstruction, arterial carbon dioxide tensions rise as a result of fatigue following a prolonged increase in the work of breathing.

Pulmonary function tests are used to document the presence of asthma, to assess the severity of airway obstruction, and to determine the response to bronchodilator therapy. Simple spirometry measures exhaled gas volume over time. The individual measurements include forced vital capacity (FVC) and forced expiratory volume in 1 second ($FEV_{1.0}$). FVC indicates the total volume of gas exhaled after a maximum inspiration, and $FEV_{1.0}$ measures the maximum volume exhaled in the first second after a maximum inspiration. $FEV_{1.0}$ is a convenient and useful measure of ventilatory capacity, but, like FVC, it is effort-dependent. Reductions in $FEV_{1.0}$/FVC below 0.75 generally indicate the presence of significant airway obstruction. These tests can be repeated after the administration of bronchodilators to assess response to therapy and to determine the relative amounts of reversible and irreversible airway obstruction. The most convenient indirect test of ventilatory capacity is the peak expiratory flow rate, which can be measured at the bedside. The most common device for measuring peak flow is the Wright peak flow meter.[47]

Other laboratory tests, such as electrocardiograms or blood eosinophil counts are nonspecific and do not provide a significant amount of additional information in routine preoperative evaluations.

Pharmacologic Therapy

Preoperative pharmacologic therapy is directed to optimizing pulmonary function, to decreasing the risk of intraoperative bronchospasm, and to reducing additional complications. In the immediate preoperative period, premedication may provide beneficial sedative effects, especially for patients with asthma who suffer from stress-induced bronchospasm. Histamine-1 receptor antagonists may reduce the risk of bronchospasm, although no clinical trials have documented clear beneficial effects. Anticholinergic agents, such as atropine, when administered intramuscularly in doses typically used for premedication, do not produce significant effects on airways; however, larger doses will block reflex-induced bronchospasm.

Longer term pharmacologic therapy should include treatment for such complications as underlying infection or heart failure, if present. In the absence of these complications, medications specific to asthma include anti-inflammatory agents to reverse chronic inflammation and bronchodilators to prevent or reverse airway obstruction.

Anti-inflammatory Agents

Glucocorticoids form one of the mainstays of therapy for asthma, primarily owing to their anti-inflammatory properties (Table 3). These agents are unique in that they reduce airway hyperresponsiveness in chronic asthma[48–50] and attenuate experimentally provoked acute attacks.[51, 52]

TABLE 3.
Pharmacologic Therapy for Acute Asthma in Adult Patients

Agent	Dosage*
Glucocorticoids	
Hydrocortisone	1–3 mg/kg, IV every 4 hr
Methylprednisolone	0.5–1 mL/kg, IV every 8 hr
β-Adrenergic agonists	
Inhaled	
Albuterol	2.5 mg (0.5 mL of a 0.5% solution, diluted with 2–3 mL NS)
Metaproterenol	15 mg (0.3 mL of a 5% solution, diluted with 2–3 mL NS)
Isoetharine	5 mg (0.5 mL of a 1% solution, diluted with a 2–3 mL NS)
Subcutaneous	
Epinephrine	0.3 mg
Terbutaline	0.25 mg
Xanthine derivatives	
Aminophylline	6 mg/kg loading dose, 0.6 mg/kg/hr continuous infusion. The infusion rate should be adjusted according to the serum theophylline level.
Anticholinergic agents	
Ipatropium bromide	1–5 mg, aerosol in saline

*IV = intravenous; NS = normal saline.

Proposed mechanisms of action include reductions in cellular infiltration and mediator release, decreases in mucosal permeability, and up-regulation of the β-adrenergic system.[53] Glucocorticoids are most often administered through the oral or intravenous routes. In the preoperative period, hydrocortisone (1 to 3 mg/kg, intravenously [IV]) takes effect 1 to 2 hours after administration. Alternatively, methylprednisolone (0.5 to 1 mg/kg/ IV) provides the advantage of fewer side effects due to minimal mineralocorticoid activity. Because of the numerous side effects associated with long-term use of glucocorticoids,[54, 55] recent attention has shifted to the use of inhaled corticosteroids.[48] Since short-term use of glucocorticoids in the preoperative period does not produce these side effects, this route of administration does not offer significant advantages over the oral or intravenous routes. The maximum effect of glucocorticoids often occurs after weeks of therapy[56]; however, reductions in nonspecific airway hyperresponsiveness can occur within 24 hours of administration.[57]

Cromolyn sodium is the prototype of another group of drugs that has served as a mainstay of chronic therapy for many years. These agents are thought to act primarily by stabilizing mast cells, and perhaps other cells as well, to prevent release of mediators of inflammation.[58] Side effects of cromolyn sodium are minimal, and interactions with other pharmacologic agents used with anesthesia are unknown. Patients who respond favorably should continue to take this medication in the preoperative period.

Nedocromil sodium is a newer drug that is thought to act similarly to cromolyn sodium. Nedocromil sodium may also inhibit release of excitatory neuropeptides from sensory nerves in response to irritant stimuli.[59] This agent, administered most frequently as an aerosol, is currently available in Europe and may provide additional protection against acute bronchoconstrictor stimuli during preoperative preparation of the patient with asthma.

Bronchodilators

Sympathomimetic agents are among the most effective forms of pharmacologic therapy in preventing and treating acute asthma. These agents act as bronchodilators by activating β-adrenergic receptors. β_2-adrenergic receptors mediate a number of processes that can be beneficial in asthma, including direct airway smooth muscle relaxation, inhibition of mediator release from inflammatory cells, enhanced mucociliary transport, a reduction in airway edema, and inhibition of cholinergic neurotransmission.[60]

Selective β_2-adrenergic agonists, such as albuterol, terbutaline, or fenoterol, minimize undesirable side effects of less selective β-adrenergic agonists (isoproterenol). These side effects, such as tachycardia and dysrhythmias, result primarily from stimulation of β_1-receptors on the heart.

Sympathomimetics can be administered as an aerosol, as an oral preparation, or parenterally via intravenous or subcutaneous injection. The advantage of the aerosol route is that high concentrations of medication can be delivered directly to the site of action in the airways, reducing the incidence of detrimental systemic side effects.

Recently, concern has centered around the question of tachyphylaxis after long-term treatment with β-adrenergic agonists.[61, 62] Tachyphylaxis, most commonly through down-regulation of β receptors, has been more easily demonstrated in animal models[63] than in human subjects with asthma, perhaps because higher doses were administered. However, tachyphylaxis was present in one study of healthy volunteers after they inhaled a high dose of albuterol.[64] Thus, although tachyphylaxis does occur, this problem does not interfere to a significant degree with the use of β-adrenergic agonists clinically in patients with asthma because the metered dose inhalers contain such a high dose.

Xanthine derivatives, such as theophylline, aminophylline (the water soluble form of theophylline), and enprofylline (used in Europe), have been used for many years in the treatment of asthma. The mechanism responsible for a reduction in airway hyperresponsiveness is controversial. Smooth muscle relaxation is generally considered the primary action of these agents. In addition, these agents may have anti-inflammatory actions.[65] When administered acutely, these effects may be mediated by the release of catecholamines.[66] In the past, the primary subcellular mechanism of action of these agents was thought to be inhibition of phosphodiesterase in airway smooth muscle, leading to increases in cyclic adenosine monophosphate and relaxation. However, this effect does not occur at clinically relevant concentrations in vivo.[67]

Clinically, xanthine derivatives cause bronchodilation in direct relation to the serum concentration of the agent.[68] For aminophylline, the therapeutic range is considered to be 10 to 20 μg/mL. When administered at higher concentrations, aminophylline produces side effects of tachyarrhythmias, hypotension, and convulsions. Perhaps because of the importance of catecholamine release in the mechanism of action of xanthines, addition of theophylline to therapy with β-adrenergic agonists provides no clear benefits in the therapy of acute asthma.[68a]

Increased attention has focused recently on the use of anticholinergic agents in the treatment of acute asthma. These agents are nonselective and block both M2 receptors on cholinergic nerves and M3 receptors on airway smooth muscle. Bronchodilation occurs through blockade of M3 receptors. The efficacy of anticholinergic agents may be limited by their ability to increase acetylcholine release as a result of blocking M2 inhibitory autoreceptors on cholinergic nerves. These agents have no known anti-inflammatory properties and are not particularly useful in the management of chronic asthma.

Traditionally, anticholinergic agents such as atropine were administered intramuscularly or intravenously. The doses of these tertiary ammonium compounds were limited by their toxic side effects. The introduction of the quaternary compound, ipratropium bromide, has allowed these agents to be delivered as an aerosol in higher concentrations and with fewer side effects.[69] Nevertheless, anticholinergic agents are generally not as effective alone as β-adrenergic agonists. [70] However, in contrast to xanthine derivatives, anticholinergic agents enhance bronchodilation when combined with β-adrenergic agonists.[70]

Intraoperative Management

Choice of Anesthetic Technique

Endotracheal intubation, by activating reflexes, provides one of the most significant stimuli for bronchospasm in the perioperative period.[71] Thus, techniques to avoid general endotracheal anesthesia in patients with asthma are generally preferable. These techniques include local sedation, peripheral nerve blocks, major regional anesthesia, and mask general anesthesia. The use of these techniques depends on the site of surgery, the presence of other complicating conditions, the expertise of the anesthesiologist, and patient preferences.

For intraabdominal surgery, epidural or spinal anesthesia offer reasonable alternatives to general endotracheal anesthesia. In unstable patients with asthma who depend on accessory respiratory muscle strength, major regional anesthesia may not be the technique of choice because high levels of motor blockade may impair ventilatory capacity. In a stable patient, one case report questioned the ability of spinal anesthesia to precipitate an episode of bronchospasm by reducing adrenal epinephrine output.[72] However, stress associated with surgery and the onset of sensory and motor blockade was also a likely triggering mechanism and could not be excluded. Thus, adequate sensory block for surgery and judicious use of sedation may minimize the risk of bronchospasm during major regional anesthesia.

Induction of General Anesthesia

Choices for induction of general anesthesia include intravenous and inhalational techniques. When other factors do not play a significant role, inhalational induction provides the best protection against bronchospasm during laryngoscopy and endotracheal intubation because of its salutory effects.

When induction with a potent inhalational anesthetic is contraindicated, a number of intravenous agents are available. Thiopental sodium is the most widely used intravenous anesthetic for induction of general anesthesia. Direct effects of thiobarbiturates on airways differ depending on the species and the system under investigation. Thiopental contracted human, rat, and dog bronchi,[73] but had no effect on baseline tone in guinea pig tracheal chains.[74, 75] In contrast, thiopental, at clinically relevant concentrations, caused dose-related constriction in guinea pig trachea, but at higher doses bronchodilation occurred.[76] Oxybarbiturates, such as methohexital, did not exert a similar effect.[77]

The clinical studies addressing this question are retrospective. One study showed an association between the use of thiopental and bronchospasm,[78] and two others could not demonstrate a significant association.[71, 79] Two of these studies were performed over 25 years ago, when anesthetic agents and techniques were much different. Thus, the risk of bronchospasm in patients with asthma treated with thiopental is still unknown.

One potential mechanism of airway constriction is the release of histamine. Although thiobarbiturates stimulate epidermal mast cells to release significant quantities of histamine,[80] histamine release from lung mast cells is negligible.[81] Oxybarbiturates do not trigger mast cell release.[80]

Without solid scientific evidence to the contrary, barbiturates do not appear to be contraindicated in patients with asthma. In selecting an agent for induction of anesthesia, an oxybarbiturate may be a reasonable alternative to a thiobarbiturate. Since endotracheal intubation presents the most significant stimulus for bronchospasm, a dose of barbiturate sufficient to attenuate this reflex would be preferable. However, the dose required to achieve this goal is uncertain.

Ketamine is the intravenous induction agent of choice in patients with asthma. Mechanisms for this beneficial effect include direct airway smooth muscle relaxation,[82–85] inhibition of vagal reflexes,[86] and increases in endogenous catecholamines.[87, 88] The use of ketamine is limited, therefore, by side effects ascribed to activation of the sympathetic nervous system.

Early clinical studies documented the bronchodilator action of ketamine.[89, 90] In the BG dog model of airway hyperresponsiveness, intravenous ketamine, in concentrations used clinically, protected against antigen-induced bronchoconstriction.[91] β-Adrenergic blockade with propranolol prevented this protective effect, suggesting that sympathomimetic actions of ketamine were responsible.

Because of cardiovascular side effects, ketamine administered in an aerosol form might provide a significant advantage. However, a small dose of aerosolized ketamine neither prevented nor reversed histamine-induced airway constriction in guinea pigs.[92]

Intravenous ketamine, therefore, is particularly useful in situations that require rapid induction of general anesthesia. Because of the cardiovascular side effects of activation of the sympathetic nervous system, ketamine generally is reserved for patients with healthy cardiovascular systems.

As an adjunct to the use of intravenous anesthetics during induction, local anesthestics are often administered to reduce the risk of bronchospasm during endotracheal intubation. Proposed mechanisms for reducing airway responsiveness include direct smooth muscle relaxation, reductions in mediator release, and inhibition of reflex pathways. Although in vitro studies demonstrated that local anesthetics have direct effects on airway smooth muscle[93, 94] and reduce mediator release,[94] these effects occurred only at concentrations above the clinically relevant range. The major mechanism in vivo, therefore, seems to be attenuation of reflexes.[95] Because endotracheal intubation provokes bronchospasm primarily by stimulating reflexes, the use of local anesthetics to prevent bronchospasm during induction of anesthesia is appropriate. Although the aerosol route of administration has been advocated, this route confers no advantage over intravenous administration[96] and may provoke bronchoconstriction, possibly by activating sensory afferent nerves. In addition, other local anesthetics, such as procaine, hexylcaine, and bupivacaine, are comparable to lidocaine in their ability to attenuate the bronchoconstriction.[97]

Maintenance of General Anesthesia

Inhalational anesthetics have traditionally been considered the most appropriate agents for maintenance of general anesthesia in patients with asthma. Halothane, enflurane, and isoflurane may prevent or reverse bronchospasm by relaxing airway smooth muscle directly, inhibiting airway reflexes, and reducing release of mediators of inflammation.

For at least 20 years, inhalational anesthetics have been known to attenuate airway reflexes.[98, 99] In the BG dog model,[100] halothane (1.5 minimum alveolar concentration [MAC]) attenuated airway constriction induced by histamine, which is thought to act through a direct action on smooth muscle and by stimulating cholinergic reflexes. Because atropine and halothane inhibited histamine-induced constriction to a similar degree and because atropine did not augment the protection afforded by halothane, the authors concluded that the major action of halothane was attenuating reflexes. Studies with vagal nerve stimulation to increase resistance in dogs without airway hyperresponsiveness demonstrated that halothane, enflurane, and isoflurane, at equivalent MAC multiples, are approximately equipotent in attenuating reflexes.[101]

The specific site of action of inhalational anesthetics in blocking reflexes includes, at a minimum, the nerve terminals. In a nerve-muscle preparation, halothane, at clinically relevant concentrations, decreased acetylcholine release in response to nerve stimulation.[99] In addition, it is likely that inhalational anesthetics block afferent reflex activity and, perhaps, nonvagal efferent activity. In another study that compared the effects of halothane on increases in lung resistance provoked by either acetylcholine or vagal nerve stimulation, halothane attenuated these responses to a nearly equivalent degree.[102] These results suggested that a direct action of halothane on smooth muscle could explain at least a part of the attenuation of vagally mediated increases in lung resistance. However, halothane attenuated a stimulus (such as histamine) almost entirely by blocking reflexes.[100] Since one difference between these two stimuli is that histamine activates afferent as well as efferent reflexes, these two studies suggest that a major action of inhalational anesthetics is blocking afferent limbs of the reflex arc.

Direct smooth muscle relaxation plays a relatively small role in contributing to the beneficial effects of inhalational anesthetics on airways in vivo. In the BG dog model, halothane (1.5 MAC) and isoflurane (1.5 MAC) provided little protection against airway constriction provoked by aerosolized methacholine.[103] Since this challenge produces bronchoconstriction primarily through direct stimulation of muscarinic (M3) receptors on airway smooth muscle, these results were consistent with the idea that in vivo the beneficial effects of inhalational anesthetics depend, for the most part, on blocking reflexes.

A direct effect of inhalational anesthetics on airway smooth muscle can be demonstrated in vitro.[99, 104–107] HOwever, these effects tend to be either small[105, 106] or nonexistent.[99] The mechanism for these direct effects is not well understood. As in cardiac muscle, some evidence supports the idea that inhalational anesthetics alter calcium kinetics, perhaps by affecting the availability of intracellular calcium stores.[107] The clinical significance of these effects has not been defined, but perhaps these direct effects are more significant in peripheral airways, where reflexes play a smaller role. In fact, inhalational anesthetics reduced canine peripheral airway responses in vivo, probably by directly relaxing airway smooth muscle.[108]

Most studies investigating the effects of inhalational anesthetics in vivo measured changes in lung resistance in the presence or absence of the anesthetic. It is now apparent that lung resistance includes the components of airway resistance as well as another component of tissue resistance. More recent studies[109, 110] showed that halothane exerts its effects at both of these levels.

A third potential effect of inhalational anesthetics is a reduction in the release of bronchoactive mediators. Halothane, in concentrations within the clinically relevant range, reduced histamine release from human foreskin cells stimulated with tubocurarine.[111] The clinical significance of these results is open to question. In vivo, halothane decreased pulmonary resistance changes following antigen challenge in dogs without significantly reducing plasma histamine concentrations.[112]

The preponderance of evidence, therefore, indicates that inhalational anesthetics are the agents of choice for maintenance of general anesthesia in patients with asthma.

The use of opioid anesthesia in patients with asthma has not received a significant amount of attention in the scientific literature. Clinical trials of opioid anesthesia in patients with asthma are lacking. Theoretically, opioids might be considered beneficial. Opiate receptors are present on sensory nerves and inhibit release of substance P or other peptides from neural tissue.[113] A similar inhibitory mechanism is evident in the respiratory tract of guinea pigs.[114] Thus, opiates, by inhibiting the release of excitatory neuropeptides in the airways, might inhibit bronchoconstriction resulting from stimulation of afferent sensory fibers. In human subjects, moderate doses of morphine (0.15 mg/kg) attenuated bronchoconstriction in response to capsaicin[115] or distilled water.[116] However, the clinical relevance of these findings is unclear because the mechanisms producing these responses are unknown.

The question has arisen as to whether patients with asthma are at increased risk of bronchospasm after the administration of high doses of morphine, which are associated with increased plasma levels of histamine.[117] Although no controlled studies have answered this question, an opioid that produces less histamine release might be preferable in cases requiring administration of high doses of opioids.

For skeletal muscle relaxation to supplement inhalational or opioid anesthesia, neuromuscular blocking agents have the potential to increase the risk of bronchospasm in patients with asthma. Some of these agents readily release histamine from mast cells found in the blood vessels. Other agents are structurally similar to acetylcholine and can bind to muscarinic receptors in the airways.

d-Tubocurarine[118] and atracurium[119] provoke histamine release from mast cells. In the past, a clear relationship between histamine release from these agents and airway constriction was lacking. Recently, intravenous atracurium (1.2 mg/kg) was shown to provoke peripheral airway constriction in BG dogs, and the response was completely abolished by pretreatment with a histamine-1 receptor antagonist.[120] A lower dose of atracurium (0.5 mg/kg) produced no response. These findings were consistent with the idea that the major mechanism of atracurium-induced airway constriction is by the release of histamine, and that, clinically, this effect can be minimized by the use of small doses or by pretreatment with antihistamines.

The structural similarities of neuromuscular blocking agents to acetylcholine might allow these agents to bind to muscarinic receptors on ganglia, at nerve terminals, or on airway smooth muscle. Gallamine, a selective antagonist of M2 autoreceptors, potentiated vagally mediated bronchoconstriction in guinea pigs.[121] Similarly, atracurium and pancuronium increased pulmonary resistance changes following vagal nerve stimulation, perhaps by antagonizing M2 autoreceptors.[101]

Anticholinesterases, such as neostigmine, are capable of provoking bronchospasm,[122] probably by interfering with the metabolism of acetylcholine at efferent nerve terminals. This potential problem is generally avoided by prior or concomitant treatment with a muscarinic antagonist.

Intraoperative Bronchospasm

Despite optimal treatment, a number of patients with asthma develop intraoperative bronchospasm. In patients undergoing local or regional anesthesia, treatment is similar to the treatment of acute asthma in the absence of anesthesia. Pharmacologic therapy includes β-adrenergic agonists, with or without xanthine derivatives, anticholinergic agents, and corticosteroids.

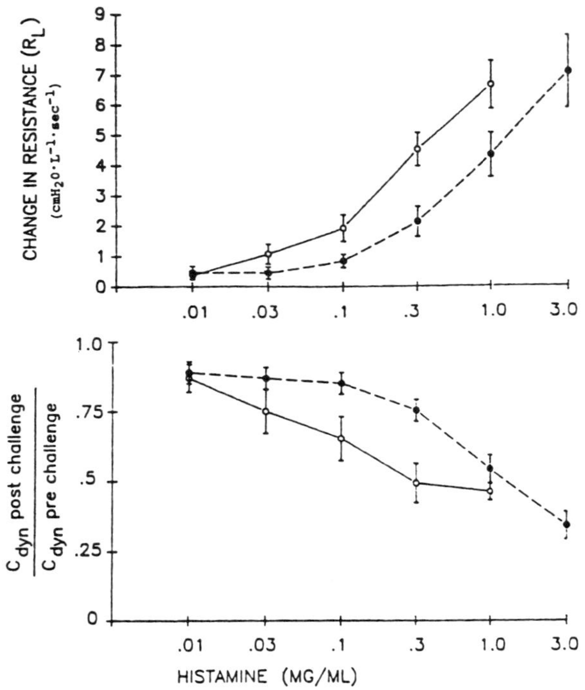

FIG 3.

Dose-response curves during thiopental/fentanyl anesthesia with *(dashed line)* and without *(solid line)* aminophylline. Note decreased resistance, *above*, in the aminophylline treated group. Note increased dynamic compliance (C_{dyn}), *below*, after histamine challenge in aminophylline-treated group. $n = 5$, mean ± standard error (SE). (From Tobias JD, Kubos KL, Hirshman CA: *Anesthesiology* 71:723–729, 1989. Used by permission.)

During general endotracheal anesthesia, management may differ to some extent. In BG dogs anesthetized with high concentrations of halothane (1.5 MAC), the addition of aminophylline did not improve the protection afforded by halothane alone[66] (Figs 3, 4). However, patients anesthetized with lower concentrations of inhalational anesthetics, or those anesthetized with opioids, may benefit from the addition of aminophylline.

Even in the presence of high concentrations of halothane, however, β-adrenergic agonists were effective at further attenuating histamine-induced bronchoconstriction[123] (Fig 5). In general, therefore, β-adrenergic agonists are the pharmacologic agents of choice for the treatment of intraoperative bronchospasm.

To minimize the cardiovascular side effects of β-adrenergic agonists, these agents are most frequently administered as an aerosol. The aerosol can be delivered via a fluorocarbon propellant generator or a jet nebulizer. A number of T-piece adaptors and connectors are available for use during general endotracheal anesthesia. As a rule, a canister, which releases a

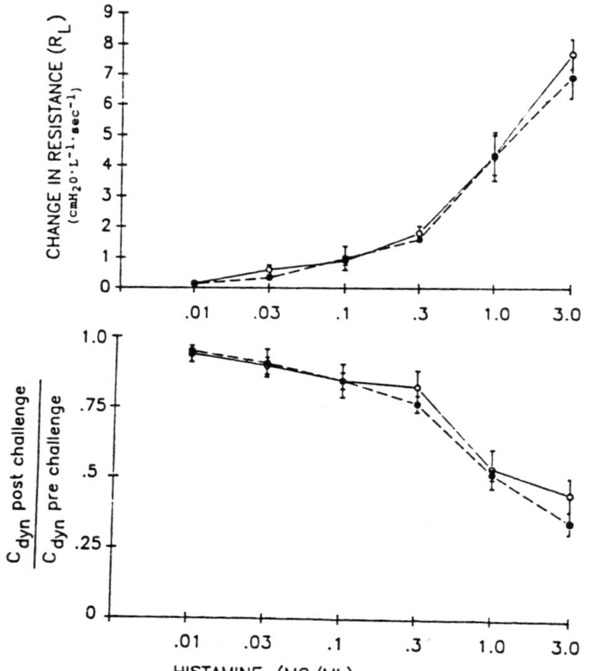

FIG 4.
Dose-response curves during halothane anesthesia with *(dashed line)* and without *(solid line)* aminophylline. Airway resistance does not change in the aminophylline treated group. $n = 5$, mean ± SE. C_{dyn} = dynamic compliance. (From Tobias JD, Kubos KL, Hirshman CA: *Anesthesiology* 71:723–729, 1989. Used by permission.)

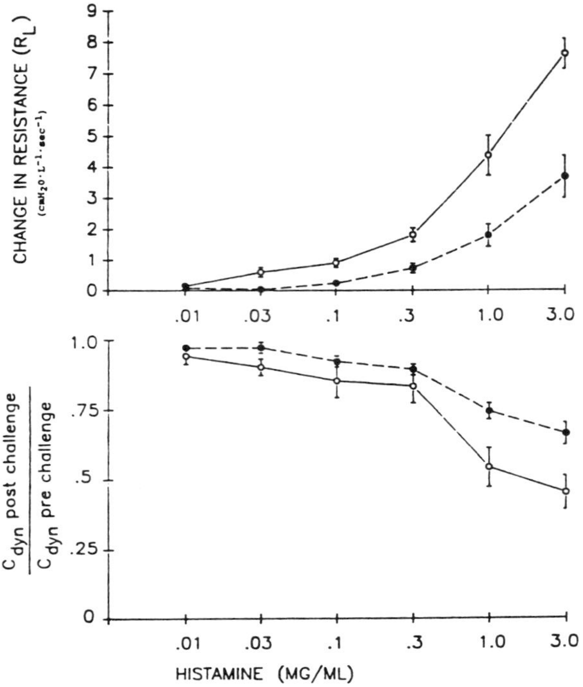

FIG 5.
Dose-response curves during halothane anesthesia with *(dashed line)* and without *(solid line)* albuterol. In contrast to aminophylline treatment, albuterol reduces airway resistance. $n = 5$, mean ± SE. C_{dyn} = dynamic compliance. (From Tobias JD and Hirshman CA: *Anesthesiology* 72:105–110, 1990. Used by permission.)

fixed amount of medication, is placed in the anesthesia circuit as close to the endotracheal tube as possible. During inspiration, pressure is applied to the canister to release the aerosol. Drug delivery is improved by use of a large endotracheal tube and by activation of the propellant during continuous gas flow.[124] A jet nebulizer is often used when fluorocarbon propellant generators are not available. An aerosol is generated by diverting a high-pressure gas stream over a liquid reservoir, drawing up the liquid by Venturi action. The chamber is connected to the inspiratory limb of an anesthesia circuit.

Other pharmacologic agents, including anticholinergic agents and corticosteroids, can be administered as described previously.

Emergence from General Anesthesia

During emergence from general anesthesia, the patient with asthma must be monitored carefully for signs and symptoms of bronchospasm. As the depth of anesthesia is reduced, stimulation becomes more likely to provoke bronchospasm. One option to avoid bronchospasm during emergence is to extubate the trachea during deep inhalational anesthesia. The potential risk with this technique is the risk of regurgitation and aspiration. For this reason, the patient is sometimes allowed to awaken fully, with careful monitoring for bronchospasm, before the trachea is extubated.

If the patient develops bronchospasm during emergence, treatment may include the pharmacologic therapy previously described. For refractory bronchospasm, continued intubation and mechanical ventilation in an intensive care unit may be necessary.

Summary

Patients with asthma provide a significant challenge to anesthesiologists involved in treating patients of all ages. Appropriate anesthetic management should be tailored to the individual patient and to the surgical procedure. With extra care, thought, and vigilance, the perioperative period can be rewarding to the patient and the anesthesiologist, alike.

References

1. Centers for Disease Control: Asthma - United States, 1980–1987. *MMWR* 39:493–497, 1990.
2. Expert Panel Report: Definition and diagnosis. Executive Summary: Guidelines for the Diagnosis and Management of Asthma. Washington DC, Public Health Service, National Institutes of Health, US Government Printing Office, DHHS Publication No 91-3042A.
3. Boushey HA et al: Bronchial hyperreactivity. *Am Rev Respir Dis* 121:389–414, 1980.
4. Cockroft DW: Airway hyperresponsiveness: Therapeutic implications. *Ann Allergy* 59:405–414, 1987.
5. Armour CL et al: The relationship between bronchial hyperresponsiveness to methacholine and airway smooth muscle structure and reactivity. *Respir Physiol* 58:223–233, 1984.
6. Armour CL et al: A comparison of *in vivo* and *in vitro* human airway reactivity to histamine. *Am Rev Respir Dis* 129:907–910, 1984.
7. Goldie R et al: *In vitro* responsiveness of human asthmatic bronchus to carbachol, histamine, β-adrenoceptor agonists and theophylline. *Br J Clin Pharmacol* 22:669–676, 1986.
8. Roberts JA et al: Comparison of *in vivo* airway responsiveness and *in vitro* smooth muscle sensitivity to methacholine in man. *Thorax* 39:837–843, 1984.
9. Roberts JA, Rodger IW, Thomson NC: Airway responsiveness to histamine in man: Effect of atropine on *in vivo* and *in vitro* comparison. *Thorax* 40:261–267, 1985.
10. Vincenc KS et al: Comparison of *in vivo* and *in vitro* responses to histamine in human airways. *Am Rev Respir Dis* 128:875–879, 1983.
11. Downes H et al: Comparison of drug responses *in vivo* and *in vitro* in airways of dogs with and without airway hyperresponsiveness. *J Pharmacol Exp Ther* 237:214–219, 1986.

12. Ludwig MS et al: Partitioning of pulmonary resistance during constriction in the dog: Effects of volume history. *J Appl Physiol* 62:807–815, 1987.
13. Cerrina J et al: Comparison of human bronchial muscle responses to histamine *in vivo* with histamine and isoproterenol agonists *in vitro*. *Am Rev Respir Dis* 134:57–61, 1986.
14. Downes H et al: Comparison of *in vitro* drug responses in airways of atopic dogs with and without *in vivo* airway hyperresponsiveness. *Pulmonary Pharmacol* 2:209–216, 1989.
15. Tobias JD, Sauder RA, Hirshman CA: Reduced sensitivity to beta adrenergic agonists in Basenji-Greyhound dogs. *J Appl Physiol* 69:1212–1219, 1990.
16. Lindeman KS, Hirshman CA, Freed AN: Functional antagonism of airway constriction in the canine lung periphery. *J Appl Physiol* 71:1848–1855, 1991.
17. Starke K, Gothert M, Kilbinger H: Modulation of neurotransmitter release by presynaptic autoreceptors. *Physiol Rev* 69:865–989, 1989.
18. Lammers J-W et al: The role of pirenzepine-sensitive (M1) muscarinic receptors in vagally mediated bronchoconstriction in humans. *Am Rev Respir Dis* 139:446–449, 1989.
19. Barnes PJ: Muscarinic autoreceptors in the airways: Their possible role in airway disease. *Chest* 96:1220–1221, 1989.
20. Fryer AD, Jacoby DB: Parainfluenza virus infection damages inhibitory M_2 muscarinic receptors on pulmonary parasympathetic nerves in the guinea pig. *Br J Pharmacol* 109:267–271, 1991.
21. Empey DW et al: Mechanisms of bronchial hyperreactivity in normal subjects following upper respiratory tract infection. *Am Rev Respir Dis* 113:131–139, 1976.
22. Richardson JB: Nerve supply to the lungs. *Am Rev Respir Dis* 119:785–802, 1979.
23. Szentivanyi A: The β-adrenergic theory of the atopic abnormality in bronchial asthma. *J Allergy* 42:203–242, 1968.
24. Barnes PJ: Neural control of human airways in health and disease. *Am Rev Resp Dis* 134:1289–1314, 1986.
25. Spina D et al: α_1-Adrenoceptor function and autoradiographic distribution in human asthmatic lung. *Br J Pharmacol* 97:701–708, 1989.
26. Lindgren BR, Ekstrom T, Andersson RG: The effect of inhaled clonidine in patients with asthma. *Am Rev Respir Dis* 134:266–269, 1986.
27. Richardson JB: Nonadrenergic inhibitory innervation of the lung. *Lung* 159:315–322, 1981.
28. Andersson RGG, Grundstrom N: The excitatory non-cholinergic, non-adrenergic nervous system of the guinea-pig airways. *Eur J Respir Dis* 64:141–157, 1983.
29. Barnes PJ: Non-adrenergic non-cholinergic neural control of human airways. *Arch Int Pharmacodyn* 280:208–282, 1986.
30. Barnes PJ: Neuropeptides and asthma. *Am Rev Respir Dis* 143:28–32, 1991.
31. Ollerenshaw SL et al: Absence of immunoreactive vasoactive intestinal polypeptide in tissue from the lungs of patients with asthma. *N Engl J Med* 320:1244–1248, 1989.
32. Lammers J-W et al: Capsaicin-induced bronchodilation in asthmatic patients: Role of non-adrenergic inhibitory system. *J Appl Physiol* 98:325–330, 1989.
33. Hogg JC, James AL, Pare PD: Evidence for inflammation in asthma. *Am Rev Respir Dis* 143:39–42, 1991.

34. Djukanovic R et al: Mucosal inflammation in asthma. *Am Rev Respir Dis* 142:434–457, 1990.
35. Liu MC et al: Evidence for elevated levels of histamine, prostaglandin D_2, and other bronchoconstricting prostaglandins in the airways of subjects with mild asthma. *Am Rev Respir Dis* 142:126–132, 1990.
36. Moreno RH, Hogg JC, Pare PD: Mechanisms of airway narrowing. *Am Rev Respir Dis* 133:1171–1180, 1986.
37. Black JL: Control of human airway smooth muscle. *Am Rev Respir Dis* 143:11–12, 1991.
38. Laitinen LA et al: Damage of the airway epithelium and bronchial reactivity in patients with asthma. *Am Rev Respir Dis* 131:599–606, 1985.
39. Flavahan NA et al: Respiratory epithelium inhibits bronchial smooth muscle tone. *J Appl Physiol* 58:834–838, 1985.
40. Frossard N, Muller F: Epithelial modulation of tracheal smooth muscle responses to antigenic stimulation. *J Appl Physiol* 61:1449–1456, 1986.
41. Hay DWP et al: Airway epithelium modulates the reactivity of guinea-pig respiratory smooth muscle. *Eur J Pharmacol* 129:11–18, 1986.
42. Johnson AR et al: Neutral metalloendopeptidase in human lung tissue and cultured cells. *Am Rev Respir Dis* 132:564–568, 1985.
43. Sugahara K et al: Epithelial permeability produced by phagocytosing neutrophils in vitro. *Am Rev Respir Dis* 133:875–881, 1986.
44. Nadel JA: Regulation of neurogenic inflammation by neutral endopeptidase. *Am Rev Respir Dis* 145:48–52, 1992.
45. Jacoby DB et al: Influenza infection causes airway hyperresponsiveness by decreasing enkephalinase. *J Appl Physiol* 64:2653–2658, 1988.
46. Gershel JC et al: The usefulness of chest radiographs in first asthmatic attacks. *N Engl J Med* 309:336–339, 1983.
47. Wright BM, McKerrow CB: Maximum forced expiratory flow rate as a measure of ventilatory capacity. *Br Med J* 2:1041, 1959.
48. Dutoit JI, Salome CM, Woolcock AJ: Inhaled corticosteroids reduce the severity of bronchial hyperresponsiveness in asthma but oral theophylline does not. *Am Rev Respir Dis* 136:1174–1178, 1987.
49. Ryan G et al: Effect of beclomethasone dipropionate on bronchial responsiveness to histamine in controlled, non steroid dependent asthma. *J Allergy Clin Immunol* 75:25–31, 1985.
50. Kraan J et al: Changes in bronchial hyperreactivity by four weeks treatment with anti-asthmatic drugs in patients with allergic asthma. A comparison between budesonide and terbutaline. *J Allergy Clin Immunol* 76:628–636, 1985.
51. Cockcroft DW et al: Allergen-induced increase in nonallergenic bronchial reactivity. *Clin Allergy* 7:503–513, 1977.
52. Fabbri LM et al: Prednisone inhibits late asthmatic reactions and the associated increase in airway responsiveness induced by toluene di-isocyanate in sensitized subjects. *Am Rev Respir Dis* 132:1010–1014, 1985.
53. Barnes PJ: Effect of corticosteroids on airway hyperresponsiveness. *Am Rev Respir Dis* 141:70–76, 1990.
54. Lofdahl CG, Mellstrand T, Svedmyr N: Glucocorticoids and asthma: Studies of resistance and systemic effects of glucocorticoids. *Eur J Respir Dis* 65:69–79, 1984.
55. Toogood JH: Complications of topical steroid therapy for asthma. *Am Rev Respir Dis* 141:89–96, 1990.

56. Darowski MJ, Hannon VM, Hirshman CA: Corticosteroids decrease airway hyperresponsiveness in the Basenji-Greyhound dog model of asthma. *J Appl Physiol* 66:1120–1126, 1989.
57. Parker SD, Brown RH, Hirshman CA: Differential effect of glucocorticoids on pulmonary responses and eosinophils. *Respir Physiol* 83:323–332, 1991.
58. Church MK, Warner JO: Sodium cromoglycate and related drugs. *Clin Allergy* 15:311–321, 1985.
59. Verleden GM et al: Nedocromil sodium modulates nonadrenergic, noncholinergic bronchoconstrictor nerves in guinea pig airways in vitro. *Am Rev Respir Dis* 143:114–118, 1991.
60. Svedmyr N: Action of corticosteroids on beta-adrenergic receptors. *Am Rev Respir Dis* 141:31–38, 1990.
61. Conolly ME et al: Resistance to β-adrenoreceptor stimulants (a possible explanation for the rise in asthma deaths). *Fr J Pharmacol* 43:389–402, 1971.
62. Avner BP, Jenne JW. Densitization of isolated human bronchial smooth muscle to β-receptor agonists. *J Allergy Clin Immunol* 68:51–57, 1981.
63. Stephan WC et al: Tachyphylaxis to inhaled isoproterenol and the effect of methylprednisolone in dogs. *J Allergy Clin Immunol* 65:105–109, 1980.
64. Holgate ST, Baldwin CJ, Tattersfield AE: β-Adrenergic agonist resistances in normal human airways. *Lancet* 2:375–377, 1977.
65. Mapp C et al: Protective effect of antiasthma drugs on late asthmatic reactions and increased airway responsiveness induced by toluene diisocyanate in sensitized subjects. *Am Rev Respir Dis* 136:1403–1407, 1987.
66. Tobias JD, Kubos KL, Hirshman CA: Aminophylline does not attenuate histamine-induced airway constriction during halothane anesthesia. *Anesthesiology* 71:723–729, 1989.
67. Bukowsky M, Nakatsu K, Hunt PW: Theophylline reassessed. *Ann Intern Med* 101:63–73, 1984.
68. Laursen LC et al: Maximally effective plasma concentrations of enprofylline and theophylline during constant infusion. *Br J Clin Pharmacol* 18:591–595, 1984.
68a. Littenberg B: Aminophylline treatment in severe, acute asthma. *JAMA* 259:1678–1684, 1988.
69. Gross NJ, Skorodin MD: Anticholinergic antimuscarinic bronchodilators. *Am Rev Respir Dis* 129:856–870, 1984.
70. Rebuck AS et al: Nebulized anticholinergic and sympathomimetic treatment of asthma and chronic obstructive airways disease in the emergency room. *Am J Med* 82:59–64, 1987.
71. Shnider SM, Papper EM: Anesthesia for the asthmatic patient. *Anesthesiology* 22:886–892, 1961.
72. Mallampati SR: Bronchospasm during spinal anesthesia. *Anesth Analg* 60:838–840, 1981.
73. Adriani J, Rovenstein EA: The effect of anesthetic drugs upon bronchi and bronchioles of excised lung tissue. *Anesthesiology* 4:253–262, 1943.
74. Fletcher SW, Flacke, Alper MH: The actions of general anesthetic agents on tracheal smooth muscle. *Anesthesiology* 29:517–522, 1968.
75. Edney SM, Downes H: Contractor effect of barbiturates on smooth muscle. *Arch Int Pharmacodyn* 217:180–196, 1975.
76. Lenox WC, Mitzner W, Hirshman CA: Mechanism of thiopental-induced constriction of guinea pig trachea. *Anesthesiology* 72:921–925, 1990.
77. Curry C et al: Contractile responses of guinea pig trachea to oxybarbiturates and thiobarbiturates. *Anesthesiology* 75:679–683, 1991.

78. Gold MI, Helrich M: A study of complications related to anesthesia in asthmatic patients. *Anesth Analg* 42:283–293, 1963.
79. Olsson GL: Bronchospasm during anesthesia: A computer aided incidence study of 136,929 patients. *Acta Anaesth Scand* 31:244–252, 1987.
80. Hirshman CA et al: Thiobarbiturate-induced histamine release in human skin mast cells. *Anesthesiology* 63:353–356, 1985.
81. Stellato C et al: General anesthetics induce only histamine release selectively from human mast cells. *Br J Anaesth* 67:751–758, 1991.
82. Cabanas A, Souhrada JF, Aldrete JA: Effects of ketamine and halothane on normal and asthmatic smooth muscle of the airway in guinea pigs. *Can Anaesth Soc J* 27:47–51, 1980.
83. Lundy PM, Gowdey CW, Calhoun EH: Tracheal smooth muscle relaxant effect of ketamine. *Br J Anaesth* 46:333–336, 1974.
84. Vitkun SA et al: Bronchodilating effects of the anesthetic ketamine in an in vitro guinea pig preparation. *Lung* 165:101–113, 1987.
85. Wanna HT, Gergis SD: Procaine, lidocaine, and ketamine inhibit histamine-induced contracture of guinea pig tracheal muscle in vitro. *Anesth Analg* 46:25–27, 1978.
86. McGrath JC, Mackenzie JE, Miller RA: Effects of ketamine on the central sympathetic discharge and the baroreceptor reflex during mechanical ventilation. *Br J Anaesth* 47:1141–1147, 1975.
87. Lundy PM, Frew R: Ketamine potentiates catecholamine responses of vascular smooth muscle by inhibition of extraneuronal uptake. *Can J Physiol Pharmacol* 59:520–527, 1980.
88. Nedergaard OA: Cocaine-like effect of ketamine on vascular adrenergic neurones. *Eur J Pharmacol* 23:153–161, 1973.
89. Corssen G et al: Ketamine in the anesthetic management of asthmatic patients. *Anesth Analg* 51:588–596, 1972.
90. Huber FC et al: Ketamine: Its effect on airway resistance in man. *South Med J* 65:1176–1180, 1972.
91. Hirshman CA et al: Ketamine block of bronchospasm in experimental canine asthma. *Br J Anaesth* 51:713–718, 1979.
92. Rock MJ et al: Effect on airway resistance of ketamine by aerosol in guinea pigs. *Anesth Analg* 68:506–510, 1989.
93. Downes H, Loehning RW: Local anesthetic contracture and relaxation of airway smooth muscle. *Anesthesiology* 47:430–436, 1977.
94. Weiss ER, Anderson WH, O'Brien KP: The effect of a local anesthetic, lidocaine, on guinea pig trachealis muscle in vitro. *Am Rev Respir Dis* 112:393–400, 1975.
95. Downes H, Gerber N, Hirshman CA: I.V. lignocaine in reflex and allergic bronchoconstriction. *Br J Anaesth* 62:873–878, 1980.
96. Downes H, Hirshman CA: Lidocaine aerosols do not prevent allergic bronchoconstriction. *Anesth Analg* 60:28–31, 1981.
97. Downes H, Hirshman CA, Leon DA: Comparison of local anesthetics as bronchodilator aerosols. *Anesthesiology* 58:216–220, 1983.
98. Hickey RF et al: The effect of halothane and cyclopropane on total pulmonary resistance in the dog. *Anesthesiology* 31:334–343, 1969.
99. Korenaga S, Takeda K, Ito Y: Differential effects of halothane on airway nerves and muscle. *Anesthesiology* 60:309–318, 1984.
100. Shah MV, Hirshman CA: Mode of action of halothane on histamine induced airway constriction in dogs with reactive airways. *Anesthesiology* 65:170–174, 1986.

101. Vettermann J, Beck KC et al: Actions of enflurane, isoflurane, vecuronium, atracurium and pancuronium on pulmonary resistance in dogs. *Anesthesiology* 69:688–695, 1988.
102. Warner DO, Brichant JF, Rehder K: Direct and neurally mediated effects of halothane on pulmonary resistance in vivo. *Anesthesiology* 72:1057–1063, 1990.
103. Hirshman CA et al: Mechanism of action of inhalational anesthesia on airways. *Anesthesiology* 56:107–111, 1982.
104. Kochi T, Hagiya M, Mizuguchi T: Effects of enflurane on contractile response of canine trachealis muscle. *Anesth Analg* 69:60–68, 1989.
105. Brichant J-F et al: Halothane, enflurane, and isoflurane depress the peripheral vagal motor pathway in isolated canine tracheal smooth muscle. *Anesthesiology* 74:325–332, 1991.
106. Sayiner A et al: Bronchodilation by halothane is not modulated by airway epithelium. *Anesthesiology* 75:75–81, 1991.
107. Tagliente TM, Evans PJ, Ben-Harari RR: Halothane- and enflurane-induced inhibition of phasic responses to carbachol in isolated guinea pig trachea. *Anesth Analg* 74:89–96, 1992.
108. Alexander CM et al: The influence of halothane and isoflurane on pulmonary collateral ventilation. *Anesthesiology* 62:135–140, 1985.
109. Vettermann J et al: Halothane decreases both tissue and airway resistances in excised canine lungs. *J Appl Physiol* 66:2698–2703, 1989.
110. Warner DO et al: Pulmonary resistance during halothane anesthesia is not determined only by airway caliber. *Anesthesiology* 70:453–460, 1989.
111. Kettlekamp NS et al: Inhibition of d-tubocurarine-induced histamine release by halothane. *Anesthesiology* 66:666–669, 1987.
112. Hermens JM et al: Inhalation anesthesia and histamine release during bronchospasm. *Anesthesiology* 61:69–72, 1984.
113. Jessell TM, Iversen LL: Opiate analgesics inhibit substance P release from rat trigeminal nucleus. *Nature Lond* 268:549–551, 1977.
114. Belvisi MG, Rogers DF, Barnes PJ: Neurogenic plasma extravasation: Inhibition by morphine in guinea pig airways in vivo. *J Appl Physiol* 66:268–272, 1989.
115. Fuller RW et al: Effect of inhaled and systemic opiates on responses to inhaled capsaicin in humans. *J Appl Physiol* 65:1125–1130, 1988.
116. Eschenbacher WL et al: Morphine sulphate inhibits bronchoconstriction in subjects with mild asthma whose responses are inhibited by atropine. *Am Rev Respir Dis* 130:363–367, 1984.
117. Rosow CE et al: Histamine release during morphine and fentanyl anesthesia. *Anesthesiology* 56:93–96, 1982.
118. Paton WDM: Histamine release by compounds of simple chemical structure. *Pharmacol Rev* 9:269–328, 1957.
119. North FC, Kettelkamp N, Hirshman CA: Comparison of cutaneous and in vitro histamine release by muscle relaxants. *Anesthesiology* 66:543–546, 1987.
120. Mehr E, Hirshman CA, Lindeman KS: Mechanism of action of atracurium on airways. *Anesthesiology* 76:448–454, 1992.
121. Fryer AD, Maclagan J: Muscarinic inhibitory receptors in pulmonary parasympathetic nerves in the guinea-pig. *Br J Pharmacol* 83:973–978, 1984.
122. Miller MM, Fish JE, Patterson R: Methacholine and physostigmine airway reactivity in asthmatic and non-asthmatic subjects. *J Allergy Clin Immunol* 60:116–120, 1977.

123. Tobias JD, Hirshman CA: Attenuation of histamine-induced airway constriction by albuterol during halothane anesthesia. *Anesthesiology* 72:105–110, 1990.
124. Crogan SJ, Bishop MJ: Delivery efficiency of metered dose aerosols given via endotracheal tubes. *Anesthesiology* 70:1008–1010, 1989.

Index

I

J

K

L

M

N

O